AMSSM Sports Medicine CAQ Study Guide

- **A resource for testing sports medicine knowledge**

- **Exam questions from previous AMSSM In-Training Exams**

- **Two complete 200-question tests with up-to-date critiques and references**

- **Modeled after the ABFM board exams**

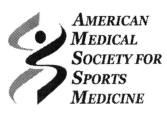

AMERICAN
MEDICAL
SOCIETY FOR
SPORTS
MEDICINE

Leading Sports Medicine into the Future

D1568640

Editors:

**Stephen Paul, M.D. • Scott Rand, M.D.
Mark Stovak, M.D. • Marc P. Hilgers, M.D.**

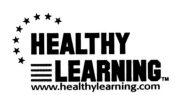

HEALTHY
LEARNING.
www.healthylearning.com

AMSSM Executive Director: Jim Griffith, MBA, CAE
AMSSM Publications Committee Chair: Andrea L. Pana, M.D., MPH

ISBN: 978-1-60679-219-3
Library of Congress Control Number: 2012935832
Cover design: Rachel Ronan, Kiwi Creative
Book layout: Roger W. Rybkowski
Front cover illustration: Hemera/Thinkstock

Healthy Learning
P.O. Box 1828
Monterey, CA 93942
www.healthylearning.com

Acknowledgments

As with any undertaking, there are many people to thank. We would like to acknowledge the board of directors of the AMSSM, as well as the leadership at Healthy Learning for having this be the first of many future joint projects. Additionally, Andrea Pana, who as chair of AMSSM publications committee provided invaluable assistance. Kristi Huelsing of Healthy Learning, who assisted with oversight in editing. I would like to thank Christine Lawless for finding appropriate ECG images. Of course, this book would not be possible without the tremendous assistance by the contributors listed who wrote and edited many of the questions from previous tests used in this version. They have enormous talent, and they represent the leaders in our field of sports medicine—especially in their talent as educators. Finally, I would like to thank my fellow editors, Scott Rand, Mark Stovak, and Marc Hilgers, who spent tireless hours reviewing the content, verifying references, and ensuring the information is up to date. Mark Stovak is currently the chair of the AMSSM fellowship committee. He and Marc Hilgers have been contributing as item writers and editors from the onset. Finally, a special thanks goes to Scott Rand, who came up with this idea to create a question book. Without Scott's dedication, time, and effort over the years, there would not be a successful In-Training Exam program, and this book would not be possible. We have all agreed, in summary, to thank our families and friends who have supported us in this project, allowing the time to spend on it and encouraging the work. Thank you.

—Stephen Paul, M.D.

Foreword

The American Medical Society for Sports Medicine is excited to partner with Healthy Learning in publishing sports medicine–related books. The first endeavor in this partnership is this test question book based on the AMSSM In-Training Exam.

AMSSM celebrated its 20th anniversary in 2011. AMSSM has grown to over 2,000 members and is leading sports medicine into the future. AMSSM members are participating in educating medical students, residents, and fellows in the area of sports medicine across the country. Clinically, our members work in a variety of settings, including primary care and multispecialty groups, urgent cares, emergency rooms, orthopedic groups, academic settings, and athletic departments amongst other practice settings. Our members' training, expertise, and experience give them a unique perspective on the practice of sports medicine.

In this first edition of AMSSM's test question book, the editors have pulled questions from previous In-Training Exams to be used as a study tool for those taking the CAQ exam. Our hope is that residency and fellowship programs may also use these questions as a tool to evaluate competency in the area of sports medicine.

AMSSM stands behind this book as an outstanding and comprehensive question book written and edited by our members experienced in the field of sports medicine.

Andrea L. Pana, M.D., MPH
AMSSM Board of Directors
Publications Committee Chair

Contents

Preface

This book represents the culmination and natural progression of the In-Training Exam for the sports medicine CAQ. It is the idea of Scott Rand. It is divided into four sections, two each with 200 questions, in test format, from previous tests given. Two sections contain the same questions with the correct answer, critique, and up-to-date references. We have maintained the spirit of the exams: provide up-to-date, easy-to-find references, mostly online. The editors have reviewed each question and checked each reference to be sure they are up to date and reflect evidenced-based practice. This book is published in e-book and paper formats to provide the optimum study tool based on the user's preference.

The intention of the book is to provide a current companion to study for the sports medicine CAQ. Additionally, it should prove useful to anyone wanting to test and seek further understanding of their sports medicine knowledge, whether in medical school, residency programs, or for fellows in primary care or orthopedic sports medicine.

Introduction

In May 2006 at the 15th AMSSM Annual Meeting in Miami, after Sean Bryan gave an update on ACGME outcomes, I remember approaching Jim Puffer, one of the founders of AMSSM and ABFM president, about creating an In-Training Exam for sports medicine fellows preparing to take the Certificate of Added Qualification (CAQ) in Sports Medicine. It would be modeled after the ABFM In-Training Exams for family medicine residencies. The idea was to provide a metric to test fellows coming in and midway through their education in preparation for the CAQ and to evaluate their progress from a program's perspective. Jim Puffer noted the start-up cost would be too great for the ABFM for only a hundred fellows. But, he lent his support in implementing this project.

With the help of Mark Lavallee, chair of AMSSM fellowship committee and the board of directors of the AMSSM, this project took off. I was also fortunate later to meet Scott Rand, a talented sports medicine physician and fellowship director, who is also gifted in computer technology. We were able to have Web-based online test software written and auditioned the first pilot test of 100 questions February 2008. The questions for this first test were written by the participating fellowship program directors. Since then, we have created 200-question tests annually online and offered them as a pretest for incoming fellows, the actual In-Training Exam for current fellows, and a recertification study test. The questions continue to be written and edited by volunteer item writers, AMSSM members who represent the leaders and educators in our field from family medicine, pediatrics, internal medicine, emergency medicine, and physical medicine and rehabilitation.

There are some special people who have been invaluable in this project along the way. Again, first Jim Puffer for his support and recommending Roger Fain, Sr. (editor) and Jason Rinaldo (psychometrician), both of the ABFM for their early assistance with this project. Chris Rand, who wrote and maintained the first software package for the online testing center; Jody Gold and Michele Lane (they represent the work behind the scenes) of the AMSSM for their incredible effort in getting this program to function. The past and current AMSSM board of directors have always been supportive of this project, in particular Kim Harmon, a past president of AMSSM, who encouraged me and supported me in getting this project to where it is today. All of the past and current item writers and educators have volunteered their time and expertise to write and edit questions for the tests. Additionally, Mark Stovak, current chair of the AMSSM fellowship committee, who helps write and organize the test each year. Finally, Scott Rand, who has been a tremendous friend and colleague throughout this project, and without him, and his talents in the technical areas, knowledge base, and writing/assembling the tests, the In-Training Exams would not have taken off.

—Stephen Paul, M.D.

1

Test 1
Questions

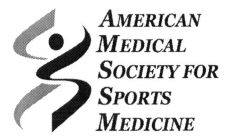

AMERICAN
MEDICAL
SOCIETY FOR
SPORTS
MEDICINE

Leading Sports Medicine into the Future

1. A 25-year-old presents to your office with popliteal artery entrapment syndrome (PAES). Which of the following is true about this condition from an anatomical, presenting signs, and diagnostic workup?

    A. It is more common under 30 years of age
    B. It occurs more commonly in females
    C. Pain at rest is pathognomonic for this disease
    D. Doppler studies show decreased velocity with knee flexion
    E. The popliteal artery derives from the deep femoral artery (profunda)

2. A 14-year-old boy nears the end of a five-minute-mile track race during an indoor track meet. He has sudden sharp pain over the left hip just proximal to the inguinal ligament. He has mild nausea and even one episode of emesis. In the office, his exam shows left low back tenderness and limited forward flexion at the waist without neurologic or radicular findings. He also has tenderness to direct and firm palpation over the left superior ilium along its anterior third. His physical exam also reveals no hernia, and the abdomen is benign. His plain radiographs and an abdominal CT in the emergency room are normal. MRI reveals a mild avulsion of the apophysis over the left superior ilium as well as some mild edema, indicating injury to the left quadratus lumborum. The plain film was read again showing the bony avulsion found on his MRI. Proper recommendations include which of the following?

    A. No running until radiologic healing is proven by plain x-ray
    B. Refer to orthopedic surgeon
    C. Conservative care, relative rest, return to running when pain has resolved and a full range of motion has returned
    D. Limit his passive hip flexion to allow healing
    E. Advise no further sprinting or racing on the track during this track and field season

3. When discussing an appropriate exercise prescription with your elderly patient, you include some of the general benefits that can be gained. Which of the following statements would you include in that discussion?

    A. Resistance training does not help maintain fat-free mass
    B. Benefits are only achievable at maximal intensity levels in the elderly
    C. Resistance training is a primary means for increasing VO_2max
    D. Strength gains cannot be maintained with once weekly exercise
    E. Age-related decline can be attenuated with regular exercise

4. A 12-year-old elite-level gymnast that is homeschooled presents to your office after three months of continued back and neck pain despite a thorough evaluation without findings and despite adequate radiologic and physical examination. After separating the child and parent, the child tells you that she just wants to spend time with her friends and she wants to go to the mall and be a normal 12-year-old. Which of the following is true?

    A. Elite-level gymnasts often present with back pain and should be pushed to "work through it" since she has a negative workup
    B. Burnout is common in elite-level child athletes as they often are subjected to excessive training loads during peak emotional and physical development times in pre-adolescence and adolescence
    C. Pressure from coaches and parents rarely leads to burnout in elite child athletes and only pushes them to work harder
    D. Respecting the child's request but not discussing it with the parent is best for the patient's recovery as the parent wants the child to continue training if the workup is negative
    E. A psychological consult is indicated as the athlete is obviously depressed

5. A 50-year-old male complains of right medial knee pain for six months after an injury sustained while playing rugby. He was diagnosed with a medial meniscal injury four months ago, underwent surgical debridement, and has recovered uneventfully, but continues to have the same medial knee pain. Pain is deep aching/burning, often nocturnal, and radiates from the vastus medialis oblique region to the medial lower leg and dorsomedial ankle and foot. Pain is worsened by sitting a laptop computer on his lap for a prolonged time. There are no weaknesses or vascular changes noted on exam. He has no success with non-steroidal anti-inflammatory drugs or conservative therapies and pushes for further diagnostic testing. Your next step in making a diagnosis is which of the following?

    A. MRI of the knee to evaluate the meniscus or other intra-articular pathology
    B. Local nerve block at the adductor canal
    C. Lumbar spine MRI to look for causes of lumbar radiculopathy
    D. Repeat arthroscopy of the knee

6. A 20-year-old female cross country runner developed right thigh pain one week ago. She describes the pain as feeling like a pulled muscle. She has not had an injury but has recently added sprint workouts to her training regimen. She is on birth control pills but no other medication. She reports normal menses, a normal diet, and one previous stress fracture of her foot in high school. She has tenderness to palpation of the distal femur but no pain with firing the quadriceps muscle. She has pain with the single-leg hop test but not with the fulcrum test. She has normal knee and hip joint exams. AP and lateral views of the right femur are negative. Which diagnosis is most likely regarding her injury?

   A. Quadriceps muscle strain
   B. Adductor longus strain
   C. Patellofemoral pain
   D. Distal femoral stress fracture
   E. Quadriceps tendonopathy

7. Which pair of objective findings is most suggestive of increased intracranial pressure?

   A. Tachycardia, low blood pressure
   B. Bradycardia, elevated blood pressure
   C. Tachycardia, elevated blood pressure
   D. Bradycardia, low blood pressure

8. In order to avoid overtraining, athletes can initiate training principles that include the use of microcycles, mesocycles, and macrocycles. Which of the following is the name for this type of training?

   A. Accommodation training
   B. Periodization training
   C. Progressive overload training
   D. Optimization training

9. You are covering a weight lifting tournament, and the competitor misses the snatch (the olympic lift in which the athlete attempts to move a loaded barbell from the floor to an overhead postion in one fluid motion). You notice through your direct observation of the lift (and subsequent review of the videotape) that the loaded barbell (which weighed around 250 pounds) came down on the athlete's neck. The athlete was able to walk off the competition platform under his own power before you could reach the individual. Off the platform, the athlete complains of a sore neck and "nothing else." He denies radicular symptoms, limb weakness, headache, or parathesias. Your exam reveals normal peripheral neurological exam (deep tendon reflex, sensation, strength) but some paracervical muscle soreness and spinous process tenderness. Which of the following is the most likely diagnosis?

   A. C3-C4 cervical subluxation
   B. Rupture of the ligamentum flava
   C. Clay shoveler's fracture
   D. Paraspinal muscle strain
   E. Thoracic outlet syndrome

10. A 29-year-old hockey player complains of one day of eye pain. The pain began suddenly while he was sharpening his skates without using eye protection. Upon exam, his visual acuity is intact, as are extraocular movements. Seidel's test is negative. Inspection shows scleral erythema and a 0.5 mm brownish stain at 12 o'clock superior to the iris. In addition to standard management and removal of this corneal foreign body, which of the following steps must be taken?

   A. Expansion of microbial coverage to include atypical organisms
   B. Patching for one week to decrease spreading inflammation
   C. Removal of products of iron oxidation from the cornea
   D. Repair of corneal perforation in the operating room
   E. Prolonged course of mydriatics

11. A 16-year-old male runner presents with a six-week history of worsening right-sided groin pain with activity. A femoral neck stress fracture is diagnosed by MRI. Conservative treatments are most appropriate initial management for which of the following types of this fracture?

   A. Superior neck fracture
   B. Tension-side fracture
   C. Compression-side fracture
   D. Displaced neck fracture

12. In which area would you not find a referred pain from sacroiliac joint dysfunction?

    A. Buttocks
    B. Hip joint
    C. Pubic symphysis
    D. Lower abdomen
    E. Lateral thigh

13. Which of the following is correct regarding the infrapatellar fat pad?

    A. The infrapatellar fat pad is located anterior to the patellar tendon
    B. Fat pad irritation is exacerbated by flexion of the knee
    C. Fad pad impingement is painful because it is a highly innervated structure
    D. Surgical excision is often necessary for definitive treatment of an irritated fat pad

14. Which of the following statements related to blood loss and anemia in athletes is false?

    A. Rupture of red blood cells occurs in the capillaries of the feet during endurance running events
    B. Hematuria in marathon runners lasts for several weeks after the marathon event
    C. Well-trained athletes with sickle cell trait perform similarly to athletes with normal hemoglobin at aerobic and anaerobic sports
    D. Iron deficiency anemia is the most common form of anemia found in athletes
    E. A drop in the hematocrit in well-trained endurance athletes can be a physiologic adaptation to exercise not requiring treatment

15. A 27-year-old female presents to your clinic, complaining of bilateral lower extremity pain that began about one month ago. She would like to run a marathon and has been training for the past three months. Initially, she felt a dull ache during the first mile of her run that she was able to run through. Gradually, the pain has increased, and she now feels it during and at the end of her run. She did try taking a week off and the pain completely subsided, but once she started running again, the pain returned. Her physical exam findings are remarkable for diffuse tenderness along the posterior medial aspect of the middle and distal tibia on both lower extremities. Her neurovascular exam is normal. You do not find focal or point tenderness and there are no abnormalities found on x-ray. You make the diagnosis of medial tibial stress syndrome (shin splints) and recommend which of the following treatments?

    A. Relative rest to allow the patient to be pain free followed by a gradual increase in exercise intensity and duration on soft, level surfaces as long as she remains aymptomatic
    B. Weight training avoiding cardiorespiratory fitness
    C. Cam-walker-style boot for four to six weeks with the application of a bone-stimulator unit at night
    D. A cool-down routine should be initiated emphasizing stretching before and after exercise

16. Which of the following statements is true regarding cubital tunnel syndrome?

    A. MRI studies are often not helpful in the diagnosis of cubital tunnel syndrome
    B. Electromyogram (EMG) and nerve conduction studies are rarely helpful in the diagnosis of cubital tunnel syndrome
    C. Patients will usually complain of paresthesias in the thumb and index finger
    D. Patients may have weakness in thumb-index finger pinch (Froment's sign) in chronic cases
    E. In throwing athletes, the first-line treatment for cubital tunnel syndrome is ulnar collateral ligament reconstruction

17. Which of the following tests is recommended during a typical high school preparticipation physical?

    A. Echocardiogram
    B. Electrocardiogram
    C. Pulmonary function testing
    D. Urine drug screen
    E. Auscultation of the heart in standing and lying position

18. Which of the following cervical spine injuries are both considered stable non-emergent fractures?

    A. Flexion teardrop fracture and clay shoveler's fracture
    B. Hangman fracture and posterior neural arch fracture
    C. Simple wedge fracture and flexion teardrop fracture
    D. Posterior neural arch fracture and simple wedge fracture

19. Which of the following statements is true regarding skin infection in athletes?

    A. Rifampin is the first line treatment for MRSA (methicillin-resistant staphylococcus aureus) infections
    B. Any skin wound that is suspicious for staphylococcus infection should be cultured
    C. The gold standard treatment of MRSA is appropriate oral antibiotics
    D. First line treatment of MRSA should be topical antibiotics
    E. Special cleaning of locker room, equipment and playing area is needed if MRSA is diagnosed in an athlete

20. Which of the following factors has most contributed to the dramatic decrease in catastrophic cervical spine injuries since 1976?

    A. Improved preparticipation physical exam screening
    B. Mental conditioning prior to games
    C. Improvement in helmet design
    D. Banning of spear tackling or primarily striking with the crown of the head

21. A 33-year-old male who is preparing for his third half-marathon is determined to improve his time at this year's race, so he decided to change several areas of his training that he thought would improve his performance, increasing his overall mileage and hill running. Unfortunately, he developed substantial lateral knee pain. His physical exam demonstrates a positive Ober's test. He responded very well to stretching and strengthening exercises. What else on the history and physical would you have expected to discover before beginning treatment?

    A. Normal lower extremity alignment
    B. Strong abductor muscles
    C. Less pain with hill running
    D. Positive Noble's test
    E. Abnormal radiographs

22. Pain originating from the facet joint complex is a common cause of back pain. The purpose of the facet joint in its protection of the lumbar intervertebral disk is best characterized as which of the following?

    A. Protection against axial rotation and loading
    B. Protection against shearing forces
    C. Protection against anterior translocation
    D. Protection against caudal translocation

23. An otherwise healthy 16-year-old male gymnast presents with a three-month history of non-radiating bilateral low back pain that worsens when he does back hand springs. On physical examination, his pain worsens with extension based maneuvers, and he has markedly decreased bilateral hamstring flexibility. There is no evidence of spondylolisthesis on plain x-rays. A bone scan with SPECT and a thin-slice CT confirm your diagnosis. Which of the following rehabilitation programs would you prescribe?

    A. Extension-biased spinal stabilization and quadriceps flexibility exercises
    B. Flexion-biased spinal stabilization and hamstring flexibility exercises
    C. Extension-biased spinal stabilization and hamstring flexibility exercises
    D. Plyometric exercise program
    E. A rehabilitation program is not indicated for this condition

24. Which of the following is correct about acute zygomatic complex fractures?

    A. Raccoon eyes are pathognomonic
    B. Unequal pupil levels
    C. They are the third-most common facial bone fractures related to sports injury
    D. Involves mandible and associated bony structures

25. You are on vacation, scuba diving in the Carribean. Just after lunch, one of your morning dive partners complains to you he is having palpitations, a headache, nausea, and abdominal pain. You briefly take a look and notice he is very anxious, maybe wheezing and has a red macular balanching rash on the trunk. You quickly confirm he is a 35-year-old experienced male diver with a history of hypertension. He denies numbness and tingling in his hands and feet. He denies fevers or chills. He states during his week he participated in four recreational dives over two consecutive days. He reported dive times and depths well within the safety parameters set by PADI (Professional Association of Diving Instructors). He takes lisinopril 10 mg a day for hypertension and has been on it for seven years. He has no allergies. He did eat some locally caught fish: tuna, mahi mahi, and other reef fish at the lunch buffet. His vitals are stable with a blood pressure of 132/86. This patient is most likely suffering from which of the following?

    A. Arterial gas embolism
    B. Pulmonary barotrauma of ascent
    C. Scombroid poisoning
    D. Decompression illness
    E. Ciguartera poisoning

26. Which statement is true regarding exercise-induced anaphylaxis?

    A. Pre-treatment with antihistamines is effective to reduce the occurrence rate
    B. Pre-treatment with NSAIDs or aspirin is effective to reduce the occurrence rate
    C. A common trigger is running within a couple of hours after ingesting a meal
    D. Initial treatment is immediate administration of anti-histamines and steroids
    E. Reccurrence is rare so affected athletes can run alone with little risk

27. A 16-year-old male football player presents to your office with acute onset of mid-thoracic back pain, which began immediately after being struck in the back during a football game the previous evening. On exam, you note an area of point tenderness immediately lateral to the midline in the mid-thoracic region of the athlete's back. Other than some moderate paravertebral muscle spasm, he has no other physical findings. Radiographic evaluation reveals a nondisplaced transverse process fracture. Which of the following are appropriate management options for this athlete?

    A. Immediate immobilization on a back board and transfer to the hospital for neurosurgical evaluation
    B. Referral for fitting of a clam-shell type back brace
    C. Use of local ice, analgesics, and antiinflammatory medication, with return to activity as tolerated
    D. MRI evaluation to assess spinal cord compromise
    E. Disqualification from participation in collision sports for a minimum of six months

28. Which of the following statements is true regarding preadolescents and well structured weight lifting programs?

    A. Strength training increases both muscle strength and hypertrophy in preadolescents
    B. Strength training increases muscle strength, but not hypertrophy in preadolescents
    C. Strength training is considered harmful to maturation, but beneficial to growth in preadolescents
    D. Strength training can have a negative impact on maturation and growth in preadolescents

29. A 16-year-old male snowboarder had an accident during the Olympic competition. It was significant enough that it was decided to transport him to the hospital. En route, he complained of left shoulder pain, but remained hemodynamically stable during transport. At the hospital, his hemoglobin remained normal and stable throughout. CT scanning with contrast revealed a grade II splenic injury. Which of the following is correct regarding his initial evaluation, management, and disposition?

    A. The spleen is rarely injured during sport
    B. Non-operative management would be preferred
    C. Splenic rupture is of minor concern in this patient
    D. Ultrasound is the preferred method of imaging in stable patients
    E. He should be vaccinated immediately

30. Which of the following exercise prescriptions should you advise against for an HIV-infected individual with mild to moderate symptoms or CD4 count < 200?

    A. Moderate exercise (40% to 60% $\dot{V}O_2$max)
    B. Weight training
    C. Intense exercise (> 75% $\dot{V}O_2$max)
    D. Three times per week

31. During the second football practice of the day on day three of the college preseason football camp, an offensive lineman is found sitting on the ground, unwilling to stand up. He states his left calf is cramping and that he feels lightheaded and exhausted. You suspect possible exertional heat stroke. Which of the following statements about this condition is true?

    A. Axillary, oral, or a rectal temperature greater than 104 degrees Fahrenheit (40 degrees Celsius) establishes the diagnosis of exertional heat stroke
    B. This condition occurs randomly without warning and cannot be predicted
    C. Cold/ice water immersion is an effective way to treat exertional heat stroke
    D. There are two patterns of presentation: sodium depletion and water depletion

32. You are evaluating an obtunded athlete who collapsed toward the end of a marathon. Physical exam is significant for a rectal temperature of 98.6 degrees Fahrenheit (37 degrees Celsius), BP 110/60, heart rate of 110, and diffusely increased muscle tone. What is the most likely diagnosis as you prepare to have your athlete transported?

    A. Heat stroke
    B. Myocardial infarction
    C. Rhabdomyolysis
    D. Exercise associated collapse

33. While treating a member of your university's women's cross country team for a fifth metatarsal stress fracture, you suspect she may have female athlete triad. Which of the following statements would help confirm the diagnosis of anorexia nervosa?

    A. Binging and purging at least twice a week for three months
    B. Menses every six to eight weeks in a postmenarchal female
    C. Normal body image
    D. A weight less than 85% of expected ideal body weight

34. Which of the following statements is true regarding metacarpal fractures?

    A. Most metacarpal fractures in athletes will eventually need a surgical procedure in order to regain full function
    B. Fifth metacarpal fractures are called "boxer's" fractures because of their common occurrence in boxers
    C. Splints and casts for metacarpal fractures should immobilize the proximal interphalangeal (PIP), metacarpophalangeal (MCP), and the wrist joint
    D. Although up to 30 degrees of angulation is acceptable for a fifth metacarpal fracture and may be treated non-operatively, fractures with malrotation should be referred for surgical reduction
    E. Fractures of the hand should be treated with prolonged immobilization since early motion leads to significant risk of non-union and poor functional outcome

35. You are participating as a volunteer physician in a preparticipation physical examination night for incoming freshman athletes at a local college. The examinations are station-based and quite busy with four physicians to evaluate 80 athletes. You see a female cross country runner with a height of 5'6"; weight 100 pounds; pulse of 45 and respirations of 18. She says she has always been thin and her mother is also thin. Her last menstrual period was more than a year ago. She has been told that the lack of menses is of no concern since she is an athlete. Physical exam is unremarkable except for the very thin stature. You recommend which of the following?

    A. Cleared for participation, but needs nutrition evaluation
    B. Not cleared for participation until nutrition evaluation
    C. Not cleared for participation until further evaluation by team physician and completion of nutrition evaluation
    D. Order labs to include estradiol, LH, FSH, and TSH, and if normal, clear her for participation

36. A 42-year-old laborer and distance runner presents to clinic with a painful click in his right hip. Pain is deep in the anterior groin. Exam shows pain with flexion combined with either internal or external rotation. Plain radiographs are normal. The test most sensitive in attempting to establish the diagnosis in this patient is which of the following?

    A. Ultrasound
    B. Computed tomography (CT)
    C. Magnetic resonance imaging (MRI)
    D. Bone SPECT scan
    E. Magnetic resonance imaging with intra-articular contrast and intra-articular local anesthetic (MRI arthrogram)

37. Which of the following is a known result of resistance training?

    A. In elderly patients, improved balance, mobility, and strength to perform ADLs
    B. Decrease in bone mass and in strength of connective tissue
    C. Decrease in lean body mass
    D. Large improvement in cardiorespiratory fitness
    E. Decrease in glucose tolerance and lipid profiles when resistance is a component of circuit training

38. A 67-year-old woman presents to your clinic with a persistent foot drop after sustaining a fibular head fracture two years ago. What type of orthotic would you prescribe?

    A. Metatarsal bar
    B. Ankle foot orthosis (AFO)
    C. UCBL (University of California-Berkeley Lab) shoe insert
    D. Thumb spica splint
    E. Hinged knee brace

39. Which of the following is not felt to improve physical performance or considered an ergogenic aid?

    A. Caffeine
    B. Creatine
    C. Anabolic steroids
    D. Alcohol

40. De Quervain's tenosynovitis involves which of the following tendon sheaths?

    A. Extensor digitorum profundus and extensor pollicis
    B. Flexor pllicis longus and abductor pollicis longus
    C. Flexor pollicis longus and abductor pollicis brevis
    D. Extensor pollicis brevis and abductor pollicis longus

41. The anterior tibialis is the main dorsiflexor of the ankle,. It originates on the anterolateral tibia and interosseus membrane and inserts on which of the following?

    A. Medial cuneiform and base of first metatarsal
    B. All three cuneiform bones, and the base of the second metatarsal
    C. Navicular bone
    D. Anterior talus

42. Which of the following statements regarding sickle cell trait athletes is true?

    A. Sickle cell trait, in contrast to sickle cell disease, has little to no mortality in athletes
    B. Any cramping, struggling, or collapse in a sickle-trait athlete must be considered sickling—a medical emergency—until proven otherwise
    C. The symptoms of exertional sickling and heat illness (heat stroke or heat cramping) are not distinguishable
    D. Acclimation to intense training, increased hydration, and increased rest afford no protection to sickling in athletes

43. Which of the following is the only immunization currently required by law for entrance into specific countries?

    A. Yellow fever
    B. Malaria
    C. E. coli
    D. Rotavirus

44. Which of the following is a property of slow twitch (type I) muscle fibers?

    A. Low mitochondrial density
    B. Rely on anaerobic metabolism
    C. Higher rate of force production
    D. Major storage fuel is triglycerides

45. A 17-year-old football player tackles an opposing player and sustains a flexion injury of his neck. He falls to the ground. The ambulance is summoned, and he is boarded and taken to the hospital. He is found to have an injury to the anterior spinal cord of his neck. Which of the following clinical findings match this lesion?

    A. Loss of motor function and position sense on the same side of the body as the lesion and loss of pain and sensation on the opposite side of the body as the lesion
    B. Bilateral lower extremity paralysis that is greater than the upper extremity paralysis; bilateral loss of pain and temperature sensation; vibratory and proprioception is intact
    C. Weakness in both upper extremities that is more severe than the weakness in both lower extremities; sacral function is spared
    D. After the period of spinal shock has resolved, the patient has no motor or sensory activity below the level of the lesion

46. A 20-year-old male soccer player presents with four months of right groin pain. It is described as a deep ache just to the side of his pubic bone and radiates down the medial thigh when he plays soccer. He also reports some paresthesias along the medial thigh after exercise and difficulty with jumping. On exam, he is weak on hip adduction and tender with stretching his adductors. You decide to order an EMG, which shows a denervation pattern of the adductor longus and brevis consistent with entrapment of which of the following nerves?

    A. Obturator nerve
    B. Ilioinguinal nerve
    C. Superior gluteal nerve
    D. Inferior gluteal nerve

47. You have been asked to coordinate preparticipation physical exams for a college with approximately 300 Division II athletes. You have the aid of some local physicians, physical therapist and athletic trainers. You elect for station-based exams. Which of the following choices is a disadvantage of station-based preparticipation physical examinations?

    A. Examinations can be limited and brief due to time constraints
    B. Many examinations can be performed in a short period of time
    C. Compared to office-base exams, it is the most cost-effective method
    D. Communication among the sports medicine team is readily available

48. The most common mechanism of injury to the carotid artery in blunt cerebrovascular injuries is due to which of the following?

    A. Direct laceration from a sharp object
    B. Hyperextension injury to the neck
    C. Flexion injury to the neck
    D. Direct blow to the neck
    E. Laceration secondary to fracture of sphenoid or petrous bones

49. A 30-year-old male with T6 paraplegia presents to the office with a desire to begin a wheel exercise program. He has been gaining weight due to a lack of activity since the injury several years ago. He wants your advice on how to safely begin an exercise program. Along with advising proper equipment, carrying water, and avoiding hot or humid days, you also advise which of the following?

    A. Wear tight leg straps to increase sympathetic tone
    B. Take 10 grams of carbohydrates every 30 minutes during exercise
    C. Empty bladder and bowels before each workout
    D. Have cervical x-rays to rule out atlantoaxial instability

50. A baseball player was hit in the upper thigh by a line drive, and he complains of swelling and pain immediately. You note a large hematoma present in the location of the injury. You begin your evaluation by palpating the borders of the femoral triangle. Which of the following structures does not form a border of the triangle?

    A. Medial border of the adductor brevis
    B. Inguinal ligament
    C. Medial border of the adductor longus
    D. Medial border of the sartorius

51. You are seeing a new patient for a preparticipation exam, and this athlete would like to be cleared to scuba dive. Which of the following statements is true regarding SCUBA diving participation?

    A. An athlete with a well-controlled seizure disorder who is on a stable dose of medication and has been seizure-free for six months is safe to be cleared
    B. An athlete with a previous spontaneous pneumothorax can be cleared for shallow dives only
    C. An athlete with sickle cell trait has no more risk of hypoxia than the average diver and is safe to be cleared
    D. An athlete with myringotomy tubes in place for three months is safe to be cleared
    E. An athlete with an active otitis media if treated with antibiotics is safe to be cleared

52. A 37-year-old male who is otherwise healthy, but minimally active physically, has signed up as a charity runner for a local marathon in August. He has been training well per Jeff Galloway's training program for first-time marathoners. He comes to see you in June before the race with concerns about hydration for prevention of heat injury. Which of the following recommendations is appropriate for fluid hydration during endurance events?

    A. Drink at each water stop along the race course
    B. Drink ad lib based on thirst
    C. Drink an adequate amount of fluids to keep urine output pale
    D. Alternate water and glucose-electrolyte solution according to a pre-planned schedule

53. Which component of the deep posterior compartment of the lower leg assists with plantar flexion of the foot?

    A. Tibialis posterior
    B. Flexor digitorum longus
    C. Soleus
    D. Tibialis anterior

54. A 15-year-old wrestler presents to the clinic with localized swelling and tenderness in the helix of the right ear. The swelling developed after a day long wrestling tournament. Which of the following statements is incorrect?

    A. The injury is caused by repeated rubbing or by absorbing repetitive blows
    B. If not treated initially, the ear will develop a deformed cauliflower-like appearance
    C. Suturing a sterile button through the ear is an acceptable treatment
    D. Repeated aspirations should be avoided
    E. Sports commonly associated with this injury are wrestling, rugby, and soccer

55. On average, VO$_2$max is lower in postpubertal females when compared to postpubertal males. Which of the following statements is true concerning reasons for this difference?

    A. Females, on average, experience a relative decrease in body fat after puberty
    B. Females, on average, have increased cardiac output compared to males
    C. Females, on average, have larger muscle fiber area compared to males
    D. Females, on average, have lower blood hemoglobin content

56. Your patient, a 43-year-old male with long-standing type 2 diabetes mellitus, wishes to begin an exercise program. Which of the following are appropriate recommendations for this patient?

    A. There is limited information regarding the benefit of exercise in type 2 diabetes
    B. There is little risk of hypoglycemia in exercising diabetic patients
    C. Patients with proliferative retinopathy are at no greater risk than those with normal funduscopic findings
    D. Hypoglycemia is more likely to occur during morning exercise
    E. The patient should undergo exercise electrocardiography before beginning an exercise program

57. Which of the following does not cause delayed onset muscle soreness (DOMS)?

    A. Lactic acid accumulation in muscle tissues
    B. Structural damage to muscle fibers
    C. Eccentric exercise
    D. Swelling on a cellular level, which may activate and sensitize afferent nerve endings around damaged muscle fibers
    E. Training at an intensity greater than customary

58. Which of the following is the main arterial blood supply to the anterior cruciate ligament in the knee?

    A. Posterior tibial artery
    B. Superior medial genicular artery
    C. Anterior tibial artery
    D. Middle genicular artery

59. A Segond fracture is pathognomonic for which ligamentous injury?

    A. Medial collateral ligament
    B. Lateral collateral ligament
    C. Anterior cruciate ligament
    D. Posterior cruciate ligament

60. A 17-year-old football player exits the game after a play due to severe right shoulder pain. Pain symptoms are completely resolved by the time he is examined on the sideline, but he describes the pain as primarily over the lateral shoulder with some radiation to the posterior arm and lateral forearm. Examination reveals no deformity or tenderness to palpation of the shoulder. He has slight weakness to the deltoid, supraspinatus and infraspinatus muscles. He has normal muscle strength on shoulder shrug, biceps, triceps, grip strength, and wrist pronation, supination, flexion, and extension. He has mild sensory changes to the lateral shoulder but normal sensation over the arm, forearm, and hand. The most likely location for the injury is which of the following?

    A. Radial nerve
    B. Posterior cord
    C. Upper trunk
    D. Lower subscapular nerve
    E. Lateral cord

61. During a preparticipation examination on one of your female high school cross country athletes, she admits to two episodes of fainting that occurred during last season's racing. Further questioning of both her and her parents reveals that these episodes occurred after she crossed the finish line, never during actual running, and are not associated with any other symptoms. She has no post-episode confusion and recovers quickly with minimal assistance. No significant cardiac history exists in her or her family. She has never had any workup for this before, and you are only able to do one test beyond a thorough history and physical examination, both of which are normal. The most helpful test at this point would be?

   A. 12-lead ECG
   B. Echocardiogram
   C. Tilt table test
   D. 24-hour event monitor

62. Two nights after a rapid ascent from sea level to an elevation of 3,500 m (11,500 feet), a non-acclimatized climber is experiencing symptoms of headache, dry cough, decreased exercise performance, tachypnea, and tachycardia at rest. In addition to descent, what is the most appropriate treatment for this climber?

   A. Dexamethasone
   B. High-flow oxygen
   C. Ibuprofen
   D. Furosemide
   E. IV fluids

63. When treating patients with osteoarthritis, what therapy program has been shown to be most effective in improving Western Ontario MacMaster (WOMAC) scores?

   A. Home exercise program to improve compliance
   B. Water therapy in a group setting
   C. Formal physical therapy for at least four weeks
   D. Supervised physical therapy followed by a home exercise program

64. What is the most common cause of airway obstruction in an unconscious athlete?

   A. Mouthguard
   B. Tongue
   C. Swelling from anaphylaxis
   D. Inhaled foreign body

65. After going up for a rebound and being poked in the eye by an opponent's finger, a high school basketball player complains of eye pain, blurred vision, and sensation of something stuck in her eye. Which intervention may increase pain while the abrasion heals?

   A. Patching
   B. Topical NSAIDs (diclofenac)
   C. Oral analgesics (acetaminophen with codeine)
   D. Erythromycin ointment
   E. Topical mydriatic agent (1% cyclopentolate)

66. Which of the following is not true regarding iron deficiency anemia (IDA) in athletes?

   A. Women are at higher risk of developing IDA than men
   B. In the initial stage of IDA, serum iron concentrations are low while the ferritin and hemoglobin levels are normal
   C. Footstrike hemolysis is a known cause of IDA
   D. Inadequate calorie consumption and menstrual losses are common causes in female athletes

67. An obese patient (BMI > 30) without other comorbidities presents to your office. To improve compliance, one strategy for the patient's exercise prescription could include which of the following?

   A. Incorporating high-impact aerobic activities
   B. Emphasizing exercising after their morning meal
   C. Strict cardiovascular prescription at 85% maximum HR for at least 30 minutes five times per week
   D. Increasing weight-bearing activities very rapidly to increase metabolism
   E. Starting with non-weight-bearing activities such as swimming and recumbent bike

68. A 17-year-old female presents after injuring her right knee. She was landing from a rebound and felt her knee "pop." She developed immediate swelling in the right knee and was unable to continue playing. On exam, the knee has a large effusion with positive Lachman and anterior drawer tests. Which of the following is true regarding her diagnosis?

    A. ACL injuries are less common in female athletes
    B. Traditional surgical reconstruction of the ACL may be performed in children regardless of physeal status
    C. The ACL is the primary restraint to posterior translation of the tibia with respect to the femur
    D. A hemarthrosis would be expected with aspiration of the injured knee
    E. Findings on standard radiography are usually specific for ACL injury

69. An avid 25-year-old male cyclist, cycling 120 miles per week, complains of left testicular pain and some perineal numbness for the past two months. He has never experienced this before and reports no recent change in his equipment, training intensity, or duration in the recent month. He reports his pain as 6 to 8 out of 10 and is relieved by standing or walking. He has discussed this with his cycling teammates, and they have advised he consider changing his seat set-up and brand to a split seat to relieve his symptoms. The likely cause of his symptoms is which of the following?

    A. Pudendal nerve compression
    B. Adductor tendinopathy
    C. Ischial periositis
    D. Scrotal ischemia
    E. Testicular torsion

70. In the absence of direct physical trauma, the activities with the highest incidence of spontaneous pneumothorax include SCUBA diving and which of the following?

    A. Soccer
    B. Weight lifting
    C. Football
    D. Swimming

71. Which of the following is not a criterion for x-ray, according to the Ottawa Ankle Rules or Ottawa Foot Rules?

    A. Pain over the navicular
    B. Positive anterior drawer sign
    C. Bone tenderness at the posterior edge of either malleolus
    D. Inability to bear weight for four steps, either immediately or in the emergency room
    E. Pain over the base of the fifth metatarsal

72. One of the new athletes to your college lists on his health history that he takes methylphenidate (Ritalin®) for his attention deficit, hyperactivity disorder (ADHD). Regarding intercollegiate athletes taking stimulant medications, which of the following is a true statement (select the best answer)?

    A. The NCAA does not ban methylphenidate (Ritalin, Concerta®) or amphetamine (Adderral) because their common use for the treatment of ADHD
    B. A medical exemption must be applied for and granted by the NCAA prior to athletic participation when stimulant medications are used for medical reasons
    C. The NCAA does not require the institution maintain, in the student-athlete's on-campus medical record, a copy of the physician's signed prescription for dispensing the medication
    D. The NCAA requires the institution to maintain, in the student-athlete's on-campus medical record, documentation from the prescribing physician detailing medical history, diagnosis, verification of that diagnosis through standard assessment, and dosing
    E. The NCAA tests for only anabolic substances and not stimulant medications

73. A 19-year-old female tennis player comes to you for her preparticipation examination. She denies any cardiac symptoms and has always kept up with her peers. There is no history of heart disease or early death in the family. Examination is unremarkable except for a systolic ejection murmur that increases with Valsalva and standing, and decreases with fist clenching and squatting. Which of the following is the most significant predictor of sudden cardiac death in this athlete?

    A. Sudden death in her brother
    B. Muscle fiber disarray on biopsy
    C. Septal thickness of > 1.8 cm
    D. Paroxysmal atrial fibrillation on Holter monitoring
    E. Resting BP 120/75, and BP 95/70 after six minutes of exercise

74. A 21-year-old female is brought to the medical tent near the finish line at your community's annual marathon after suddenly collapsing moments after completing the race. Her mental status is normal, and her temperature is 103.6 degrees Fahrenheit (38.9 degrees Celsius). She reports feeling slightly lightheaded and has difficulty standing up. Your intial treatment strategy should include which of the following?

    A. Provide the patient with walking assistance until she no longer feels it is difficult to stand or walk
    B. Place the patient in a supine position so that both her legs and pelvis are elevated
    C. Provide IV fluid replacement with 5% dextrose in half normal saline
    D. Provide IV fluid replacement with 5% dextrose in normal saline
    E. Provide active cooling with ice water tub immersion until her temperature drops below 104 degrees Fahrenheit (38.0 degrees Celsius)

75. Which of the following statements is correct?

    A. Congenital sensorineural deafness is associated with long QT syndrome
    B. Albuterol should be encouraged in patients with suspected congenital prolonged QT interval
    C. Taking ciprofloxacin prolongs the QT interval
    D. Athletes with known prolonged QT can be cleared to run the 110 m hurdles, but not to run the 1,500 m in track and field

76. Hypertension is the most common cardiovascular disease that the sports medicine physician will encounter. There are many aspects of both the patient and his chosen sporting activity to consider when selecting a pharmaceutical intervention in the management of the hypertensive athlete. Select the choice that represents the best antihypertensive for the given athlete?

    A. White female biathlete (cross country ski and riflery): metoprolol
    B. White male Olympic weight-lifter: hydrochlorothiazide
    C. Black female swimmer with a history of cholinergic urticaria: lisinopril
    D. White male lacrosse player: valsartan
    E. White female marathoner with a prior history of thyrotoxicosis-related atrial fibrillation: diltiazem

77. In patients with chronic pulmonary disease, endurance training is often beneficial with improved pulmonary function and less symptoms. Which of the following is true regarding pulmonary rehabilitation?

    A. The American Thoracic Society (ATS) recommends a specific strength training program
    B. Successful rehabilitation requires optimal medical management, including pharmacotherapy
    C. Pulmonary rehabilitation resembles cardiac rehabilitation with similar applications
    D. In pulmonary rehabilitation, the patient is encouraged to exercise to maximal effect without relying on oxygen supplementation

78. Factors associated with increased risk of primary exertional headaches include which of the following?

    A. Exercise in cold weather
    B. Dehydration
    C. Intense exercise at sea level
    D. Age above 40 years
    E. Previous head trauma

79. A 16-year-old female soccer player receives a direct blow to the mouth from an opposing player's elbow. She immediately comes to the sideline and is noted to have bleeding from her mouth. In her hand, she is holding an intact, avulsed tooth. Which of the following management options will help to ensure the best outcome?

    A. Gently wipe away blood and tissue remnants from the tooth with sterile saline-moistened gauze, preserve in saline, and refer to dentist immediately
    B. Clean the tooth with sterile saline, protect it in dry sterile gauze, and follow up with dentist within eight hours
    C. Reimplantation of the avulsed tooth and immediate referral
    D. Preserve the tooth in milk and ensure follow-up with her dentist within eight hours
    E. Discard the tooth and salvage and stabilize the underlying tissue with a protective mouth guard

80. During a masters race in mid-March, one of the runners collapses and dies shortly thereafter. While running a marathon, which of the following is the most common cause of sudden death in older athletes (> 35 years old)?

    A. Hyponatremia
    B. Neurocardiogenic syncope
    C. Cerebral vascular accident
    D. Poorly controlled diabetes mellitus
    E. Coronary artery disease

81. A tight end receives a blow with a helmet to the right side of the chest wall while stretched out for a pass. He complains of right sided pleuritic chest pain and progressive dyspnea. On exam, you note contusion and a step-off of the rib. The right lung field is hyperresonant, and there are decreased breath sounds on the right. There is asymmetry in inspiration with the right chest wall not moving. Which of the following are the best indications for emergent, on-field, needle thoracostomy?

    A. Trachea deviated left and BP 124/82
    B. Trachea deviated left and BP 90/40
    C. Trachea midline and BP 162/94
    D. Trachea deviated right and BP 162/94
    E. Trachea deviated right and BP 90/40

82. An 18-year-old male baseball pitcher presents with a one-month history of fatigue and weakness in his throwing arm. His symptoms gradually worsen with increasing pitch counts and will resolve with rest. He reports normal sensation in his hands, but reports his right hand will feel cool after he has finished pitching. You suspect subclavian artery compression. Which of the following provocative maneuvers may recreate his symptoms if he has subclavian artery compression?

    A. Roos stress test
    B. Tinel's test at the wrist
    C. Spurling's maneuver
    D. Inability of the patient to make a circle with the index finger and thumb

83. A patient presents to your office unable to dorsiflex his great toe. Which of the following is true?

    A. The extensor hallucis longus, which inserts on base of the distal phalanx of the great toe, is the muscle responsible for extending the great toe
    B. The motor function for this is from L4 and L5
    C. The muscles that allow this action are all contained in the lateral compartment of the lower leg
    D. The muscles that allow this action are inervated by the tibialis anterior nerve

84. When evaluating anterior knee pain, the defining characteristics of patellar tendinitis include which one of the following?

    A. There are findings on imaging that are "pathognomonic" for patellar tendinitis
    B. Surgery is more effective than rehabilitation
    C. Patellar tendinitis is common and rarely requires treatment
    D. Training errors are the most common cause

85. You accept responsibility to cover a local football game in a stadium. Which of the following choices is your top priority for this or any other athletic event?

    A. Investigate EMS coverage
    B. Confirm AED availability
    C. Coordinate the entire sports medicine team in advance
    D. Review the chain of command with covering physicians
    E. Require an ATC to be present

86. Of the following, which is not an appropriate indication for the use of a sugar tong splint?

    A. Colles' fracture
    B. Prevention of supination
    C. Elbow immobilization
    D. Prevention of pronation
    E. Scaphoid fracture

87. A day after being struck with a pitched ball on the ulnar aspect of the left wrist and hand, a professional baseball player develops "pins and needles" in the small and ulnar half of his ring fingers. He finds it extremely difficult to grab the bat to participate in batting practice. After x-rays demonstrate no acute abnormalities of the left wrist and hand, he is diagnosed with Guyon's canal syndrome. What two bones form Guyon's canal?

    A. Pisiform and triquetrum
    B. Pisiform and hamate
    C. Hamate and lunate
    D. Triquetrum and lunate

88. An important aspect of the preparticipation physical exam is the blood pressure reading. Which of the following statements is true regarding blood pressure readings in children?

    A. The JNC 7 classification of hypertension in adults can be also be used for children under age 18
    B. Stimulant use is rarely a cause for blood pressure elevation in children under age 18
    C. One isolated elevation in a child's blood pressure greater than 95th percentile should fully restrict sports participation
    D. Blood pressure charts based on sex, age, and height percentile should be used for children under age 18

89. Which of the following statements about fibula fractures is true?

    A. The best x-ray view to identify whether there is any widening between the talus and fibula is the AP view
    B. A proximal fibula fracture (Maisonneuve) occurs most commonly secondary to an inversion mechanism
    C. A proximal fibula fracture (Maisonneuve) is usually unstable and requires orthopedic surgical referral and intervention
    D. A proximal fibula fracture (Maisonneuve) is usually stable and can be treated in a non-weight bearing cast
    E. A proximal fibula fracture (Maisonneuve) occurs most commonly from a direct blow to the proximal fibula

90. A mother brings her 15-year-old son in for evaluation of curvature of the back noted by the athletic trainer at his school. He has no complaints about back pain and a normal neurological exam. After your evaluation, to include a scoliosis radiographic evaluation, you identify that he has dextroscoliosis with a Cobb angle of 15 degrees. His Risser classification is Risser 3. On further exam, his leg lengths are equal. Which of the following is an appropriate recommendation for follow-up evaluation?

    A. Follow up with evaluation in six months
    B. Refer for physical therapy
    C. Refer to a pediatric spine surgeon
    D. Order a lumbar MRI
    E. Only follow up as needed if symptomatic

91. In the majority of people, the median nerve courses between the two heads of which one of the following muscles in the forearm?

    A. Supinator
    B. Pronator teres
    C. Flexor carpi ulnaris
    D. Pronator quadratus

92. A female volleyball player is in clinic for a preparticipation evaluation. Her history is negative except for frequent right ankle sprains. Her exam shows a positive anterior drawer and mild weakness of her peroneal muscles. In addition to having her do an ankle rehabilitation program, you recommend she use which of the following prophylactic devices to most effectively reduce her rate of recurrence?

    A. High top shoes
    B. Ankle brace
    C. Medial shoe wedge
    D. Ankle elastic wrap

93. The most common nerve injury in glenohumeral shoulder dislocations is which of the following?

    A. Suprascapular nerve
    B. Axillary nerve
    C. Long thoracic nerve
    D. Radial nerve
    E. Musculocutaneous nerve

94. A 34-year-old African-American Florida native is visiting her cousin in Colorado in early January. Temperatures are near record lows (−80 degrees Fahrenheit, −62 degrees Celsius). While her cousin is at work, she decides to go out snowshoeing with cotton socks and bindings that are a bit tight. After about five minutes, she notices numbness in her toes. She comes in to urgent care with white, cold, and firm toes. Further questioning reveals that she has smoked one pack of cigarettes per day since age 18. The definitive treatment is which of the following?

    A. Vigorously rub the toes with warm hands to stimulate circulation
    B. Warm the toes by immersion in a 104-degree Fahrenheit (40-degree Celsius) whirlpool
    C. Immediately amputate the affecte d toes
    D. Wrap the affected toes with warm blankets
    E. Use a small heater to warm the toes

95. Which of the following is true regarding children and sports activity?

    A. Preteen athletes most commonly injure lower limbs, whereas teenagers injure upper limbs
    B. Salter-Harris II fractures generally require surgical intervention
    C. Joint dislocations and ligamentous injuries are more common than buckle and other types of fractures
    D. Physes close on average at 14.5 years in girls and 16.5 years in boys
    E. Non-union fractures are common in the immature skeleton

96. In order to improve athletic performance, endurance athletes may train at altitude. Which of the following is true about this technique?

   A. Sleeping and training at altitude provide the best performance improvement
   B. Altitude training only improves performance for athletes of lower fitness levels
   C. The altitude required to create benefit is 3,000 m (9,800 feet) or greater
   D. Athletes with iron-deficiency status can gain significant benefits from this training technique
   E. The training effect can persist for three weeks after returning to previous living altitude

97. A three-phase bone scan can aid in the diagnosis of complex regional pain syndrome. Which of the following diagnostic findings would be the most helpful?

   A. Focal increased activity on bone scan
   B. Diffuse increased activity with juxta-articular accentuation uptake on delayed images
   C. Normal bone scan in late stage of syndrome
   D. Focal changes on phases 1 and 2

98. Which of the following statements is correct in regards to the diagnosis of a pubic ramus stress fracture?

   A. Female soldiers are more susceptible to pubic rami stress fractures than male soldiers
   B. Plain films are the imaging study of choice to diagnose pubic rami stress fractures
   C. The hop test is not helpful in the clinical diagnosis of a pubic ramus stress fracture
   D. Pubic rami stress fractures are caused by the abductor and sartorius muscles pulling on the lateral aspect of the pubic ramus
   E. "Flamingo view" plain radiographs are useful in the diagnosis of a pubic ramus stress fracture

99. Concerning the prevalence of exercise-induced bronchoconstriction (EIB) in athletes, _____% of all asthmatics have airways hyperreactive to exercise, and _____% of cross country skiers are reported to have EIB?

    A. 50% to 90% and 50%
    B. 25% to 50% and 15%
    C. > 90% and 25%
    D. > 90% and < 10%

100. A thumb spica cast is the treatment of choice for which of the following fractures?

    A. Boxer's fracture
    B. Colles' fracture
    C. Scaphoid fracture
    D. Lisfranc fracture
    E. Hangman's fracture

101. Skeletal muscles that function as a group to stabilize the scapula against the posterior thoracic wall during upper extremity overhead activities include which of the following?

    A. Levator scapulae, rhomboid major, rhomboid minor, and serratus anterior
    B. Supraspinatus, infraspinatus, subscapularis, and teres minor
    C. Thoracic paraspinals, trapezius, latissimus dorsi, and posterior intercostals
    D. Deltoid, triceps brachii, pectoralis major, and pectoralis minor

102. A high school football player presents to your clinic with his parents. They seek information about nutrition and supplements for athletes. Which of the following statements is true regarding nutrition and high intensity exercise?

    A. Fat is broken down to glycogen during exercise
    B. With regard to training in a hot, humid environment, thirst is a sensitive and reliable indicator of dehydration and estimating fluid loss
    C. Due to the increased demand on an athlete's body, protein supplements are necessary in addition to a healthy diet
    D. An athlete's diet should consist of about 60% carbohydrates

103. Which of the following is true of hypertrophic cardiomyopathy?

    A. Hypertrophic cardiomyopathy (HCM) is a genetic disorder with an autosomal recessive pattern of inheritance
    B. HCM is characterized by right ventricular wall thickness of > 5 mm
    C. The murmur associated with HCM is exacerbated by the Valsalva maneuver
    D. Most patients have detectible signs of HCM before sudden death
    E. The best initial test for diagnosis is cardiac CT

104. In response to intense exercise, catecholamine release will occur. These hormones can lead to several effects in the athlete. Which of the following is due to alpha receptor effect?

    A. Vasoconstriction
    B. Cardiac acceleration
    C. Lipolysis
    D. Bronchodilatation
    E. Increased myocardial contractility

105. A 21-year-old senior female softball player presents to the clinic with left-sided abdominal pain. She says she first noticed the pain after hitting a double and sliding head-first into second base in last night's game. She was able to finish the inning, but felt like she had trouble taking a deep breath and removed herself from the game. Today, she says she is breathing okay, but still has pain with deep inspiration. She has pain with trunk rotation and bending, and bruising in the antero-lateral abdomen of the left side. She has bilateral breath sounds equal in nature, and she is tender to palpation along her ribs and the abdominal wall of the left side. A chest x-ray and vital signs are normal. Her pain has likely resulted from which of the following?

    A. Rib fracture
    B. Costochondritis
    C. Internal oblique strain
    D. Splenic hematoma

106. An afebrile patient with acute low back pain notices pain going down the posterior-lateral aspect of her right thigh and leg. It is noted on your exam that she has the following: (+) straight leg raise test, a slight sensory deficit over the lateral aspect of the right lateral foot, a diminished Achilles tendon reflex and weakness with plantar flexion of the great toe. It is also noted that it is hard for her to walk on her toes. Which nerve root is most likely affected?

    A. L3
    B. L4
    C. L5
    D. S1
    E. L2

107. A 16-year-old male long jumper lands awkwardly with his right knee hyperextended, collapsing in the pit. He experiences acute swelling of the right knee immediately. He has a past medical history of resolved bilateral jumper's knee and prominent tibial tubercles diagnosed two years ago. There is anterior deformity and swelling immediately distal to the patella. Which of the following statements is true regarding tibial tubercle apophyseal fracture?

    A. Patients with type II and III fractures of the tibial tubercle are able to actively extend the knee against gravity several degrees
    B. Negative Lachman testing immediately after injury eliminates rupture of the anterior cruciate ligament as a possibility
    C. Fracture at the tibial apophysis can be comminuted, displaced, or involve the tibial articular surface
    D. Osgood Schlatter's disease is not associated with tibial tubercle fracture

108. Which of the following statements is true regarding stretching and flexibility?

    A. Stretching has been proven to decrease rates of muscle injuries
    B. Stretching is most beneficial if performed 30 minutes prior to exercise
    C. Ballistic stretching should be avoided by all individuals, as it predisposes to muscle injury
    D. Increasing muscle temperature with light cardiovascular exercise is as adequate as stretching to increase muscle flexibility prior to exercise

109. Lisfranc injuries involve a disruption in which of the following joints?

    A. Inter-phalangeal joint
    B. Metatarsal-phalangeal joint
    C. Tarsal-navicular joint
    D. Tarsal-metatarsal (T-MT) joint

110. You are performing a preparticipation exam on one of your patients, who happens to be a student at the high school you cover. Of the following items, which one would require further evaluation?

    A. Mononucleosis three years ago
    B. Mildly enlarged liver
    C. Non-palpable spleen
    D. Small tattoo
    E. History of appendectomy

111. Which of the following is a property of anabolic steroids?

    A. They increase the actions of glucocorticoids and help metabolize ingested proteins, converting a negative nitrogen balance into a positive one
    B. They give the athlete a state of euphoria and decreased fatigue that allows the athlete to train harder and longer
    C. Anabolic effects increase the number of muscles in the body for larger size and strength and better performance
    D. They may induce hypotension, lung tumors, and delayed closure of growth plates
    E. Androgenic effects will not increase or decrease libido along with other side effects like gynecomastia

112. Which of the following best describes the correct effect of cryotherapy in treatment of injuries?

    A. Cryotherapy increases tissue metabolism
    B. Cryotherapy decreases the pain threshold
    C. Cryotherapy decreases pain post operatively
    D. Cryotherapy increases motor perfusion
    E. Cryotherapy increases nerve conduction

113. With a scaphoid fracture, non-union is a common complication. Which fracture location order shows the correct risk for non-union, from most likely to least likely?

    A. Proximal pole, distal pole, waist
    B. Waist, distal pole, proximal pole
    C. Proximal pole, waist, distal pole
    D. Distal pole, waist, proximal pole
    E. Waist, proximal pole, distal pole

114. A storm is approaching during a high school football game you are covering. You notice what appears to be a lightning strike in the distance but still have clear skies overhead. The most correct evaluation of the situation is which of the following?

    A. Since the most severe storms are only dangerous in the spring, you decide the players, coaches, and others are safe
    B. You should watch for a funnel cloud, as that would present the most likely danger. You, therefore, will take action when the funnel cloud is spotted
    C. You know that with the clear skies overhead that immediate danger is unlikely and continue to watch for further changes in the weather
    D. You realize that lightning can strike in a large radius surrounding any storm and decide to take the next appropriate step

115. A 45-year-old tennis player presents with six weeks of low back pain with radiation to the left big toe made worse with bending over to tie his shoes. He wants to do physical therapy, and you write a prescription for which of the following back programs to reduce his current symptoms of pain?

    A. McKenzie exercises
    B. Williams exercises
    C. Back school
    D. Lumbar traction

116. A fit 58-year-old male with bright red rectal bleeding and known hemorrhoids presents to your office following a canoeing marathon. Which of the following options is appropriate?

    A. Treat his hemorrhoids conservatively, avoid constipation, and watch for further bleeding
    B. Ask to see him in the office for a rectal exam and guaiac assessment, and follow his case clinically if the guaiac test is negative
    C. Ask him to call the office if the bleeding recurs (no other assessment is needed)
    D. A colonoscopy should be recommended

117. An 18-year-old returns from a trip to Colorado with ankle pain and an antalgic gait. She was treated initially for a severe ankle sprain after eversion injury during snowboard lessons. Ankle radiographs reveal a lateral process fracture of the talus that is typical in snowboarding injuries, and a CT scan verifies the non-displaced position of the small fragment. Appropriate treatment consists of which of the following?

    A. Ankle rehabilitation and return to activity if the CT scan shows a Hawkin's sign
    B. Ankle splint, weight bearing as tolerated, and aggressive ankle rehabilitation
    C. Non-weight-bearing in a cast for four to six weeks followed by progressive weight bearing and ankle rehabilitation
    D. Walking cast for four to six weeks, then ankle rehabilitation
    E. Emergent orthopedic consultation because of tenuous blood supply to the talus

118. Which of the following statements are correct in the management of sports-related concussion?

    A. There are three classifications of concussion according to the Zurich 2008 Summary and Agreement Statement of the 3rd International Conference on Concussion in Sport
    B. Tonic posturing occurring with a sports-related concussion is generally benign and requires no further management beyond the standard treatment of the underlying concussive injury
    C. Loss of consciousness less than 30 seconds is a sign that would classify a concussion as complex
    D. A concussed athlete in high school and/or college may begin a return to play protocol when symptoms decrease from sideline evaluation

119. Which of the following is the most appropriate long-term treatment option for fibromyalgia?

    A. Aerobic exercise
    B. Lidocaine patches
    C. Cyclobenzaprine
    D. Ibuprofen
    E. Hydrocodone

120. A 16-year-old female basketball player presents with five days of sore throat, fever, and fatigue. On exam, she has an exudative pharyngitis and posterior cervical lymphadenopathy. She has a playoff game scheduled for the weekend and wants to know if she can play. Which of the following tests is the most sensitive and could assist with the decision to allow the athlete to play?

    A. Heterophile antibody–latex agglutination (monospot)
    B. Viral capsid antigen IgM
    C. Viral capsid antigen IgG
    D. Complete blood count

121. You are one of several first responders on the scene of an unresponsive 17-year-old female with witnessed collapsed during basketball practice. CPR is begun, EMS activated, and the AED placed. Shock is advised. The next step should be which of the following?

    A. Three consecutive shocks followed by resumption of CPR
    B. One shock, then check pulse/rhythm and immediately reshock if advised
    C. One shock, then resume CPR for five cycles before rechecking rhythm
    D. Two rescue breaths and five cycles CPR before proceeding with shock

122. A 17-year-old male high school baseball pitcher presents to your sports medicine clinic for review of an MRI ordered by another physician. The pitcher has pain in his throwing shoulder. The MRI demonstrates bone marrow edema and cortical flattening suggestive of a Hill-Sachs lesion in the proximal humerus with subchondral sclerosis in the posterosuperior aspect of the glenoid. You would anticipate which of the following physical exam findings based on the imaging study?

    A. Visible atrophy of the supraspinatus and infraspinatus with muscular weakness on testing
    B. Posterior shoulder pain with passive abduction and external rotation of the affected shoulder
    C. Marked weakness of shoulder internal rotators
    D. Enlarged cervical and peri-clavicular lymph nodes

123. A 19-year-old basketball player, exchange student from Italy, has an episode of unexplained syncope during practice. The patient adamantly denies any previous cardiac history and believes he was just dehydrated. He does admit, however, that a cousin died suddenly at age 20 of cardiac causes. An ECG is obtained. Which abnormality would be suggestive of arrythmogenic right ventricular dysplasia?

    A. Normal ECG
    B. T-wave inversion
    C. Prolonged QT interval
    D. Q waves with ectopy
    E. Pre-excitation

124. A 15-year-old high school football player was hit on his blind side as he was running with the football. He landed on the side carrying the football, and the tackler landed on top of him. After needing assistance to the sideline, he became tachycardic, hypotensive, and there was a clear change in his mental status. He was transported to the nearest hospital where he was reevaluated. The patient is initially stabilized with IV hydration. However, the patient's pain is persistent. Which of the following testing types is going to take the longest to produce results?

    A. CT abdomen and pelvis
    B. Peritoneal lavage
    C. MR abdomen
    D. Plain films of abdomen and chest
    E. Abdominal ultrasound

125. A 40-year-old male distance runner presents for a routine physical. As part of the physical, you obtain a urine sample, which shows 1+ protein on a dipstick test. Which of the following would support a diagnosis of exercise-induced proteinuria?

    A. Regular creatine supplementation
    B. A history of completing an intense speed training workout just prior to the physical
    C. A history of a 150-mile bike race two weeks prior to the physical
    D. A history of uncontrolled type 2 diabetes mellitus
    E. A 20-year history of distance running with over 40 marathons in the past 10 years

126. A college springboard diver, while entering the water, felt pain at medial aspect of right thumb. Position of thumb during entry was hyperextended and abducted. On exam, she had tenderness and mild swelling along the medial aspect of first MCP, but with solid end point. Which of the following is the most appropriate initial management of choice for this injury?

    A. Immediate surgery
    B. No necessary intervention
    C. Taping
    D. Short arm thumb spica splint with wrist in slight extension, thumb in abduction
    E. Short arm thumb spica splint with wrist in slight flexion, thumb in abduction

127. A 55-year-old female is a regular participant in her aggressive aerobics class at the park district community center five days per week. She presents with subjective pain with motion over the most lateral portion of the proximal right femur for two to three weeks. Her right hip joint motion is smooth, without pain, and symmetric passively and actively when compared to the left hip. There is tenderness to palpation over the most lateral portion of the proximal right femur. She responds to treatment with a conservative program consisting of icing, deep tissue massage using a foam roller, over-the-counter analgesics, and an injection into the painful area. Which of the following is the proper diagnosis?

    A. Iliopectineal bursitis
    B. Ischial bursitis
    C. Greater trochanteric bursitis
    D. Pes anserine bursitis

128. A 23-year-old mountain bike racer flips over his handlebars and lands on the posterior superior portion of his right shoulder. Evaluation in the medical tent demonstrates significant weakness with resisted extension of the shoulder when tested at 90 degrees flexion, 30 degrees lateral to the coronal plane, and with hand pronated (empty can test) as well as an inability to initiate abduction of the involved arm. The patient also has weakness with resisted external rotation. There are no sensory deficits to light touch or pin prick over the shoulder, arm, thorax, or back. Which nerve has most likely been injured?

   A. Axillary nerve
   B. Subscapular nerve
   C. Suprascapular nerve
   D. Dorsal scapular nerve

129. A 13-year-old female with a history of Legg-Calve-Perthes disease as a child presents to your clinic with worsening chronic left hip and groin pain. She reports occasional catching or locking. On exam, she has pain with passive range of motion and reduced internal rotation and abduction. On MRI of the hip, you expect to find which of the following?

   A. Osteochondritis dissecans of the femoral head
   B. Labral tear
   C. Normal hip
   D. Arthritis

130. The use of a TENS (transcutaneous electric nerve stimulation) unit does which of the following?

   A. Results in increased dorsal horn cell activity
   B. Most likely relieves pain via endorphin release with high frequency, low intensity modalities
   C. Is relatively contraindicated for a patient with an implantable cardiac defibrillator (ICD)
   D. Has been proven to reduce fracture pain
   E. Results in local analgesia that is typically long-lasting (> one hour) after stimulation is stopped

131. A 27-year-old male complains of pain and numbness in his palm and fourth and fifth fingers after his recent karate tournament. There is a tender mass in his hypothenar area and an abnormal Allen's test. You suspect damage to which of the following structures?

   A. Thrombosis of ulnar artery
   B. Thrombosis of radial artery
   C. Thrombosis of median artery
   D. Thrombosis of common palmar digital artery

132. A 16-year-old male high school athlete presents to the ER after being hit in the testicle by a racquetball in the groin during a competitive match with his father. Patient was unable to finish the competition because of nausea, vomiting, and difficulty walking due to pain. Examination revealed a tender and swollen right testicle and scrotal hematoma measuring 2 cm in diameter. A scrotal US with Doppler revealed a testicular parenchymal fracture and intact testicular blood flow. His parents are very concerned about the patient's future fertility since he is their only child. The most appropriate next step would be which of the following?

   A. Oral antibiotics
   B. Rest, pain control and ice packs on groin for 24 to 48 hours
   C. Urology consult for surgery to repair the testicular integrity
   D. Percutaneous drainage of the hematoma for pain control
   E. Scrotal MRI

133. The erector spinae and abdominal musculature stabilize the spine in a strength ratio of 1.3:1. The muscles you palpate in the erector spinae when the athlete has low back pain include?

   A. Iliocostalis, longissimus, spinalis
   B. Longissimus capitis, semispinalis capitis, splenius capitis
   C. Semispinalis thoracis, multifidus, rotatores thoracis
   D. Interspinalis lumborum, lateral intertransversi, quadratus lumborum

134. A high school senior kicker was involved in a calamitous play during a kickoff return. Upon rushing the field to examine him, you immediately noticed what initially appeared to be a fracture. Your exam showed this to be an anterior dislocation of the knee. Although difficult, you were able to successfully reduce and stabilize the joint. After the reduction, you reevaluated his knee on the sideline. Which of the following items would concern you the most during that exam?

    A. The difficult reduction of his anterior dislocation
    B. Gross multidirectional instability on exam
    C. Non-progressive dorsiflexion weakness on neurologic exam
    D. Difficulty obtaining palpable pulses from the foot

135. A 16-year-old male presents to your clinic for a preparticipation physical evaluation. His best corrected visual screen reveals < 20/40 vision in his right eye and 20/20 vision in his left eye. He states he lost vision in this eye after he was struck in the fourth grade by a baseball. The remainder of his history and physical are unremarkable. He should be excluded from participation in which of the following sports?

    A. Football
    B. Wrestling
    C. Ice hockey
    D. Lacrosse

136. Which of the following statements is true regarding Legg-Calve-Perthes disease?

    A. Legg-Calve-Perthes disease occurs most commonly in girls in the first decade of life
    B. Most patients with Legg-Calve-Perthes disease will have excruciating hip pain, which results in a unilateral limp
    C. The most common exam findings are of reduced internal rotation and abduction of the hip
    D. Long-term sequelae of untreated Legg-Calve-Perthes disease are rare
    E. With Legg-Calve-Perthes disease, an older child has a better prognosis than a younger child

137. You are asked to be the physician for a local summer league junior softball tournament. Which of the following factors are true in relation to the risk for heat illness?

    A. Children's sweat rates are equal to adults and, therefore, are at no greater risk
    B. Children usually stop before they get too hot and, therefore, are at no greater risk than adults
    C. Children don't absorb fluids as readily as adults and, therefore, are at greater risk than adults
    D. Children have increased heat production per kilogram of body mass and are at greater risk than adults

138. The most effective treatment for a symptomatic dorsal carpal ganglia is which of the following?

    A. Nothing, as most ganglia resolve spontaneously and do not require treatment
    B. Aspiration with corticosteroid injection
    C. Aspiration without corticosteroid injection
    D. Surgery

139. What is the role of calcium in muscle contraction?

    A. Calcium binds troponin, moving tropomysin and allowing crossbridge linkages and contraction
    B. Calcium binds troponin, allowing for release of ATP and therefore initiating contraction
    C. Calcium binds tropomysin, moving troponin and allowing crossbridge linkages and contraction
    D. Calcium binds tropomysin, allowing for release of ATP and therefore initiating contraction

140. You are performing the preparticipation physical examination for one of the new soccer recruits for the college. He is an 18-year-old male who had his first generalized tonic-clonic seizure eight months ago. He was appropriately evaluated; testing confirming the diagnosis of idiopathic epilepsy, and was started on valproic acid. He has tolerated the medication well and has been seizure free for seven months. He resumed his workouts but has not returned to competitive soccer before this time. With regard to his participation with the college soccer program, your recommendations and counseling would be which of the following (select the best answer)?

    A. There is no known risk for increasing seizure frequency with contact or collision sports, and since his seizures are well controlled, he may be cleared to participate
    B. Persons with history of seizure should not be active in strenuous activities, even if their seizures are well controlled as physical activity lowers the seizure potential and activity speeds clearance of anti-seizure medications
    C. There is still a significant risk of seizure, so he should not participate in any contact or collision sports (in addition, he should not participate in sports such as archery, riflery, swimming, diving, and weight or power lifting)
    D. Valproic acid is a banned substance by the NCAA. Although he is well controlled and is cleared to participate in soccer on this medication, an exception based on your request must be granted by the NCAA before he can participate with the team
    E. Because he has been seizure-free for more than six months, you can recommend stopping the valproic acid today (as long as he is seizure-free with non-contact sport activities for the next two weeks, he can be released for full activity)

141. After completing heat acclimation, which of the following changes would be a physiologic change in an athlete after exercising in a heat environment?

    A. An increase in plasma aldosterone
    B. A significant decrease in the percent dehydration during exercise
    C. A right shift of the sweat osmolality
    D. A significantly higher plasma lactate concentration

142. In order to prevent exercise-induced bronchospasm during competition, athletes with documented asthma would benefit from which of the following treatments?

    A. Pre-medicate with beta-adrenergic agonist
    B. Pre-medicate with oral corticosteroids
    C. Pre-medicate with inhaled corticosteroids
    D. Pre-medicate with antihistamines
    E. Pre-medicate with nasal steroids

143. Which of the following structures is the primary static stabilizer for preventing lateral subluxation of the patella?

    A. Medial patellofemoral ligament
    B. Vastus medialis obliquus (VMO)
    C. Medial patellotibial ligament
    D. Superficial oblique retinaculum

144. A 26-year-old African-American female presents to the medical treatment tent you are staffing at a large cross country ski race in upper Wisconsin. She is complaining of painful edematous purple lesions on her face. She is in excellent health, an avid cross country runner from southern Illinois. She denies pregnancy or any medical problems. She does not seem to be in any acute distress. She and her friends have been taking "nips" out of a pocket flask containing Blackberry brandy. Which of the following is true?

    A. She has classic pernio (or chilblain)
    B. She should immediately stop the race and be transported to the main medical tent 10 km away via ambulance
    C. She can go back out after applying protective UV cold barrier ointment on her face
    D. She should quickly rewarm her face by sitting next to the propane gas warmer in the tent
    E. It is best to warm her face slowly, using cool water and then slowly applying heated water to prevent further tissue damage

145. A college football player sprains his ankle at the bottom of a pileup. When considering diagnosis of syndesmotic ankle sprain, which of the following is true?

    A. Imaging shows < 5 mm of clear space and > 10 mm of tibiofibular overlap
    B. One mechanism of injury is a blow to the back of the externally rotated ankle while prone
    C. Anterior drawer, talar tilt, and squeeze testing are negative
    D. If interosseous sprain is strongly suspected and distal fibular pain is present, the Ottawa Ankle Rules do not apply, as x-rays are not needed

146. Which of the following measurements of left ventricular wall thickness on 2D-echocardiogram at the end of diastole is considered left ventricular hypertrophy in a 70 kg male?

    A. > 6 mm
    B. > 9 mm
    C. > 12 mm
    D. > 15 mm

147. There are several different types of muscle stretching techniques. Using a partner to stretch the hamstring passively, then pushing against the partner by contracting the muscle isometrically, and then stretching farther in the same range of motion is an example of which of the following?

    A. Static stretching
    B. Dynamic stretching
    C. Ballistic stretching
    D. Proprioceptive neuromuscular facilitation

148. A 21-year-old type 1 diabetic athlete begins training for a 50-mile bike ride with a partner. She uses an insulin pump and is experienced with running cross country in high school. During her first 30-mile ride, she experiences symptoms of hypoglycemia at 25 miles and almost falls before stopping. She is confused, and her blood sugar level is 40. Which of the following is the most appropriate immediate action?

    A. Eat a banana or sports bar
    B. Administration of glucagon by her partner
    C. Drink a carbohydrate sports drink then quickly resume riding to reach a safe destination
    D. Drink eight ounces of water to improve volume status

149. A 17-year-old male presents to your office with a chief complaint of heel pain. If this patient has Sever's disease, which of the following items collected during the history and physical examination would you expect?

    A. Skeletal maturity
    B. Normal foot radiograph
    C. Pain worse in the morning
    D. Tight gastrocnemius-soleus muscle complex
    E. Normal foot alignment

150. The "clunk test" evaluates shoulder pathology caused by which of the following?

    A. Impingement
    B. Tendinopathy
    C. Labral tears
    D. Sliding biceps tendon
    E. Instability

151. Which of the following statements is true regarding proximal biceps tendon rupture?

A. A complete rupture results in formation of "Popeye" deformity with a large bulge in the proximal arm

B. Must be treated with surgery within two weeks of injury in order to preserve function

C. The typical mechanism of injury is forceful extension against excessive resistance

D. Plain x-rays should be obtained to rule out avulsion of the bony origin

E. The weakness caused by proximal biceps tendon rupture is significantly less than the weakness caused by distal biceps tendon rupture

152. Which of the following statements is true regarding hip flexor injury?

A. X-ray to rule out hip flexor origin avulsion is needed in adolescents with the possible diagnosis of hip flexor pain and tenderness over the ischial tuberosity

B. A hop test with pain in the ipsilateral groin is indicative of a hip flexor strain

C. Patients with large, palpable defects in the rectus femoris rarely need surgery

D. Hip flexor strains are commonly accompanied by a tingling sensation in the anterior thigh because of irritation of the lateral femoral cutaneous nerve

E. Significant weakness is usually seen on exam with most hip flexor strains

153. An 800 m open water swim is part of a short-course triathlon with over 800 registered athletes. It will be held in a shallow, protected lake that is usually calm but has been notorious for sudden weather changes. The race was cancelled the prior year because of excessive wave chop and poor visibility, and a duathlon (bike and run race) was held in its place. Since that time, you have implemented some changes to improve safety in the case of any adverse events. Which of the following is an adequate safety measure for this race?

A. Local volunteer swim club members will be on hand at the finish to deal with common minor conditions

B. A "mass start" will begin the swim to assure the race finishes at an early time

C. There will be one certified lifeguard for every 50 swimmers in this non-ocean race

D. There will be large, highly visible buoys positioned 1000 m or so apart and secured in a manner that will limit their movement in the most severe wave conditions in that body of water

E. A highly mobile, powered watercraft will be "on call" in the area to facilitate any emergency plan that is implemented

154. A 12-year-old girl with no previous hip problems suffers an injury immediately after landing in the sand pit following setting her personal record in the long jump. She now has pain and tenderness deep within the hip over the proximal and medial femur. There is pain with passive internal and external rotation of the involved hip and with active hip flexion. The examination of the other hip is normal. The most accurate diagnosis is avulsion of the apophysis over which of the following?

    A. Ischial tuberosity
    B. Anterior superior ischial spine
    C. Anterior inferior ischial spine
    D. Lesser trochanter
    E. Greater trochanter

155. Which of the following is listed as a minor criterion of Marfan syndrome?

    A. Ectopia lentis
    B. Dilation of the ascending aorta
    C. Lumbosacral dural ectasia
    D. Scoliosis > 20 degrees
    E. High-arched palate

156. A 26-year-old female triathlete comes in to see you in consultation at your sports medicine clinic. She asks for your nutrition recommendations to complement her current training regimen. For optimal post-exercise recovery, you recommend that she take which of the following?

    A. Low glycemic index carbohydrates and protein (in a ratio of 3:1), and no fat within 30 minutes of completing her workouts
    B. High glycemic index carbohydrates and protein (in a ratio of 3:1), and some fat within 30 minutes of completing her workouts
    C. Low glycemic index carbohydrates and fat (in a ratio of 3:1) within 30 minutes of completing her workouts
    D. High glycemic index carbohydrates and fat (in a ratio of 3:1) within 30 minutes of completing her workouts
    E. Low glycemic index carbohydrates and protein (in a ratio of 3:1), and some fat within 30 minutes of completing her workouts

157. Which of the following has been reported in association with creatine use in an otherwise healthy athlete?

   A. Muscle cramping
   B. Cardiac complications
   C. Weight loss
   D. Renal complications
   E. Constipation

158. The number of disabled athletes competing in sports has substantially increased over the years. Athletes with spinal cord injury (SCI) often have difficulty regulating body temperature during training or competition in both warm and cold environments. These conditions necessitate understanding which of the following true statements?

   A. In cold weather, SCI athletes are predisposed to hypothermia from paralysis and decreased muscle mass below the level of the lesion and a reduced ability to generate body heat by shivering
   B. In warm weather, impairment of sweating and control of peripheral blood flow below the level of the lesion (decreased surface area for cooling via evaporation) decreases the risk of hyperthermia
   C. Proper clothing, hydration and avoidance of activities during extreme temperatures are not as important because decreased peripheral sensation allows increased exposure time without significant detriment
   D. Athletes participating in cold weather sports need not be concerned about inspecting extremities to avoid frostbite if properly dressed for the activity

159. A 42-year-old female runner presents to your office with a history of multiple joint pain that started after her return from a sprint distance triathlon in Michigan last week. Her diet, menses, and weight are unchanged. She runs about 15 to 20 miles a week, swims three miles per week and bikes 50 miles a week. She denies a fever but does feel flushed at times. No history of autoimmune condition in her family. Her vitals are normal and afebrile. She has a normal musculoskeletal exam outside of subjective joint soreness. Her skin exam shows an abdominal rash, which is 6 cm in diameter, appearing as an annular homogenous erythema with a central purpura. The test you would most likely order **first** is which of the following?

    A. CBC
    B. Lyme titre
    C. ANA
    D. Rheumatoid factor
    E. Thyroid stimulating hormone

160. The most common site from which nosebleeds arise is which of the following?

    A. Sphenopalantine artery
    B. Anterior ethmoidal artery
    C. Kiesselbach's plexus
    D. Posterior ethmoidal artery

161. A professional basketball player comes to you, his team physician, during the off-season to discuss his medical history in light of his contract renewal option. He is medically healthy except for seven documented concussions over the course of his eight-year career. He had one concussion that included brief loss of consciousness. In no instance was he held out of competition for longer than one week. Which of the following would be a true statement to consider when advising him medically about retirement?

    A. Assessment of each prior concussion, particularly severity, should not influence his decision
    B. There is a higher risk of concussion after sustaining more than two concussions in a seven-year period
    C. Subsequent concussions could possibly resolve faster than prior ones
    D. A recently performed, normal MRI would lessen concerns
    E. There is potential risk for neurocognitive deficits

162. A 23-year-old professional snowboarder falls while making a jump. He lies on the snow and does not get up. When ski patrol reaches him, he is conscious and complaining of back pain. He is boarded and collared and transported to the nearest hospital. He is neurologically intact. A plain film radiograph shows a compression fracture of T12. Which of the following is the appropriate next step in his course of treatment?

   A. Obtain a CT scan to further assess the fracture
   B. Place the patient in a TLSO brace and perform follow-up x-rays in two weeks
   C. Consult the neurosurgeon for surgical correction of the fracture
   D. Consult interventional radiology for kyphoplasty of the fracture

163. A volleyball player presents with right shoulder pain after attempting to spike the ball in practice. The player is holding her arm in slight abduction and external rotation. The humeral head is palpated anteriorly. Before proceeding, it is important to first evaluate which of the following?

   A. Supraclavicular nerve by testing sensation over the clavicular area
   B. Axillary nerve by testing sensation over lateral aspect of the shoulder
   C. Radial nerve by testing sensation over inferolateral arm
   D. Medial cutaneous nerve by testing sensation over medial aspect of arm

164. A 17-year-old woman notes on her preparticipation physical that she has had regular menstrual periods over the past four years until the last 10 months. During the last 10 months, she has had no menstrual periods. Her history reveals no obvious causes for this other than her participation in cross country and track. Her physical exam is unremarkable. Which of the following statements is the best statement that reflects her condition?

   A. She is suffering from exercise-related amenorrhea and should be counseled about starting on calcitonin to prevent osteoporosis
   B. She is suffering from oligomenorrhea and should be counseled to gain weight so that her menstrual cycles return to normal
   C. She is normal for her age and should wait one year to see if her menstrual cycle returns to normal
   D. She is suffering from an eating disorder and should be counseled to seek a mental health consultation
   E. She is suffering from amenorrhea and should be counseled to have laboratory testing to determine the cause

165. A 33-year-old female runner has increased her running regimen for an upcoming marathon. She has had only three menstrual periods in the last six months. Her pregnancy test is negative. The most likely etiology of her menstrual dysfunction is which of the following?

    A. Increased testosterone
    B. Increased LH
    C. Decreased GnRH
    D. Increased prolactin

166. A 22-year-old male wrestler presents to your clinic after falling awkwardly in a match approximately four hours earlier in the day, injuring his left wrist. The patient appears uncomfortable and states the pain has been getting worse since the time of the injury despite ice and immobilization. On exam, he has swelling and is tender over the distal radius. His neurovascular exam is intact, but he is unwilling to allow extension of his wrist or fingers because of pain. An x-ray is done and shows a minimally displaced extra-articular fracture of the distal radius. Which of the following complications of this injury is most likely at this time?

    A. Stretch injury of the median nerve
    B. Compartment syndrome
    C. Malunion
    D. Complex regional pain syndrome

167. You are evaluating a 27-year-old recreational tennis player. She felt some searing chest wall pain on her dominant side while extending for a forehand shot three days ago. On her exam today, you notice substantial bruising along the anterior chest wall, suggesting some soft tissue injury. You begin by palpating the pectoralis major muscle. Of the following points, which one is helpful when trying to palpate the pectoralis minor?

    A. Sternum
    B. Clavicle
    C. Ribs 2 through 6
    D. Humerus
    E. Coracoid process

168. Which of the following regarding injury prevention is correct?

    A. Single-hinge knee braces can prevent knee injuries in American football
    B. Lace-up braces for ankles can reduce recurring ankle injuries in athletes with previous ankle injuries
    C. Headgear (scrum caps) can decrease the incidence of concussions in rugby
    D. Eyewear with corrective lenses can prevent injury to the orbit

169. According to the ATLS guidelines, which of the following is the estimated minimum systolic blood pressure with a palpable radial pulse?

    A. 40 mm Hg
    B. 100 mm Hg
    C. 80 mm Hg
    D. 120 mm Hg

170. A 19-year-old female basketball player tries to deflect a pass and sustains a hyperextension injury to the PIP joint of her middle finger. Her finger dislocates dorsally. You reduce the dislocation on the sideline. Radiographs taken after the game are negative for bony injury and show good alignment. Which of the following is the most appropriate next step?

    A. No further treatment is necessary
    B. The finger should be splinted in full extension
    C. The finger should be splinted in 20 to 30 degrees of flexion
    D. The finger and hand should be placed in a short arm cast

171. What has been shown to give patients—with moderate to severe symptomatic knee osteoarthritis—better pain relief according to the glucosamine/chondroitin arthritis intervention trial (GAIT)?

    A. Glucosamine with chondroitin
    B. Glucosamine
    C. Chondroitin
    D. Placebo
    E. Glucosamine with chondroitin and MSM

172. Which of the following statements about open and closed kinetic chain exercises is correct?

    A. Open kinetic chain exercises occur when the distal aspect of the extremity is fixed and cannot move
    B. Closed kinetic chain exercises typically involve functional weight-bearing activities
    C. Knee extensions and straight leg raises are examples of closed kinetic chain exercises
    D. During open kinetic chain exercises, motion occurs simultaneously at all joints comprising the kinetic chain
    E. Closed kinetic chain exercises produce shearing forces, while open kinetic chain exercises produce compressive forces

173. A 20-year-old basketball player falls on a pronated right hand. He was initially treated by the athletic trainer, noted to have prominence of the ulnar head and loss of supination. The trainer reduced it with supination of the forearm. You see him in the training room, he has full range of motion, neurovascular exam is intact, radiographs do not show fracture, dislocataion, or widening of the distal radioulnar joint (DRUJ). This injury should subsequently be treated in which manner?

    A. Thumb spica splint for two weeks
    B. Short arm cast for four weeks
    C. Long arm cast for six weeks
    D. Ulnar gutter splint

174. Where is the purest area for sensory testing of the radial nerve on the hand located?

    A. Dorsal web between the thumb and the index finger
    B. Radial side of the hand
    C. Dorsum of the wrist
    D. Thenar eminence

175. A climber in the Himalayas crests 2,500 m (approximately 8,200 feet) and experiences headache, nausea, fatigue, significant confusion, and ataxia. The most appropriate treatment option for this condition is which of the following?

    A. Rapid descent
    B. Corticosteroid (prednisone)
    C. Calcium channel blockers
    D. Non-steroidal anti-inflammatories

176. Which of the following is an absolute contraindication to collision sports participation?

    A. Torg-Pavlov ratio < 0.8
    B. Recurrent cervical cord neuropraxia
    C. Healed-displaced-stable fracture of C3-C7 at posterior ring
    D. Clay shoveler's fracture
    E. Healed herniated nucleosis pulposis

177. A 13-year-old female soccer player sustains a groin strain when performing a sliding tackle in a game. Her evaluation in the emergency room is remarkable for an avulsion of the lesser trochanter with 1 cm displacement. Appropriate management would include which of the following?

    A. Refer immediately for surgical management
    B. Start physical therapy
    C. Place on crutches and make her non-weight bearing
    D. Rest for one week and clear for sports when her pain has resolved

178. Which of the following is true regarding commotio cordis?

    A. Little League baseball now requires the batter to wear chest protectors for prevention in children under 12
    B. The apparent mechanism for death is ventricular fibrillation induced by an abrupt blunt precordial blow during a specific time in the cardiac cycle
    C. Baseballs thrown at 20 mph, a blow in the left area of the heart, and blunt impacts are associated with more deadly outcomes in commotio cordis
    D. With rapid defibrillation, cardiac support, and AED maneuvers, greater than 25% of individuals may survive commotio cordis
    E. Impact must occur within the QRS of the cardiac cycle in order for ventricular fibrillation to occur and cause commotio cordis

179. Which of the following statements regarding exercise testing in individuals with coronary artery disease (CAD) or risk factors for CAD is true?

    A. Excessive ST depression of > 2 mm horizontal or downsloping is an absolute indication to terminate an exercise test
    B. Recommendation to get a graded exercise test for a 25-year-old with type 1 diabetes (diagnosed with IDDM for at least 10 years)
    C. During an exercise test, a change of less than or equal to 12 beats per minute from peak exercise HR to HR two minutes into recovery is strongly predictive of mortality
    D. MET level or exercise duration is not an important predictor of adverse cardiac events after MI

180. A female runner with knee pain presents after running a 10K and has a mildly swollen knee. Which of the following is true?

    A. Voshell's bursitis is an inflamed bursa between the medial collateral ligament and the tibia and may be treated with rest, anti-inflammatory medicines, and cross training
    B. Bursitis in the knee should be drained and sent for culture for proper antibiotic coverage
    C. Pes anserine bursitis is less often associated with pes planus than prepatellar bursitis
    D. Voshell's bursa is one of two bursas in the body that can become infected, most commonly by staphylococcus aureus
    E. Prepatellar bursitis often presents as medial knee pain that is more common after long periods of sitting and long trips

181. A 15-year-old rugby player presents with a left fourth finger injury. She is unable to flex the DIP, and there is fullness along the flexor tendon. Which of the following is the appropriate course of treatment?

    A. Ice and NSAIDs
    B. Early surgical intervention
    C. Custom splint during games
    D. Buddy taping to left third finger

182. Regarding pediatric injury and Salter-Harris fractures, which of the following creates the greatest risk to joint integrity?

    A. Salter-Harris Type I
    B. Salter-Harris Type II
    C. Salter-Harris Type III
    D. Salter-Harris Type IV
    E. Salter-Harris Type V

183. It is well known that the weather can play a significant role in the outcomes at endurance races. Which wet bulb globe temperature (WBGT) is the threshold that would warrant a black flag warning on race day?

    A. 78 degrees Fahrenheit (25.6 degrees Celsius)
    B. 88 degrees Fahrenheit (31 degrees Celsius)
    C. 82 degrees Fahrenheit (27.8 degrees Celsius)
    D. 85 degrees Fahrenheit (29.4 degrees Celsius)

184. A 25-year-old male presents with thumb pain after a fall while skiing. On exam, his MCP joint is grossly unstable and MRI reveals a Stener lesion. Optimal management of this injury requires which of the following?

    A. Thumb splinted in extension for four weeks
    B. Thumb spica splint for six weeks
    C. Short arm cast for six weeks
    D. Surgical repair

185. A 20-year-old male patient presents to your office with a history of anterior shoulder dislocation which occurred during a pick-up basketball game last week. This was the athlete's first such injury, and the report from the emergency department stated that the dislocation was reduced without difficulty. Which of the following findings would lead you to recommend surgical evaluation for the patient?

    A. Persistent anterior capsular pain one week after the injury
    B. Decreased range of motion on your initial examination
    C. Positive apprehension test on your initial examination
    D. Avulsion of the anterior capsulolabral complex on radiographic evaluation

186. At a college tennis tournament, you are caring for a 22-year-old male tennis player from Italy who passed out in the middle of his match. He denies chest pain. You order an ECG, which shows some T-wave inversions in leads V_1 to V_3 and an incomplete right bundle branch block. When asked about family history, he recalls his grandfather died at a young age of some heart problem. You are most worried about sudden cardiac death in this patient from which of the following?

    A. Coronary artery disease
    B. Hypertrophic cardiomyopathy
    C. Prolonged QT syndrome
    D. Arrhythmogenic right ventricular dysplasia

187. A volleyball player complains of shoulder pain with overhead activity. She denies any new trauma to the shoulder. Physical examination shows pain with impingement testing, but no anatomical deformities are visualized. Normal strength of the rotator cuff is noted, and radiographs are negative for fracture and dislocation. Which of the following is the most likely diagnosis?

    A. Subacromial bursitis
    B. Hill-Sachs lesion
    C. Complete rotator cuff tear
    D. Acromioclavicular (AC) separation

188. Which of the following is a current American Heart Association (AHA) recommendation regarding cardiac evaluation during the preparticipation exam?

    A. Auscultate for heart murmur during provocative maneuvers
    B. Palpate bilateral brachial pulses
    C. Obtain bilateral brachial blood pressure with the athlete standing
    D. Perform electrocardiogram on all athletes

189. A female cross country runner complains of right-sided heel pain. She states the pain has been present for two weeks. Initially, the pain only occurred with long runs, but now hurts most of the time. On exam, pain is elicited by squeezing the heel. X-rays confirm the diagnosis. Which of the following statements about this condition is true?

    A. Surgical intervention is required
    B. Posterior night splints should be used
    C. She should be sent for injection therapy
    D. Patient can expect to return to activity in four to six weeks
    E. Extracorporal shock wave therapy should be used

190. A 23-year-old thin marathon runner is diagnosed with a stress fracture of the second metatarsal bone. She recently recovered from a similar stress fracture of the contralateral extremity. Which of the following is most important in the management for this patient?

    A. Arch supports to correct pes planus and evaluation of running shoes
    B. Increased training as tolerated after appropriate respite period
    C. Proper screening for female athlete triad
    D. A bone scan to differentiate stress fracture from stress reaction
    E. Intramedullary screw fixation for an elite athlete

191. Which of the following statements is true regarding pronator syndrome?

    A. The most common cause is mechanical compression by the pronator teres
    B. Athletes with pes planus are at increased risk for pronator syndrome
    C. Athletes with pronator syndrome are at increased risk for ankle sprains
    D. An MRI is often helpful in making the diagnosis
    E. Pronator syndrome is caused by compression of the radial nerve

192. Which of the following statements is true concerning the respiratory system during pregnancy?

    A. Tidal volume decreases
    B. Vital capacity is unchanged
    C. Minute ventilation is unchanged
    D. Reserve volumes increase

193. A 36-year-old female recreational soccer player presents with insidious onset of left posterior heel pain and a limp. She is wearing flip-flops because shoes make the pain worse. Examination reveals swelling and erythema of the posterior heel. There is no palpable defect in the Achilles tendon, and a Thompson test is negative. The most likely diagnosis is which of the following?

    A. Stress fracture of the calcaneus
    B. Plantar fasciitis
    C. Achilles tendon avulsion
    D. Sural neuritis
    E. Retrocalcaneal bursitis

194. Which item would a sports medicine physician want in a game bag to help emergently reduce a symptomatic posterior sternoclavicular dislocation in the field?

    A. Trainer's Angel
    B. Towel roll
    C. Towel clamp
    D. Sling and swathe

195. A 54-year-old male presents to your office today, complaining of bilateral knee pain. He was diagnosed with osteoarthritis in both his knees after he was referred by his primary care provider to see an orthopedic surgeon. He was given a prescription for an anti-inflammatory medication and told that he may need knee replacement surgery some day. He does not like taking medications and has come to see you regarding non-pharmacologic treatment options. Which of the following statements regarding exercise and osteoarthritis is true?

    A. Aerobic exercise should be discouraged because it will increase the patient's pain
    B. This patient's x-ray findings are moderate to severe; therefore, exercise is unlikely to be helpful
    C. Strengthening exercises may be helpful in preventing osteoarthritis and may also alter disease progression
    D. Aquatic exercise has not been shown to be beneficial for patients with osteoarthritis

196. Which of the following statements is true regarding nail disorders in athletes?

    A. The risk of ingrown toenails can be minimized by having the athlete wear shoes that are snug and minimize the sliding of the foot inside the shoe
    B. Trimming the toenails in a curved arc just distal to the free edge will minimize the risk of ingrown toenails
    C. Any collections of dark fluid beneath the nail bed should be immediately drained with a red-hot paper clip
    D. The persistence of a linear black band or streak running the length of the nail warrants further evaluation
    E. The treatment of choice for onychomycosis is a topical antifungal

197. Which of the following statements is true regarding scapular fractures?

    A. Reduction of an isolated displaced glenoid neck fracture is usually not necessary to achieve a good clinical outcome
    B. Non-surgical treatment is an option for glenoid fractures that involve 50% or less of the articular surface
    C. Non-operative treatment of glenoid fractures consists of immobilization with a sling and swathe for at least two weeks
    D. Non-operative treatment of glenoid fractures consists of immobilization with a sling for at least two weeks
    E. Sports-related injury is responsible for almost half of the cases of scapular fractures

198. A college athlete presents with fever, myalgias, and rhinorrhea for three days. Which of the following treatments are banned by NCAA standards?

    A. Phenylephrine
    B. Pseudoephedrine
    C. Antipyretic agents
    D. Ephedrine
    E. Antihistamines

199. A 55-year-old female presents to your clinic after a fall during a hike earlier in the day. You obtain an x-ray and see a fracture through the surgical neck of the proximal humerus. Which motor function corresponds to the nerve that may have been damaged as a result of this injury?

    A. Abduction of the arm
    B. Wrist extension
    C. Finger abduction
    D. Wrist flexion and abduction

200. A 20-year-old endurance athlete presents to your clinic complaining of a generalized, itchy, papular rash that occurs only during exercise. You would recommend that he do which of the following?

    A. Use unscented laundry detergent
    B. Take a hot shower the night before a long run or try an antihistamine tablet one hour prior to exercise
    C. Use topical steroids on the rash during exercise
    D. Use sunscreen with PABA (para-aminobenzoic acid) at least half an hour prior to exercise

2

Test 2
Questions

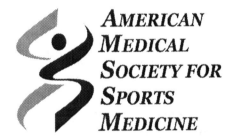

AMERICAN
MEDICAL
SOCIETY FOR
SPORTS
MEDICINE

Leading Sports Medicine into the Future

1. A 25-year-old male tennis player has noted loss of strength and power in his backhand stroke. He denies injury, and only mild pain with range of motion, specifically cross-arm adduction of his dominant arm. Exam reveals infraspinatus atrophy and weakness with external rotation. You diagnose infraspinatus syndrome, involving which of the following nerves?

    A. Long thoracic nerve
    B. Dorsal scapular nerve
    C. Radial nerve
    D. Suprascapular nerve
    E. Axillary nerve

2. An 18-year-old male novice crew athlete presents to the athletic training room with a one-week history of low back pain. He just started crew about three weeks ago and is trying to keep up with the strength and conditioning as well. He points to the lumbosacral junction as the point of maximal pain. His pain is more right-sided and occurs when he pulls back the oar. He denies groin pain. He denies numbness or tingling, radicular signs and symptoms, bowel or bladder incontinence. Ibuprofen does help him somewhat; however, the symptoms return the next day in the boat. On physical exam, he has full range of motion and 5/5 strength on forward flexion and extension. His DTRs are +2/4 bilaterally. His leg lengths are equal. His straight leg raise is negative. FABER is positive on the right and negative on the left. FADIR is negative bilaterally. His lumbosacral and thoracolumbar junctions are equivocal. He has no gluteal tenderness to the point. What is your working diagnosis, and what is the best treatment option for the patient?

    A. Sacroiliac dysfunction: perform a corticosteroid injection, continue to evaluate
    B. Lumbar radiculopathy: obtain a plain film and subsequently an MRI
    C. Sacroiliac dysfunction: improve lumbar core strength and stability with ATCs, osteopathic manipulation (if available)
    D. Femoral neck stress fracture: stop crew, and remain non-weight-bearing
    E. Piriformis syndrome: exercise program with ATCs

3. A 35-year-old third base coach is hit below the right breast by a line drive and collapses to the ground. He is in obvious pain and has difficulty speaking more than three words between breaths. He is transported by EMS for evaluation. His heartrate is 120, and breath sounds are decreased on the right side. Which other factor indicates need for urgent needle or tube thoracostomy?

   A. A 10-pack-per-year history of smoking
   B. Chest x-ray showing 1 cm of pleural space at the right apex
   C. CT scan indicating a 20% pneumothorax
   D. Tracheal deviation to the left

4. Which of the following is a physiologic change associated with aging?

   A. Skin, tendon, and ligamentous elasticity increases
   B. Basal metabolic rate and caloric needs increase
   C. VO_2max remains unchanged
   D. Muscle mass decreases due to loss of type II muscle fibers

5. A recreational diver develops stupor, confusion, focal weakness, visual loss, and seizures 10 minutes after ascent. What is the most likely diagnosis?

   A. Middle ear barotrauma
   B. Diving migraine
   C. Oxygen toxicity
   D. Arterial gas embolism
   E. Spinal cord decompression syndrome

6. A 20-year old male basketball player collapses and dies suddenly during a recreational basketball game. He was evaluated by a physician prior to participation in division I college athletics, and family reports the doctor noted no cardiac problems and "cleared him" for all sports. His height was 6'7". The family reports his grandfather was also tall and died of "heart problems" in his 60s. Which of the following is the most likely cause of death?

   A. Hypertrophic cardiomyopathy
   B. Coronary anomalies
   C. Myocarditis
   D. Aortic dissection
   E. Arrhythmia

7. A tennis player you previously diagnosed with ulnar neuropathy and referred for surgical decompression returns six months post-surgery with complaints of recurrent paresthesias of the hand in an ulnar distribution. Exam reveals no tenderness with a normal Tinel's at Guyon's canal. Imaging demonstrates normal bony structures of the wrist and hand. Review of the patient's surgical records and physical exam reveal that the patient underwent a submuscular transposition of the ulnar nerve. Which of the following would most likely explain the patient's persistent symptoms?

    A. Hypermobility of the ulnar nerve at the cubital tunnel
    B. Accessory anconeous epitrochlearis muscle compressing the ulnar nerve
    C. Compression by the medial head of the triceps
    D. Compression in the distal upper arm by the Arcade of Struthers

8. A 46-year-old workers' compensation case manager presents to your clinic, complaining of pain over her lateral elbow. After appropriate workup, the diagnosis of lateral epicondylitis is made. Which of the following comments is correct in regards to evidence-based medicine?

    A. Topical anti-inflammatory medications (NSAIDs) are as effective as placebo
    B. Oral NSAIDs are as effective as placebo
    C. A corticosteroid injection is as effective as a wait-and-see approach at 52 weeks
    D. For six weeks, a corticosteroid injection is more effective than physiotherapy

9. A 16-year-old male is found to have an elevated blood pressure at a mass preparticipation physical exam (PPE) to participate in high school football. Which of the following is the next-best step in management for this athlete?

    A. Restrict him from playing this season if the blood pressure was above 140/90
    B. Restrict him from playing this season if the blood pressure was above the 95% for his age, sex, and height
    C. Restrict him from playing this season if the blood pressure falls within the stage 2 (moderate) category of hypertension
    D. Arrange for the patient to receive follow-up care with his personal physician to obtain three different readings on three different days
    E. Start the patient on an antihypertensive medication in order to control his blood pressure, and allow him to play

10. Which of the following patient conditions is not an absolute contraindication to starting an exercise program?

    A. Unstable angina
    B. Severe symptomatic aortic stenosis
    C. Left main coronary artery stenosis
    D. Uncontrolled symptomatic heart failure

11. Which of the following statements is true?

    A. Panner's disease occurs in children ages four to eight and is a self-limiting condition managed by conservative treatment
    B. Panner's disease is a defect of the wrist in gymnasts and most commonly needs casting
    C. Panner's disease occurs as a result of a traumatic injury that usually requires surgical repair
    D. Panner's disease is a congenital problem involving the hips and usually presents with a limp
    E. Panner's disease involves the medial elbow

12. A right-hand-dominant 16-year-old female tennis player complains of chronic aching pain distal to the lateral epicondyle of the elbow. Her symptoms are worse after tennis practice. She denies any numbness or tingling. On exam, she has weakness with supination and wrist extension. Pulses and neurological exam are within normal limits. The remainder of the hand exam is unremarkable. She has entrapment of which nerve?

    A. Posterior interosseous nerve
    B. Anterior interosseous nerve
    C. Superficial radial nerve (Wartenberg's disease)
    D. Ulnar nerve

13. When covering an athletic event, it is recommended that the team physician do all of the following except?

    A. Assess the playing conditions of the venue
    B. Introduce yourself to the opposing team medical staff, and review emergency protocols
    C. Choose a location in the stands that allows good visibility of the game action
    D. Meet with ambulance personnel and assess their capability and available equipment
    E. Document the care provided

14. A 19-year-old lacrosse player first presented to the training room with a two-day history of persistent left axillary pain and swelling. He noted the pain was exacerbated by weight lifting activities. He denied fevers, chills, rash, left arm numbness, or constitutional or respiratory symptoms. There was no recent history of direct trauma. His symptoms persisted for two days despite ibuprofen and a significant reduction in upper extremity resistance training (he remained active in lacrosse practice). He has no known sick contacts and denied recent unprotected intercourse. No change in hygiene or deodorant. He denies leg swelling or shortness of breath. Physical exam reveals localized area of swelling and tenderness in the left axilla with some firmness on palpation. No increased warmth. Distal pulses were strong. When supine, prominent superficial venous structures were noted in both extremities and were slightly more dilated in the left upper extremity. Which of the following is the presumed diagnosis?

    A. Superficial phlebitis
    B. Pectoralis major tear
    C. Labral tear
    D. Effort-induced thrombosis
    E. Lymphangitis

15. Which of the following statements is true about what happens during muscle contraction?

    A. Actin filaments on the thick filament bind to the myosin thin filament
    B. Sarcomere length increases during a concentric muscle contraction
    C. During muscle action and contraction calcium binds to myosin
    D. During muscle action and contraction ATP binds to myosin, allowing the thin and thick filaments to slide past each other
    E. When muscle stimulation increases intercellular calcium levels decrease and there is less calcium available for the actin and myosin filaments

16. A 67-year-old male runner presents to the office complaining of right knee pain for several months. He denies mechanical symptoms. An MRI demonstrates osteoarthritis and a degenerative meniscal tear. Which of the following treatments is least likely to result in significant long-term reduction of pain?

   A. NSAID medication
   B. Activity modification
   C. Physical therapy
   D. Arthroscopic debridement
   E. Acetaminophen

17. The most reliable magnetic resonance imaging (MRI) finding, signifying osteitis pubis that is chronic and has likely been present for greater than six months, is which of the following?

   A. Subchondral sclerosis
   B. Fluid in the symphysis pubis joint
   C. Subchondral bone marrow edema
   D. Periarticular edema of the symphysis pubis joint
   E. Symphyseal disc extrusion

18. Encouraging patients to lead an active lifestyle is important to reduce the risk of developing a variety of different medical conditions including obesity, diabetes, and hyperlipidemia. There is also strong medical evidence to show that physical activity reduces the risk of development of which of the following types of cancer?

   A. Breast cancer
   B. Melanoma
   C. Prostate cancer
   D. Ovarian cancer

19. A 35-year-old experienced male diver with a history of hypertension has just returned from a week of recreational scuba diving in the Carribean and comes to your office. He reports feeling ill the last couple of days with episodes of nausea, vomiting, and tingling in his hands and feet. He states that when he washes his hands in cold water, it feels oddly warm. He denies fevers, chills, or diarrhea. He states during his week-long stay that he stayed in a resort and participated in four recreational dives over two consecutive days. He reported dive times and depths well within the safety parameters set by PADI. His last dive was over 36 hours before his departure. His symptoms started on the last day of his trip. He denies using any alcohol or drugs around the times of his dives. He takes lisinopril 10 mg a day for HTN and has been on it for seven years. He has no allergies. He denies eating any sushi or raw fish, but did eat some locally caught fish (i.e., eel). His vitals are stable with BP 132/86. Rest of exam is remarkably normal, including full neuro exam. This patient is most likely suffering from which of the following?

    A. Arterial gas embolism
    B. Pulmonary barotrauma of ascent
    C. Scombroid poisoning
    D. Decompression illness
    E. Ciguartera poisoning

20. A 21-year-old male ice hockey player is struck in the mouth by a hockey puck during a game. After initially being evaluated by the team athletic trainer, the player is escorted off the ice for you to evaluate his injury. The patient is alert and oriented. Your examination reveals a single dental fracture. The exposed surface of the fractured tooth appears to be yellow with a discrete, central pink-red focus, exhibiting a slow seepage of blood. The athletic trainer has retrieved the fracture fragment for you. Assuming no cervical injuries, concussion, or other fractures, the best next step in treatment is which of the following?

    A. Apply a wax dressing to the exposed surface of the fractured tooth, have the athlete wear a mouthpiece, and allow him to return-to-play
    B. Restrict the athlete from continued participation, referring him to see his dentist the next day
    C. Restrict the athlete from continued participation, referring him to see a dentist immediately for urgent evaluation, root canal, and/or crown (cap) placement
    D. Place the fractured tooth fragment in cold milk, allow him to return to play, and refer the athlete to see a dentist immediately following the conclusion of the game for splinting
    E. Restrict the athlete from continued participation, and attempt to reapproximate the fractured tooth fragment as soon as possible, taking care to achieve anatomic reduction

21. A 12-year-old competitive female gymnast presents to your office after sustaining an inversion injury to her right foot 10 days earlier. At that time, she saw her athletic trainer in the training room and was advised to ice, elevate, and rest the ankle. Her father reports that she has been very diligent in following these instructions. However, her ankle remains swollen and painful, and she reports difficulty bearing weight. On physical exam, you find exquisite tenderness over the lateral malleolus, the anterior talofibular ligament, the talar dome, and the midfoot section. The remainder of the exam is unremarkable.

    X-rays of the ankle reveal no acute bony abnormality. The decision is made to make her nonweightbearing in a pneumatic boot for two weeks.The patient returns to you after two weeks of nonweightbearing, complaining that the pain in her ankle is still present. Physical exam reveals marked tenderness over the distal tip of the fibula with no remaining tenderness over the ATFL, the talar dome, or the midfoot section. At this time you order an MRI, which supports your suspicion of which of the following?

    A. Complete rupture of the deltoid ligament
    B. Salter-Harris I fracture of the lateral malleolus
    C. Munchhausen syndrome
    D. Sever's disease

22. Which of the following is true regarding children and sports activity?

    A. Preteen athletes most commonly injure lower limbs, whereas teenagers injure upper limbs
    B. Salter-Harris II fractures generally require surgical intervention
    C. Joint dislocations and ligamentous injuries are more common than buckle and other types of fractures
    D. Physes close on average at 14.5 years in girls and 16.5 years in boys
    E. Non-unions fractures are common in the immature skeleton

23. An otherwise healthy 12-year-old boy presents to the office for evaluation of left foot pain. He states that it occurred while training for soccer. He states the pain is worse with activity and totally resolves by the next day. No night pain. On exam, he has mild point tenderness over the proximal fifth metatarsal. You confirm your diagnosis with foot radiographs that show a fragment of bone running parallel to the fifth metatarsal diaphysis bilaterally. Initial treatment would include which of the following?

    A. Supportive shoes with a narrow toe box
    B. Short leg cast in 30 degrees of plantar flexion
    C. Holding the child out of activities that cause pain
    D. Referral to a surgeon to correct the deformity

24. A right-hand-dominant 20-year-old college baseball pitcher feels a pop in his elbow while throwing followed by medial elbow pain. He experiences persistent pain and decreased throwing velocity. On exam, he has pain and mild opening on valgus stress of the elbow. Which of the following is the test of choice?

    A. MRI
    B. CT scan
    C. Ultrasound
    D. MRI arthrogram

25. Regarding training at altitude, which of the following statements is true?

    A. Maximal aerobic power is reduced by 5% for every 100 m above 1500 m elevation in normal individuals
    B. Acclimatized individuals demonstrate lower peak lactate levels at altitude than at sea level for a given workload
    C. Reduction in maximal aerobic power is less severe in endurance trained athletes
    D. Living at lower elevations but training at higher elevations introduces the greatest physiological adaptation to altitude

26. A 20-year-old female soccer athlete complains of pain and pressure over the anterior aspect of her shin with exercise. Physical exam that is performed just after exercise reveals a tense anterior compartment, weakness in great toe extension and ankle dorsiflexion, as well as decreased sensation in the first toe web space. Which nerve is involved?

    A. Superficial peroneal nerve
    B. Sural nerve
    C. Deep peroneal nerve
    D. Tibial nerve
    E. Obturator nerve

27. Of the following, identify the false statement regarding acute patella dislocations?

    A. Often associated with hemarthrosis or effusion
    B. Requires disruption of the medial patella restraints
    C. Frequently associated with chondral injury or loose bodies
    D. Rarely responds to non-operative treatment

28. A sophomore female college soccer player tests positive for amphetamines on an NCAA drug test. She requests a medical exemption for the positive result because her physician prescribes Ritalin for her ADHD. The medical exemption will be approved only if which of the following is the case?

    A. The athletics medical administrator has medical records proving that Ritalin is prescribed by her primary care physician or team physician
    B. The athletics medical administrator has medical records proving that she has undergone standardized testing for ADHD and is prescribed Ritalin by her team physician or primary care physician
    C. She makes an appointment to undergo standardized testing for ADHD, tests positive for ADHD, and the team physician or her primary care physician prescribes Ritalin and she sends the records to the NCAA
    D. Her primary care physician and/or team physician has medical records proving that she has a documented improvement in ADHD symptoms with Ritalin and that they prescribe the Ritalin

29. Which of the following training interventions, if used alone, has been proven to be most effective in reducing injuries, including ACL tears in athletes?

    A. Eccentric hamstring strength training
    B. Plyometrics
    C. Warm-up stretching
    D. Flexibility training

30. A severe varus injury to the knee can result in an injury to which of the following nerves?

    A. Femoral
    B. Common peroneal
    C. Tibial
    D. Sural
    E. Deep peroneal

31. You are covering a marathon on a slightly warm day. You are presented with a male runner who collapsed shortly after crossing the finish line about one minute ago. You are able to determine that he is conscious and has no mental status changes. His racing bib did not indicate any underlying medical conditions. His temperature was 101 degrees Fahrenheit (38 degrees Celsius). He was able to orally rehydrate. His pulse was 142. His blood pressure was not elevated, and demonstrated a 26 mm Hg systolic drop between supine and standing. There are no recent illnesses reported. The runner completed the race and sprinted to the finish for a personal best, and decided during the race to skip a few water stops to keep his record time. He reported no nausea or vomiting. Which of the following is the best statement regarding this scenario?

    A. The runner is withholding information
    B. The runner is hyponatremic
    C. The runner has experience exertional heat illness
    D. The runner suffered an episode of exercise-associated collapse

32. Which of the following is thought to play the most significant role in the increased risk of anterior cruciate ligament (ACL) injury for female athletes?

    A. Cyclical hormonal changes
    B. Decreased femoral notch width
    C. Imbalances in neuromuscular control
    D. Shoe-playing surface interactions
    E. Greater participation in high-risk sports

33. A 25-year-old female presents to your office with the chief complaint of right thigh pain. She is training for her first marathon and shows you her detailed training log. It documents a gradual increase in her running intensity and length of training runs. She ran on a park trail and was comfortably running eight miles. Three weeks prior to her appointment, friends from her local running club encouraged her to run a half marathon road race with them. Upon finishing the race, she became aware of a nagging pain in her thigh. She presumed it was "just a strain" and continued on her usual training schedule. The thigh pain significantly limited the length of her runs, and by the time she presents to your office, she is having pain with walking.

    On exam, she is limping, favoring her right leg. Range-of-motion testing of the hip and knee is full and pain-free both actively and passively. Palpation of the right thigh reveals a poorly localized area of pain in the midshaft of the femur. There is no difference in circumferential measurement of the right and left thighs. Strength testing of the right quadricep with resisted straight leg raise does not exacerbate her pain. Radiographs performed in the office of the right hip and femur are negative. What is the most likely diagnosis?

    A. Quadriceps tear
    B. Anterior superior iliac spine (ASIS) avulsion fracture
    C. Femur stress fracture
    D. Myositis ossificans

34. An 18-year-old Division I wrestler presents for skin checks at the NCAA National Championships. He reports having been diagnosed three days prior with primary orolabial herpes. He was started on acyclovir 200 mg by mouth five times daily. He denies any current constitutional symptoms or new lesions since his diagnosis. On physical examination, there is a cluster of well-dried lesions on the left lower lip and chin area. In accordance with NCAA regulations, which of the following is the most appropriate return-to-play decision?

A. Allow the wrestler to participate because he is currently asymptomatic
B. Allow the wrestler to participate since he has not developed new lesions for the past 72 hours
C. Allow the wrestler to participate if he covers the lesions
D. Disqualify the wrestler because of an inadequate treatment course
E. Disqualify the wrestler because of an inappropriate dosage of systemic antiviral

35. A 12-year-old male soccer player presents to your clinic with right anterior hip pain after feeling a pop in this area after taking a strong shot to score a goal. His radiographs reveal an avulsion of the anterior inferior iliac spine apophysis. The muscle that attaches here is which of the following?

A. Sartorius
B. Rectus femoris
C. Gracilis
D. Tensor fascia lata

36. A collegiate level rower presents to your office after exercise-associated syncope. Your workup includes detailed personal and family histories and further cardiovascular testing, including ECG and 2D-echocardiogram with color Doppler. Which of the following most favors the diagnosis of athlete's heart rather than hypertrophic cardiomyopathy?

A. Left ventricular cavity dilation
B. Altered echocardiographic parameters in first degree relatives
C. EGG patterns including extremely elevated voltages, Q waves, and negative T waves
D. Maintenance of wall thickness after deconditioning
E. Marked left atrial enlargement

37. A senior high school athlete with college aspirations comes to your clinic for a pre-participation physical exam. He states that he was syncopal while running on a hot day, preparing for the upcoming football season. He was seen at the emergency room, but he was only given intravenous fluids since he was felt to be dehydrated. He recovered well and has not had another syncopal episode. Since he had syncope with exertion, you decide to get an ECG, which is shown below. Which of the following is the best diagnosis?

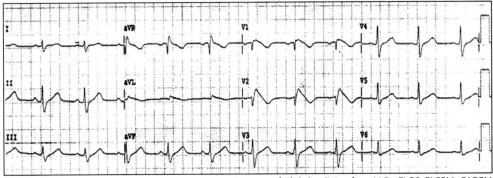

Courtesy of Christine E. Lawless, M.D., FACC, FACSM, CAQSM

   A. Hypertrophic cardiomyopathy (HCM)
   B. Arrythmogenic right ventricular dysplasia (ARVD)
   C. Brugada syndrome
   D. Long QT syndrome
   E. Wolff-Parkinson-White syndrome (WPW)

38. A 13-year-old male year-round soccer player presents for evaluation with a two-month history of knee pain. He denies any trauma or initial injury and reports that the pain initially was only after games and practices. Gradually, it began to bother him more toward the end of practice sessions, and now it starts to hurt within a few minutes of exercise. He localizes the pain to the inferior pole of the patella. This is most consistent with which of the following diagnoses?

   A. Quadriceps tendinitis
   B. Osgood-Schlatter's disease
   C. Anterior fat pad syndrome
   D. Sindig-Larsen-Johannson disease

39. A 19-year-old offensive lineman sustained an injury to his right foot during a tackle. He developed forefoot swelling, ecchymosis, and has pain with weight-bearing. On physical examination, there is tenderness at the first MTP joint with limited range of motion. Routine standing AP and lateral foot radiographs are unremarkable. He was diagnosed with "turf toe." Which of the following is the most common mechanism of injury?

   A. Hyperflexion of first MTP joint
   B. Hyperextension of first MTP joint
   C. Plantarflexion of forefoot
   D. Valgus force to first MTP joint
   E. Inversion of ankle

40. Toward the middle of the season, a college soccer player suffers a lateral and syndesmosis ankle sprain, which prevents her from returning to play. Which of the following psychological issues needs to be addressed as it pertains to rehabilitation of her injury?

   A. Encourage a fear of reinjury so as to motivate the athlete in her rehabilitation program
   B. Share the basics about the injury, and encourage the athlete to look it up on the Internet to get a better understanding
   C. Foster an obsession with the question of return to play
   D. Prepare the coach for the injury recovery process, and encourage that the athlete not be isolated from the team

41. A volleyball player presents with right shoulder pain after attempting to spike the ball in practice. The player is holding her arm in slight abduction and external rotation. The humeral head is palpated anteriorly. Before proceeding, it is important to first evaluate which of the following?

   A. Supraclavicular nerve by testing sensation over the clavicular area
   B. Axillary nerve by testing sensation over lateral aspect of the shoulder
   C. Radial nerve by testing sensation over inferolateral arm
   D. Medial cutaneous nerve by testing sensation over medial aspect of arm

42. Which of the following is not true of hepatitis B infection?

    A. Concurrent HDV infection increases risk of fulminent infection
    B. Enteric precautions will be necessary to avoid transmission
    C. Sexual contact increases the risk of transmission
    D. E-antigen-positive status is of concern for possible transmission
    E. Symptoms begin two to four months post exposure

43. Which of the following statements is true regarding exertional headache?

    A. Factors associated with increased risk of exertional headaches include hot weather and high altitude
    B. Exertional headaches are always benign
    C. Exertional headaches most commonly occur in young women
    D. The typical duration of exertional headaches is seconds to minutes
    E. The athlete typically describes the pain from exertional headache as "the worst headache of my life"

44. Which of the following is a normal ECG response to exercise?

    A. Increase of T-wave amplitude
    B. Depression of the J point
    C. Increase of the QRS duration
    D. ST-segment depression

45. In 2009, the NCAA recommended that all athletes with a diagnosis of attention deficit disorder be started on a non-stimulant medication unless contraindicated. Which of the following medications would be an appropriate initial therapy within those guidelines?

    A. Methylphenidate (Ritalin)
    B. Dextroamphetamine (Adderall®)
    C. Atomoxetine (Strattera®)
    D. Lisdexamfetamine (Vyvanse®)

46. You are performing a preparticipation physical exam on a 17-year-old male football player. In the process of questioning him about his history of concussion and neurological injuries, he reports an event last season when he had a few hours of weakness and numbness in his arms and legs after being tackled. He reports that he had negative C-spine x-rays at that time. He also had an MRI, but does not recall the findings. As part of your discussion with this athlete and his parents about this episode of transient quadriparesis (also referred to as transient neurapraxia and cervical cord neurapraxia), which of the following options would most represent an absolute contraindication to returning to contact sports?

   A. This was his second episode of transient quadriparesis
   B. His Pavlov-Torg ratio was less than 0.8
   C. He was found to have associated intervertebral disk disease with some degenerative changes
   D. He was found to have an associated type II Klippel-Feil deformity involving the interspace at C3

47. A 16-year-old with Down syndrome presents to the clinic with his parents. They are concerned with the patient's increasing weight. When considering an exercise program for this individual, you need to consider which of the following?

   A. A normal VO_2max is commonly found in individuals with Down syndrome
   B. There is no evidence supporting exercise as an intervention to improve fitness in Down syndrome individuals
   C. Low exercise tolerance exists in the majority of Down syndrome individuals
   D. There is a normal muscle tone in individuals with Down syndrome

48. You diagnose a patient with rotator cuff dysfunction. Which of the following would be least beneficial in the rehabilitative treatment of rotator cuff syndrome and dysfunction?

   A. Eccentric strengthening of the biceps
   B. Stretching of the posterior glenohumeral joint capsule and increasing internal rotation range-of-motion
   C. Scapular retraction postural training, with periscapular strengthening and stretching
   D. Strengthening of the teres minor, subscapularis, and infraspinatus, followed by strengthening of the supraspinatus
   E. Scapular protraction postural training, with stretching of the scalenes

49. You are asked to set up a drug testing protocol for your school. You design a program that involves random testing, education, and rehabilitation. During the urine drug testing procedure, you ensure a chain of custody, which is defined as which of the following?

    A. The record of a prescribing physician, who has given an athlete a banned substance for medical reasons
    B. The witnessed observation of an athlete giving a urine sample
    C. The order of procedures done during the testing
    D. The physical barrier needed to ensure the athletes are kept in line
    E. The chronological documentation showing the disposition of a sample from collection to testing

50. Your patient sustains an injury to his proximal forearm, and after exam you suspect pronator syndrome. Which of the following exam findings would support this suspicion?

    A. Decreased sensation over the lateral forearm
    B. Pain at night
    C. Positive Tinel's over the radial forearm
    D. Weakness of flexor pollicis longus

51. The placement of a methoxy group at position 8 of the quinolone antibiotics' chemical structure, as in gatifloxacin and moxifloxacin, has eliminated which of the following potential side effects of this class of antibiotic?

    A. Tendinopathy
    B. Seizures
    C. QTc prolongation
    D. Phototoxicity
    E. Alterations in blood glucose levels

52. Which of the following statements regarding carbohydrates and exercise is true?

    A. The optimal carbohydrate concentration in rehydration solutions is 6% to 8%
    B. Carbohydrate loading before a marathon is only recommended for novice runners
    C. Carbohydrate ingestion only has value in events lasting less than one hour
    D. Glycogen synthesis can be enhanced by ingesting a combination of carbohydrates and fats shortly after exercise

53. During a session of free preparticipation physical exams offered at your local high school, you see a freshman who had a tibial osteotomy early in childhood. She is new to organized sports. After surgery, there had been no mention of the ACL, bracing, or care during sports participation. She has had no symptoms involving her knee. There is no knee effusion. Your full examination includes an abnormal Lachman test and a positive pivot-shift test, indicating absence of the anterior cruciate ligament. There is also a scar from her previous corrective tibial osteotomy. Concerning clearance for sports, you should do which of the following?

    A. Clear her to play sports without restrictions since she has had no symptoms over the years since her osteotomy
    B. Disqualify her from any fitness or athletic activities
    C. Prescribe physical therapy
    D. Refer her to an orthopedic surgeon experienced in handling teens with no anterior cruciate ligament
    E. Provide a brace and clear her to play sports

54. A 65-year-old male with past medical history of diabetes, who was recently seen in your office to discuss an exercise presciption prior to intiating a new exercise program, now presents to your office with a one-week history of left hip pain and numbness and tingling of the lateral thigh. The symptoms are aggravated by walking and relieved by sitting. Physical examination is normal with the exception of a sensory deficit on the lateral thigh area. Which of the following nerves is involved?

    A. Obturator nerve (L2-L4)
    B. Femoral nerve (L2-L4)
    C. Superior gluteal nerve (L5)
    D. Lateral femoral cutaneous nerve (L2-L3)
    E. Genitofemoral nerve (L1-L2)

55. A 22-year-old male presents complaining of pain following being hit in the nose about one hour ago. On exam, you find a soft and fluctuant mass that is seen at the nasal septum bilaterally. Which of the following statements is true of this patient's injury and treatment?

    A. Once drained, there is no risk of reaccumulation or need for nasal packing
    B. Hematoma does not occur without associated nasal fracture
    C. If treatment is delayed, there is increased risk for infection or abscess formation
    D. Hematoma formation is most commonly unilateral
    E. Treatment can be delayed up to 72 hours without increased risk for complication

56. In an adult heart transplant recipient, the donor heart is completely denervated. Which of the the following is correct concerning the heart rate during exercise following a heart transplant?

    A. The heart rate during exercise following a heart transplant is determined by circulating plasma catecholamines alone
    B. Complete denervation of the heart prior to transplant is followed by complete functional reinnervation after transplant
    C. The heart rate control mechanisms are exactly the same as prior to transplant
    D. Partial functional reinnervation allows some heart rate control by sympathetic and parasympathetic stimuli
    E. Increased sensitivity of myocardial adrenergic receptors completely replaces the role of sympathetic and parasympathetic innervation in determining heart rate during exercise

57. A 12-year-old right-hand-dominant male baseball pitcher presents with right upper extremity pain after pitching his most recent game. He reports feeling severe pain after throwing a fastball, with immediate loss of strength in that arm. He admits to some vague discomfort for a week or so before the injury, and confesses that he "may have thrown more than 85 pitches" in the previous game, with only one day of rest between games. His father tells you that playoffs are in two weeks. After examination and radiographs (with comparison views), you determine he has "Little League shoulder" and recommend which of the following?

    A. Complete rest from throwing for 6 to 12 weeks
    B. One week rest, with return in time for playoffs
    C. Moving to the catcher position for the next game, and return to pitching when pain-free
    D. Ice, a rotator cuff rehabilitation program, and allow pitching with a pitch count of < 60 pitches per game through the playoffs
    E. Referral for surgical evaluation of rotator cuff tear

58. A 17-year-old female volleyball player presents for her first college preparticipation exam. You note that she is 6'4' tall with long thin limbs, arachnodactyly, scoliosis, and a pectus excavatum. Which of the following would be considered a major eye criterion in assisting in making the clinical diagnosis of Marfan syndrome?

    A. Ectopia lentis
    B. Flat cornea
    C. Myopia
    D. Retinal detachment

59. The most common cause of sudden death in older athletes (> 35 years old) while running the marathon is which of the following?

    A. Hyponatremia
    B. Neurocardiogenic syncope
    C. Coronary artery disease
    D. Trauma
    E. Cerebral vascular accident

60. A 14-year-old male is hit in the left eye with a softball. He complains of blurry, double vision. On exam, he has numbness of his left cheek and is unable to look up with his left eye. The athlete still wants to play. Which of the following should you do next?

    A. Cover the left eye with a shield, and send the athlete to the emergency room
    B. Cover the left eye with a pad, and send the athlete to the emergency room
    C. Have the athlete wear sports goggles and return to play
    D. Cover the left eye with a pad, and return the athlete to play

61. Which of the following responses during cardiopulmonary exercise testing would most likely indicate myocardial ischemic dysfunction?

    A. Decrease in systolic blood pressure
    B. Increase in systolic blood pressure
    C. Decrease in diastolic blood pressure
    D. Increase in diastolic blood pressure

62. A 21-year-old right-handed female collided with the shortstop during a softball game and injured her left elbow when she fell. She presents to you two days after the injury with lateral elbow pain. On exam, she is tender directly over the radial head and has some limitations in range of motion (ROM) with most pain during pronation/supination. An anterior and posterior fat pad are noted on her lateral x-ray from her initial four views of the left elbow, which showed overall normal alignment and no displaced fractures or fracture fragments. What single factor among the following choices would be an indication for orthopedic referral to discuss ORIF for this elbow?

    A. Limited ROM in first two days following injury
    B. Mechanical block to motion
    C. <2 mm displacement of radial head fracture
    D. No dislocation or ligamentous injury
    E. Posterior fat pad sign on lateral x-ray

63. A 15-year-old male competitive soccer player falls to the ground during a tournament you are covering. He was running maximally without difficulty, but then loses muscle tone and falls to the ground in prone position. You do not remember witnessing any head trauma or collisions to the chest during the game. The trainer signals you to the field, and en route, you notice convulsions lasting two to five seconds. Rolled onto supine position with cervical spine protected, he is unresponsive to verbal and painful stimuli, not breathing spontaneously, and has no radial or carotid pulse.

You initiate rescue breathing and chest compressions while the trainer retrieves the AED and activates EMS. You perform CPR, and the AED delivers shocks twice. With pulse regained, the athlete is transported to the hospital, and he is admitted to you.

On admission, his urine drug screen, urine specific gravity, and serum sodium were normal. His cardiac enzymes, potassium, glucose, and liver enzymes are elevated. Further research reveals that he has had previous episodes of exertional syncope at ages six, seven, and 11, for which the ECG, echocardiogram, treadmill exercise test, and EEG were normal. Newborn screen for sickle cell was normal, and previous fasting glucose was normal. He has had no history of seizures nor syncopal episodes at rest. He had no history of abnormal heart sounds on exams. He does not taking any medication or supplements. There is no family history of sudden cardiac arrest or premature cardiovascular disease. Which of the following is the next appropriate step to arrive at a diagnosis?

A. Cardiac MRI
B. Three-hour 100 g glucose tolerance test
C. Video EEG
D. Psychiatric evaluation
E. Myocardial biopsy

64. Which of the following is the most common cause of airway obstruction in an unconscious athlete?

A. Mouthguard
B. The tongue
C. Swelling from anaphylaxis
D. Inhaled foreign body

65. A six-year-old soccer player twists his ankle and presents to you three hours later with a tender, swollen lateral ankle and limited weight bearing. Which of the following is true?

    A. Patients of this age more commonly have sprains than fractures
    B. The Ottawa Ankle Rules have been validated for patients of this age
    C. Salter I fractures are usually evident on plain radiographs at this time
    D. Sever's disease is the most likely diagnosis
    E. Childhood obesity is not associated with a greater risk of ankle injury

66. You are seeing a 13-year-old in follow-up one week after being kicked by a horse. He was transferred to an emergency department from the scene and was diagnosed with simple fractures of the sixth and seventh ribs and a right pulmonary contusion. He briefly received supplemental oxygen but did not require mechanical ventilation and was discharged from the hospital after two days. After seeing the patient, you are concerned that he is suffering from the most common complication of a pulmonary contusion. The clinical scenario most supportive of your suspicion would be which of the following?

    A. Severe respiratory distress and hemoptysis productive of copious amounts of bright red blood
    B. Orthopnea, pulsus paradoxus, muffled heart tones, and a friction rub auscultated over the precordium
    C. Hypoxia and diffuse, bilateral hazy ground-glass opacities on chest radiography
    D. Tympany on percussion of the affected side, tracheal shift to the contralateral side, and diminished breath sounds on the affected side
    E. Fever, tachypnea, cough productive of purulent sputum, and focal rhales

67. A 16-year-old male high school wrestler presents to the ER after being accidentally kicked in the groin during a competition. Patient was unable to finish the competition because of nausea, vomiting, and difficulty walking due to pain. Examination revealed a tender and swollen right testicle and scrotal hematoma measuring 2 cm in diameter. A scrotal ultrasound with doppler revealed normal parenchymal echo pattern and intact testicular blood flow. His parents are very concerned about the patient's future fertility since he is their only child. The most appropriate next step would be which of the following?

    A. Oral antibiotics
    B. Exploration of hematocoele
    C. Rest, pain control and ice packs on groin for 24 to 48 hours
    D. Scrotal MRI
    E. Microsurgery to diagnose/repair possible injury to vas deferens since this cannot be seen in the diagnostic studies

68. In order to diagnose the presence of a posterior tibialis injury, which of the following signs or symptoms would be present?

    A. Poorly defined burning, tingling, or numbness sensation on the plantar surface, inferior to the medial malleolus and the plantar aspect radiating to the toes
    B. Pain on toe-off or forefoot weight bearing
    C. Pain with resisted dorsiflexion and eccentric inversion
    D. Pain with passive pronation and active supination

69. When there is suspicion of a basilar skull fracture, one is told to look for Battle's Sign. Which of the following best describes Battle's Sign?

    A. Ecchymosis around the eyes
    B. Ecchymosis over the zygomatic arch
    C. Ecchymosis at the base of the neck
    D. Ecchymosis of the mastoid process

70. Which of the following is correct regarding the tendon of the long head of the biceps muscle?

    A. The tendon traverses anteriorly across the glenohumeral joint and attaches to the coracoid process
    B. As the tendon traverses the intertubercular sulcus, it is held in place by the tendon of the pectoralis minor muscle
    C. Superiorly, the tendon is covered by the coracohumeral and superior glenohumeral ligaments
    D. The tendon remains extra-articular throughout its course

71. Which of the following statements is true regarding fungal infection in athletes?

    A. The most common cause of "jock itch" is candida
    B. Most cases of tinea pedis involve the toe web spaces
    C. An NCAA collegiate wrestler diagnosed with tinea corporis at a pre-meet skin-check, may be cleared for participation, as long as the lesions can be adequately covered
    D. Classical tinea corporis lesions present as weeping, red scaly patches surrounded by satellite lesions

72. Which of the following has been shown to have the greatest risk reduction of cardiovascular disease?

    A. Resistance training
    B. Mild cardiovascular exercise
    C. Moderate cardiovascular exercise
    D. Vigorous cardiovascular exercise

73. An inability to supinate the forearm could be due to an injury to which of the following pairs of nerves?

    A. Suprascapular/axillary
    B. Musculocutaneous/median
    C. Axillary/radial
    D. Radial/musculocutaneous
    E. Median/ulnar

74. An 18-year-old college athlete sustains a traumatic injury to his lower leg during a football game. The physical exam reveals gross angular deformity of the lower leg and no sensation to the first dorsal web space. In addition to a fracture, which of the following is the most likely diagnosis?

   A. Acute compartment syndrome of the anterior compartment
   B. Acute compartment syndrome of the deep posterior compartment
   C. Acute and chronic compartment syndrome of the anterior compartment
   D. Acute compartment syndrome of the lateral compartment
   E. Acute compartment syndrome of the lateral and superficial posterior compartment

75. A football player presents to your clinic with a long thoracic nerve injury on the right that has resulted in weakness of the muscle this nerve innervates. Which of the following do you expect to see on physical exam?

   A. Lateral winging of the right scapula
   B. Medial winging of the right scapula
   C. Weakness with internal rotation of the right humerus
   D. Weakness with right shoulder shrugs
   E. Weakness with abduction of the right shoulder

76. A 50-year-old female patient presents to your office with exertional pain in her right calf. She has noted the pain during exercise for the past several weeks. Which of the following historical and physical findings would you expect with a diagnosis of popliteal artery entrapment syndrome?

   A. Diminished foot pulses at rest
   B. Pain more closely associated with volume of exercise rather than intensity of exercise
   C. Slow resolution of symptoms at conclusion of exercise
   D. Normal pulses that disappear or decrease with plantar flexion or dorsiflexion of the foot
   E. Markedly elevated compartment pressure

77. An 18-year-old female long distance runner has recently been diagnosed with her second tibial stress fracture and reports her last menstrual cycle occurred six months ago. You rule out other causes for amenorrhea and get a DEXA scan, which reports "low bone density below the expected range for age." Which of the following options is the first aim of treatment for this athlete?

    A. Begin an antidepressant to treat emotional issues and/or unhealthy thought processes that maintain her disorder
    B. Treat low bone density below the expected range for age with a bisphosphonate
    C. Restore regular menstrual cycles with hormone replacement therapy or oral contraceptive pill
    D. Optimize nutritional status by increasing energy intake and/or reduce energy expenditure

78. An afebrile patient with acute low back pain notices pain going down the posterior-lateral aspect of their right thigh and leg. It is noted on your exam that she has the following: positive straight leg raise, a slight sensory deficit located on the lateral aspect of the right foot, a diminished ankle jerk, and weakness with plantar flexion of the great toe. It is also noted that it is hard for her to walk on her toes. Which nerve root is mostly likely the cause of her symptoms?

    A. L3
    B. L4
    C. L5
    D. S1
    E. L2

79. Which of the following is true regarding eye protection in sports?

    A. Soft contacts or daily wear glasses can provide some eye protection
    B. Lensless eyeguards provide adequate protection
    C. Highly farsighted athletes may be more prone to retinal detachment injuries
    D. Radial keratotomy (RK) surgery can strengthen a cornea after healing
    E. Well-fitted, certified polycarbonate lenses provide adequate protection in sports

80. A 12-year-old male pitcher collapses shortly after being struck in the chest by a baseball. Which of the following is true regarding commotio cordis (CC)?

    A. The use of chest protectors is proven to decrease the likelihood of CC
    B. Impact occurs during the QRS complex in the cardiac cycle
    C. Initial arrhythmia is atrial fibrillation
    D. Defibrillation is highly successful in reverting CC events
    E. Age appropriate safety balls have been proven to reduce CC events

81. A 20-year-old male college basketball player presents for a preparticipation exam. He reveals that he is HIV+. He is asymptomatic, on appropriate medications, and has normal laboratory findings. If his health status remains stable, your recommendations should include which of the following?

    A. He discontinues playing basketball, and his previous teamates are tested for HIV
    B. He continues playing basketball, and his previous teamates are tested for HIV
    C. He discontinues playing basketball and his previous teamates should not be tested for HIV
    D. He continues playing basketball, and his previous teamates are not tested for HIV

82. The four bones that make up the proximal carpal row of the wrist are which of the following?

    A. Capitate, hamate, trapezium, trapezoid
    B. Scaphoid, lunate, trapezoid, pisiform
    C. Lunate, triquetrum, scaphoid, pisiform
    D. Scaphoid, lunate, triquetrum, hamate

83. Which of the following is a contraindication to hyaluronic acid viscosupplementation?

    A. Hip osteoarthritis
    B. Pregnancy
    C. Knee osteoarthritis
    D. Rheumatoid arthritis
    E. Glenohumeral osteoarthritis

84. Which of the following statements is true based on the image provided?

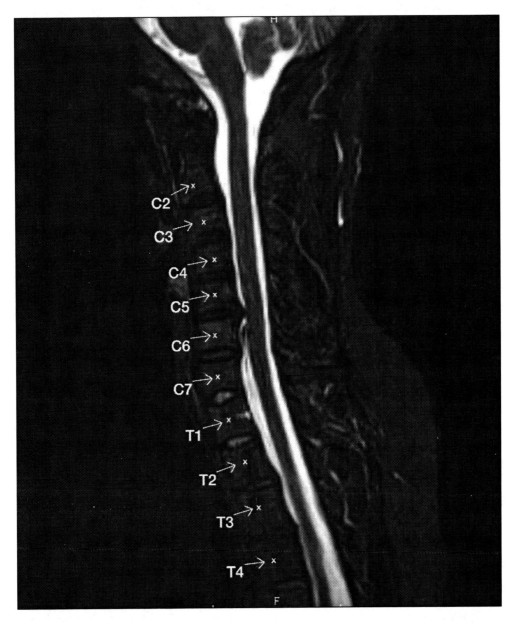

A. The patient is likely to present with complaints of numbness and tingling of the fourth and fifth digit
B. Testing the wrist flexors and finger extensors is likely to present with weakness
C. Reflex testing of the triceps will indicate an increased response
D. The patient may complain of pain and tingling to deltoid and shoulder
E. Atrophy of the thenar eminence may be a presenting symptom

85. A 12-year-old black male with sickle cell disease presents to your office for a preparticipation physical exam. He has had no recent hospitalizations, blood transfusions, or sickle cell crisis. He can be cleared for participation in which of the following sports?

    A. Football
    B. Baseball
    C. Soccer
    D. Basketball

86. Which of the following is true regarding the use of cryotherapy and heat in the treatment of athletic injuries?

    A. Cryotherapy and heat both decrease tissue metabolism
    B. Cryotherapy produces vasodilation and heat produces vasoconstriction
    C. Cryotherapy and heat can both decrease muscle spasm
    D. Cryotherapy and heat both increase soft tissue swelling
    E. Cryotherapy increases nerve conduction, and heat decreases nerve conduction

87. A right-hand-dominant 16-year-old female volleyball player has an x-ray in the emergency room showing an acute fracture of the middle third of her right clavicle. The distal fragment is displaced superiorly 0.8 cm with shortening of about 20 mm. Pulses and neuro exam are within normal limits. Management should include which of the following?

    A. Routine surgical fixation
    B. Immobilization in sling for four to six weeks
    C. Immobilization in figure-of-eight brace for four to six weeks
    D. Emergent surgical consultation

88. You are dealing with an athlete who just sustained a penetrating chest trauma from falling on a sharp object. The object was removed by a teammate and now you are concerned the victim has an open tension pneumothorax. Which of the following is the definitive method of treating this condition?

    A. Dressing affixed on three sides to create a flap valve
    B. Fully occlusive dressing
    C. Occlusive dressing with intercostal chest drain
    D. Intercostal chest drain with dressing affixed on three sides

89. A soccer player presents with injury to the mandible from an elbow. You identify post-traumatic malocclusion, focal swelling, and tenderness over the mandible. On examination, you find defects of the dental occlusal surface, alveolar ridge disruptions, and anesthesia in the distribution of the anterior aspect of the chin and lower lip. You suspect a mandible fracture and injury to which of the following nerves?

    A. Anterior cutaneous nerve
    B. Mental nerve
    C. Infraorbital nerve
    D. Facial nerve
    E. Supratrochlear nerve

90. A 54-year-old male presents to your office, complaining of bilateral knee pain. He was diagnosed with osteoarthritis in both his knees after he was referred by his primary care provider to see an orthopedic surgeon. He was given a prescription for an anti-inflammatory medication and told that he may need knee replacement surgery some day. He does not like taking medications and has come to see you regarding non-pharmacologic treatment options. Which of the following statements regarding exercise and osteoarthritis is true?

    A. Aerobic exercise should be encouraged because it may decrease the patient's pain
    B. This patient's x-ray findings are moderate to severe, therefore, exercise is unlikely to be helpful
    C. Strengthening exercises may be harmful and alter the disease progression
    D. Aquatic exercise has not been shown to be beneficial for patients with osteoarthritis

91. A 19-year-old female basketball player tries to deflect a pass and sustains a proximal, interphalangeal (PIP) dorsal dislocation of her middle finger that you reduce on the sideline. Later, radiographs are negative for fracture and show good alignment. Which of the following is true for this injury?

    A. Delayed complications include Boutonniere deformity
    B. The injury can result in extension lag at the DIP joint
    C. Immediate orthopedic consult to prevent proximal migration of flexor profundus
    D. Delayed complications include swan neck deformity deformity

92. A 24-year-old female runner is being seen by you in your sports medicine clinic for two weeks of gradually worsening radial sided right wrist pain. She is six weeks post-partum after a normal spontaneous vaginal delivery of a relatively uncomplicated pregnancy. There has been no known trauma otherwise. Her pain is worse when she lifts her newborn, and she reports some wrist stiffness. Your examination reveals tenderness to palpation over the radial styloid and in the approximated soft tissues. There is a positive Finkelstein's test. The most likely involved structure(s) is (are) which of the following?

A. The tenosynovial compartment associated with the abductor pollicis longus and extensor pollicis brevis
B. The tenosynovial compartment associated with the extensor carpi radialis longus and extensor carpi radialis brevis
C. The tenosynovial compartment associated with the extensor pollicis longus
D. The tenosynovial compartment associated with the flexor carpi radialis
E. The first carpal-metacarpal joint and its joint capsule

93. A 70-year-old unconditioned male comes into your office wanting to start working out again. He has a resting heart rate of 70 beats per minute, no medical problems, and takes a multivitamin every morning. His time is limited, so he wants to optimize his training. He has a heart monitor (exercise cardiotachometer), which consists of a wrist monitor that communicates with a strap that is placed around his chest. He wants to know what his heart rate range should be for cardiovascular fitness. You tell him that based on the ACSM guidelines, his range for target heart rate should be which of the following?

A. 60 to 70 beats per minute (bpm)
B. 75 to 90 bpm
C. 95 to 110 bpm
D. 115 to 130 bpm

94. A 16-year-old basketball player presents with eye pain after his teammate pokes him in the eye. You suspect he has a corneal abrasion and begin your discussion of antibiotic and non-steroidal drops while you examine him. The finding on exam that would cause you to send him to the emergency room for evaluation of possible globe injury is which of the following?

A. Abrasion of more than 50% of cornea surface
B. Abrasion related to a fractured contact lens
C. Multiple vertical abrasions
D. Abrasion with a positive Seidel's sign

95. Which of the following components of concussion assessment is the least sensitive in detecting a concussion?

    A. Anterograde amnesia
    B. Postural instability
    C. Retrograde amnesia
    D. Loss of consciousness
    E. Orientation

96. The two types of bursitis that are associated with an infectious component and for which aspiration for culture and antibiotics should be considered as part of the management are the olecranon and which of the following?

    A. Trochanteric bursitis
    B. Prepatellar bursitis
    C. Subacromial bursitis
    D. Iliopsoas bursitis

97. The most common activity associated with exercise-induced urticaria has been which of the following?

    A. Running
    B. Swimming
    C. Bicycling
    D. Weight lifting

98. A nine-year-old overweight boy limps into your office with complaints of left knee pain for over three weeks. He does not participate in sports but plays computer strategy games for several hours a day. He denies any trauma to his knee, and his knee exam is normal. He has no fever or chills or night pain. Which of the following diagnostic tests do you order?

    A. Aspiration of knee joint for fluid analysis
    B. Erythrocyte sedimentation rate and CBC
    C. No further workup; tell his family that his knee is normal
    D. X-rays of his hips: AP and frog leg

99. A college female lacrosse player comes to see you as she has been feeling tired more than usual the days after her games. Her history, physical, and lab work are otherwise unremarkable. She does tell you that she has been on a low carbohydrate diet to help lose weight. You tell her which of the following?

A. Limiting her carbohydrates will help her fatigue and improve her physical and mental performance

B. Her carbohydrate consumption should be 6 to 8 g/kg of body weight daily

C. She should not eat after her games as this may upset her stomach and delay her recovery time

D. Carbohydrates provide 9 calories per gram

100. Which of the following sports reports the highest incidence of incontinence during participation?

A. Softball

B. Gymnastics

C. Golf

D. Swimming

101. A 15-year-old high school basketball player is seeing you in the training room to look at her ankle. She suffered an inversion ankle injury two weeks ago that was confirmed on the game tape when reviewed by the athletic trainer. This is her fourth episode with this ankle in three years. The next-most recent sprain was three months ago. She says she was "nearly 100%" recovered from that episode when this one occurred. She also states that she is not progressing as well as she normally does when she "tweaks" this ankle. In particular, she states that there is no pain, but the ankle feels like it is giving out especially when jumping or cutting. Her anterior drawer and ankle inversion tests are definitely normal. The ankle hasn't been helped by the new active ankle brace the athletic trainer obtained to replace her old one that she has used since her last sprain. Current treatment has consisted of ice, rest, and gentle range of motion. Which of the following statements is true regarding her injury?

A. Ankle instability should only be assessed with plain radiographs

B. Aggressive early functional rehabilitation should be tried first

C. The etiology of her recurrent injuries has to do with her age

D. The primary ligament involved is the deltoid ligament

E. Ankle instability cannot occur without increased mechanical laxity

102. During pregnancy, which of the following components of the woman's respiratory system decreases during pregnancy?

    A. Tidal volume
    B. Vital capacity
    C. Minute ventilation
    D. Reserve volume

103. A 45-year-old premenopausal African-American female comes into your office requesting a physical for initiation of an exercise program. She denies exertional symptoms of cough, headache, chest pain, reflux, dyspnea, near-syncope, or syncope. She is a non-smoker. Her BP is 124/84. Her BMI is 29.8. Physical exam is notable for lack of cardiovascular abnormalities or evidence of neurological injury. In regards to her exercise prescription, which of the following is the most appropriate initial step?

    A. Obtain an exercise stress test
    B. Obtain an electrocardiogram to rule out left ventricular hypertrophy or conduction abnormality
    C. Check for other major cardiovascular risk factors
    D. Rule out valvular disease with an echocardiogram
    E. Write a prescription using the FITT (frequency, intensity, time, and type) method

104. Which of the following statements is true regarding the use of protective equipment?

    A. Requiring the use of protective equipment rarely changes the epidemiology of injury for a given sport
    B. Protective equipment may cause an increase in absolute numbers (e.g., injuries per 1,000 participants) of some injuries after adoption by a given sport
    C. Laws requiring use of protective equipment (e.g., bicycle helmet laws) have proven to be cost-effective, increasing protective equipment usage and decreasing sports-related injuries
    D. Athletes and coaches are usually eager to adopt the usage of protective equipment
    E. Health care providers should always campaign for the use of protective equipment

105. A 16-year-old springboard diver complains of three weeks of lower back pain. The pain has progressed from activity-related pain now to pain at rest. X-rays of the lumbar spine are negative. You advise which of the following?

    A. Rest from diving and obtain CT scan
    B. Rest from diving and obtain MRI
    C. Continue diving
    D. Rest from diving

106. Which of the following statements about open and closed kinetic chain exercises is correct?

    A. Open kinetic chain exercises occur when the distal aspect of the extremity is fixed and cannot move
    B. Closed kinetic chain exercises typically involve functional weight-bearing and sport-specific activities
    C. Knee extensions and straight leg raises are examples of closed kinetic chain exercises
    D. During open kinetic chain exercises, motion occurs simultaneously at all joints comprising the kinetic chain
    E. Closed kinetic chain exercises produce shearing forces, while open kinetic chain exercises produce compressive forces

107. PIN syndrome involves a dysfunction of the posterior interosseus nerve branch of the radial nerve. A patient with PIN syndrome will report which of the following symptoms in the affected extremity?

    A. Altered sensation in the little and ring finger
    B. Decreased ability to make a fist
    C. Altered sensation of the dorsum of the wrist
    D. Decreased ability to extend the wrist

108. Which of the following biomechanical loading techniques, when done repetitively, is most effective in the treatment and management of patellar tendinopathy?

    A. Concentric
    B. Eccentric
    C. Isometric
    D. Isotonic

109. You are performing a preparticipation exam on one of your patients who happens to be a student at the high school you cover. Which of the following items would require further evaluation?

    A. Mononucleosis three years ago
    B. Mildly enlarged liver
    C. Non-palpable spleen
    D. Small tattoo
    E. History of appendectomy

110. When performing a preparticipation exam on a 14-year-old high school athlete trying out for football, a single testicle is detected. You must advise him and his mother about the implications of a single testicle and sports. Which of the following is correct?

    A. A protective cup eliminates the risk of loss of the testicle in contact collision sports
    B. Sperm banking is available and, while costly, is an option to preserve fertility if a single testicle is injured or lost later
    C. Athletes with an undescended testicle are managed the same as a player with a single testicle
    D. Due to the high risk in contact collision sports of losing a single testicle, the use of a cup is required

111. A 40-year-old drummer presents with left wrist pain that developed one day after a four-hour concert. He has maximal tenderness 7 cm proximal to radial styloid with Finkelstein's test exacerbating pain at that location. There is also subtle swelling over the point of maximal tenderness. The most likely diagnosis is which of the following?

    A. De Quervain's tenosynovitis
    B. Carpal tunnel syndrome
    C. CMC arthritis
    D. Intersection syndrome
    E. Posterior interosseous nerve (PIN) entrapment

112. Which of the following statements is true about herpes gladiatorum and herpes rubeiorum?

    A. Lesions are caused by herpes simplex virus type 2
    B. Return to play guidelines are lesions dry, crusted, covered, and antiviral treatment for 48 hours before competition
    C. No prodromal symptoms precede the painless clusters of small vesicles on an erythematous base
    D. Prophylaxis therapy in athletes with outbreaks in the past year is valacyclovir 500 mg twice daily

113. You are seeing a 21-year-old football player in the athletic training room on Monday evening. He is complaining of a severe occipital headache with neck pain. He reports that he had a mild hyperextension injury in the game this past Saturday while making a tackle. His neck hurt for a brief instant and then it subsided, and he completed the game, as it was the fourth quarter. He denied loss of consciousness or other neurologic symptoms and reported nothing to the athletic trainer. His neck stiffness and headache started Sunday morning and have persisted. He has no migraine history. He takes no supplements, and his only medication has been Aleve® for his headache. He denies fever, rash, cough, nausea, and photophobia. On examination, his range of motion is limited by pain with lateral flexion and rotation to the right, limiting his motion by 50%. He has a negative Spurling's test bilaterally. His neurological exam is grossly normal, but on further review he has a Horner's sign on the right. He is sent to the emergency room and cervical spine radiographs are normal. The most appropriate next step would be which of the following?

    A. Lumbar puncture
    B. Head CT
    C. Neck CT
    D. MRI of the brain
    E. MRA of the neck

114. A 21-year-old male golfer comes to you for his preparticipation physical exam. He denies having any previous cardiac symptoms or difficulty working out with his teammates. The only finding on exam is a systolic ejection murmur that increases with standing and lessens with laying down. Which of the following is not considered a major risk factor for sudden cardiac death in this athlete?

    A. Sudden death in his younger brother
    B. Nonsustained ventricular tachycardia during ambulatory ECG monitoring
    C. Maximal wall thickness > 30 mm
    D. Genotype assessment in genetic testing
    E. Drop in systolic blood pressure > 15 mm HG from peak recorded to end of exercise on treadmill stress test

115. Which of the following may reduce lower limb soft tissue injuries in runners?

    A. Stretching
    B. Long, gradual increase in training program for novice runners
    C. Patellofemoral (PFPS) type braces for anterior knee pain
    D. Running shoes fitted for foot type
    E. Not using insoles as opposed to using custom biomechanical insoles

116. A college football player jumps up to catch a high pass and is hit hard and tackled from behind. He plays several more downs before leaving the field, complaining of right flank and back pain. Which of the following is true regarding his probable injury?

    A. His injury has clearly identifiable signs and symptoms
    B. Renovascular hypertension is a frequent complication of this injury
    C. The degree of hematuria is indicative of the severity and extent of injury
    D. CT scan with contrast is the procedure of choice in identifying the full extent of urologic injury
    E. Athletes with solitary kidney are at high risk for kidney loss in contact sports

117. Pronation of the subtalar joint is an important part of the biomechanics of the walking and running gait. Which of the following accurately describes the component motions of pronation?

    A. Forefoot abduction, hindfoot inversion, and plantarflexion
    B. Forefoot adduction, hindfoot eversion, and plantarflexion
    C. Forefoot abduction, hindfoot eversion, and dorsiflexion
    D. Forefoot adduction, hindfoot inversion, and dorsiflexion
    E. Forefoot abduction, hindfoot inversion, and plantarflexion

118. A 35-year-old male aerobics instructor is seen in your clinic because he has had several months of lower abdominal and groin pain. He reports that over the past two months the pain has increased, exacerbated by coughing or laughing. He reports no acute injury and no prior muscle strains. He stopped all physical activity for the past four weeks. An inguinal hernia is not appreciated on physical exam. Plain films, MRI, and bone scan do not show any bony anomalies. Which of the following would be considered the best initial treatment plan for this athlete?

    A. Corticosteroid injection to the conjoined tendon sheath
    B. Reassurance and rest
    C. Non-weight-bearing and crutches for six weeks given patient may have occult stress fracture
    D. Conservative treatment with a comprehensive rehabilitation program to improve core strengthening and posterior abdominal wall weakness

119. A female cyclist presents to you for $\dot{V}O_2$max testing. She has heard that a high $\dot{V}O_2$max is predictive of aerobic fitness. You know that $\dot{V}O_2$max is determined by measuring pulmonary ventilation and the difference in directly measured fraction of oxygen in expired and inspired air: $\dot{V}O_2 = V_e (FiO_2 - FeO_2)$. The pulmonary ventilation is increased primarily during exercise by increases in the respiratory rate and increase in which of the following?

    A. Total lung capacity
    B. Residual volume
    C. Functional residual capacity
    D. Vital capacity
    E. Tidal volume

120. A female cross country runner presents early in the season, complaining of heel pain. She states the pain has been present for two weeks. Initially, the pain only occurred with long runs, but now it hurts most of the time. On exam, pain is elicited by squeezing the heel. X-rays are initially unremarkable. Repeat x-rays obtained two weeks later, however, confirm the diagnosis. Which of the following statements about this condition is true?

    A. Surgical intervention is required
    B. Patient should be counseled that healing is expected to take 10 to 12 weeks and may end her season
    C. Patient is at increased risk of plantar fascia rupture
    D. Patient can expect to return to activity in four to six weeks
    E. Patient's body habitus is not a factor in this diagnosis

121. A 45-year-old construction worker presents to see you regarding right-sided neck pain. The pain began five days ago, and has not improved. He does describe regular physical labor at work most recently working in a small space, which has caused him to maintain some awkward positions. He has been unable to work since the injury. He has tried some Tylenol with little relief. He has rare radiating pain into the top of his shoulder on the right but otherwise no numbness or weakness. He had a minor MVA with neck pain five years ago, but that resolved in one week without any long-term issues. Exam reveals limited range of motion to flexion and lateral bending to the left, a negative neurologic exam and a Spurling's test which reproduces pain in right paraspinal area without radiation. He has some palpable muscle spasm along the right cervical paraspinal musculature. Which of the following is the best diagnostic/treatment option?

    A. Request plain x-rays including oblique views
    B. Place him in a cervical collar, and give him a note off of work for 14 days
    C. Prescribe ibuprofen 600 mg TID, which has been shown to be effective for acute neck pain
    D. Discuss the benefits of early mobilization, and refer to physical therapy

122. The primary prophylactic medical treatment for prevention of acute mountain sickness is which of the following?

    A. Dexamethasone
    B. Calcium carbasalate
    C. Acetazolamide
    D. Scopolamine patch
    E. Nifedipine

123. At the finish line of the local marathon, a runner stops by your medical station, having completed the race and then stands to get his picture taken. He states he is lightheaded, and doesn't feel like he can walk to his car. You subsequently determine he has exercise-associated collapse (EAC), and in your management you remember that EAC is due to which of the following?

    A. Depletion of muscle glycogen, commonly known as "hitting the wall"
    B. Pooling of venous return in the lower extremities contributing to postural hypotension
    C. Altered cerebral circulatory autoregulation
    D. Common premature atrial contractions that reduce systemic filling pressure
    E. Reduced glomerular filtration rate (GFR)

124. Shoulder abductors can be paralyzed due to a lesion, affecting which of the following pairs of nerves?

    A. Axillary/musculocutaneous
    B. Thoracodorsal/upper subscapular
    C. Suprascapular/axillary
    D. Radial/lower subscapular
    E. Suprascapular/dorsal scapular

125. A 40-year-old female presents to your first-aid station during a 20-mile fundraising walk, complaining of confusion, lethargy, and dizziness. She says that she has been drinking water regularly and eating energy bars along the walk and has used the portable toilets at each scheduled rest stop. Which of the following is the most likely cause of her symptoms?

    A. Dehydration
    B. Hypoglycemia
    C. Hypokalemia
    D. Hyponatremia

126. Which of the following findings should always be considered pathologic on a screening ECG of an asymptomatic athlete?

    A. First-degree A-V block
    B. Sinus bradycarida
    C. QTc of > 460 ms in a male
    D. Left ventricular hypertrophy
    E. Sinus arrhythmia

127. You are at a high school football game, evaluating your starting running back. Earlier in the game, he was tackled from behind and ended up lying over the football at the bottom of a pile of tacklers. He is now complaining of abdominal pain and left shoulder pain. You are concerned about which of the following?

    A. Myocardial infarction
    B. Liver laceration
    C. Sickle cell crisis
    D. Shoulder dislocation
    E. Splenic injury

128. Which of the following statements is correct when referring to athletes with spinal cord injury?

    A. There is decreased incidence of overuse injuries above the spinal cord lesion
    B. Spinal-cord-injured patients have a normal ability to maintain body temperature in cold environments but not in hot environments
    C. There is a potential for reduced perception of exertion due to nociceptive input below the spinal cord lesion
    D. There is increased sweating below the spinal cord lesion
    E. There is normal bone mineral density in lower extremity

129. A 16-year-old African-American basketball player with hypertrophic cardiomyopathy and an implantable cardiac defibrillator (ICD) is cleared by cardiology to play. While providing medical coverage for a game where you have an automated external defibrillator (AED), this athlete collapses while running. You begin an assessment and find he is not breathing and has no pulse. You should do which of the following?

    A. Wait to see if the ICD will fire
    B. Place an AED on the chest to get a rhythm analysis, and shock if advised
    C. Begin CPR and await EMS. An AED is contraindicated in a collapsed athlete with an ICD
    D. Avoid doing CPR because the ICD may shock you

130. You are performing a preparticipation physical on a 15-year-old high school freshman, accompanied by his mother, who is trying out for the football team. During the history, you find the student had a brief syncopal event during conditioning drills one year ago. He says he got light-headed and passed out for a few seconds, but with some rest was able to continue the workout. You ask the mother about family history of syncope, and she tells you that there are several people in her extended family that pass out all the time, but it is "no big deal." You obtain an ECG on the student that shows a prolonged QTc interval. He wants to be able to participate in some form of athletic activity. Based on the findings of the ECG, which of the following sports (if any) would you clear him to play this year?

    A. Basketball
    B. Golf
    C. Wrestling
    D. Table tennis
    E. He is not clear to participate in any organized sports

131. Repetitive valgus extension overload to the medial epicondyle can lead to medial epicondylitis. Which of the following are involved in this injury?

    A. Origins of the pronator teres, palmaris longus, flexor carpi ulnaris
    B. Biceps brachii, flexor carpi ulnaris, pronator teres
    C. Origin of pronator teres, extensor carpi ulnaris
    D. Insertion of pronator teres and flexor carpi ulnaris

132. According to the *Preparticipation Physical Evaluation* (4th ed.), which of the following is a "yes, may participate" as opposed to a "qualified yes"?

    A. Kidney, absence of one
    B. Liver, enlarged
    C. Ovary, absence of one
    D. Spleen, enlarged
    E. Eye, loss of one

133. Ankle dislocations at the tibiotalar joint mortise without fracture occur with motor vehicle accidents, falls, and sports injuries. The most common position at the time of dislocation is which of the following?

    A. Maximal dorsiflexion with an external rotation force
    B. Maximal plantar flexion with an external rotation force
    C. Maximal plantar flexion with an axial load and forced inversion
    D. Maximal dorsiflexion with an axial load and forced inversion
    E. Neutral position with a direct medial to lateral blow to the tibia

134. A 15-year-old student-athlete presents prior to a high school track meet with symptoms of a viral upper respiratory illness accompanied by a temperature of 101 degrees Fahrenheit (38 degrees Celsius). Which of the following recommendations should you give to the athlete?

    A. If he has no respiratory compromise, he can participate in the meet
    B. Body effects of his elevated temperature are independent of the effect of environmental temperature
    C. Cardiac output and aerobic capacity are adversely affected in febrile athletes, and he should not participate
    D. There is no risk for orthostatic hypotension when exercising while febrile
    E. Fever has no effect on endurance or strength

135. Which of the following is not consistent with a diagnosis of complex regional pain syndrome?

    A. Focal increased activity on bone scan
    B. Diffuse increased activity with juxta-articular accentuation uptake on delayed images
    C. Pain out of proportion to physical findings
    D. Transient cyanosis and skin mottling in the affected limb

136. A 58-year-old female golfer presents with pain in the lumbar spine after a particular swing. She has point tenderness over L1 and limited range of motion. She does not have sensory or motor deficits on exam. A radiograph shows a compression fracture of L1 with approximately 50% loss of height. A CT scan should be ordered to rule out which of the following types of fracture?

    A. Compression fracture
    B. Middle column and burst fractures
    C. Spondylolysis
    D. Spondylolisthesis

137. A 54-year-old male former football player presents to your office complaining of low back pain. He has a prior history of acute low back pain due to "a herniated disc" four years ago, which was successfully treated with a short course of oral corticosteroids, physical therapy, and a home exercise program. Your patient had been doing well until about six months before seeing you, when he began to experience a vague, poorly localized low back pain, radiating to both his thighs. He reports that these symptoms are constant although he has "good days and bad days." His symptoms do seem to be worse after prolonged sitting. Which of the following clinical features is most consistent with a correct diagnosis of lumbar spinal stenosis?

    A. A positive Hoover's test
    B. Low back pain worse with lumbar forward flexion than with lumbar extension
    C. Low back pain alleviated when leaning over an object while standing
    D. Leg and calf pain that recurs predictably after walking four city blocks
    E. Low back pain worse with walking uphill than with walking downhill

138. An 18-year-old first semester college soccer player with type 1 diabetes mellitus uses an insulin pump to control her glucose. Since she plays a contact sport, she removes her pump prior to exercise. She notices that she is very high (300 finger stick glucose) after practice but acceptable (110) prior to practice. She monitors her glucose every 30 minutes in practice. In order to help her with this problem of elevated post-exercise glucose, you recommend which of the following?

    A. She should increase her pre-exercise insulin rate by 50% for an hour prior to exercise
    B. She should stop playing soccer and participate in a sport in which she can wear her pump at all times
    C. She should increase her food intake prior to exercise
    D. She should look for the onset of glucose increase and give herself 50% of basal rate bolus
    E. She should avoid all sugar prior to and during exercise

139. You are admitting a 28-year-old male after being hit by a car while cycling. Among his other bumps and bruises, he has an unstable hip fracture. While the orthopedic surgeon is preparing for an open reduction internal fixation of the patient's hip, you want to start the patient on prophylaxis against deep venous thromboembolism and pulmonary embolism. Which of the following is the best regimen to begin along with intermittent pneumatic compression devices?

    A. Unfractionated heparin daily
    B. Low molecular weight heparin daily
    C. 325 mg aspirin daily
    D. Warfarin daily
    E. No anti-coagulation is necessary

140. If an athletic event is suspended or postponed due to lightning activity, it is important to establish criteria for resumption of activities. Which of the following is a reasonable guideline for when it is generally safe to resume activity?

    A. If the sky is blue and there is no rain, it is fine to resume activities no matter how long it has been from the last lightning or thunder
    B. Activity may be resumed when flash activity in the area is slowing down
    C. Wait at least 30 minutes after the last lightning flash or sound of thunder
    D. Wait until the storm is at least five miles from your location
    E. Indoor pool activities may continue despite thunder and lightning activity outside the building

141. Which phase of the throwing motion is characterized by hyper-external rotation of the shoulder, eccentric stresses on internal rotators and shoulder adductors, and leads to the subscapularis activating to begin internal rotation of the shoulder?

    A. Windup
    B. Early cocking
    C. Late cocking
    D. Acceleration
    E. Follow-through

142. A 16-year-old recreational snowboarder presents with a history of a fall on an outstretched hand, which occurred one day prior to presentation. He was seen in the emergency room and radiographs demonstrate a 1.5 mm displaced fracture at the proximal anatomic section of the scaphoid. On examination, he has mild swelling and scaphoid tenderness on the affected side. Which of the following is the most appropriate next step in management?

    A. Strict immobilization in a well-molded short arm thumb spica cast
    B. Strict immobilization in a well-molded long arm thumb spica cast
    C. Application of a short arm thumb spica splint and re-image in two weeks
    D. Referral for screw fixation by an orthopedic hand specialist
    E. Referral for MRI evaluation of the affected wrist

143. A female softball pitcher is hit in the left chest with a line drive. She is initially gasping for air due to the sudden impact but regains her breath and does not lose consciousness. On exam, she is noted to have tenderness, ecchymosis, and unilateral enlargement of the left breast. Which of the following studies is (are) always indicated in this situation?

    A. None needed if she has no further shortness of breath
    B. Mammogram
    C. Chest x-ray
    D. ECG
    E. Chest x-ray and ECG

144. Which of the following drugs would be an appropriate choice as initial first line medication for long-term asthma control in a patient with persistent asthma?

    A. Inhaled albuterol
    B. Inhaled salmeterol
    C. Oral theophylline
    D. Inhaled fluticasone
    E. Oral montelukast

145. Patients with fibromyalgia may benefit from exercise programs. Which of the following types of programs would help improve physical capacity the most?

    A. Aerobic exercise
    B. Strength training exercises
    C. Muscle lengthening exercises
    D. Flexibility training exercises
    E. Resistance training

146. A high-mileage competitive runner presents with complaints of posterior lateral knee pain. His pain has gradually progressed from an occasional irritant to a persistent pain while running. He denies pain at rest and reports no history of trauma. His recent training history includes an increase in mileage and a significant increase in the amount of running on hilly terrain. You have previously diagnosed the patient as an overpronator. Examination demonstrates tenderness to palpation of the area just anterior and posterior to the lateral collateral ligament with the patient sitting in a cross-legged (figure-of-four) position. Which of the following is the most likely diagnosis?

    A. Medial meniscus tear
    B. Medial collateral ligament injury
    C. Popliteal cyst
    D. Posterior tibialis tendonopathy
    E. Popliteus tendonopathy

147. A 22-year-old male senior soccer player presents to your office with a two-year history of right hip pain. The pain is not present during activities of daily living but is becoming increasingly more painful and limiting with running, kicking, jumping, and cutting movements. He points to the area of pain as the right groin. There is occasional painful clicking but no low back pain or paresthesias. Exam shows pain deep to the anterior groin that is non-palpable but present with internal log roll and with flexion, adduction, and internal rotation motions. Hip flexion strength is good, and no pain is reported with manual testing. There is no pain with flexibility testing, and flexibility is good during the Thomas test. There is no palpable pain over the trochanter. Standard AP pelvis/cross-table lateral radiographs show a normal head-neck junction of the femur, no degenerative joint disease, but a large crossover sign (figure-of-eight sign). The most likely diagnosis for this patient is which of the following?

    A. Hip flexor strain
    B. Cam impingement
    C. Pincer impingement
    D. Trochanteric bursitis

148. A mother of a post-puberty female athlete wants to discuss Vitamin D with you. She is interested in the benefits and dangers of Vitamin D. You explain that Vitamin D does which of the following?

    A. With calcium supplementation, it has been shown to reduce stress fractures
    B. It can be toxic and should not be taken in doses higher than 1,000 IU per day
    C. It is rarely (< 5%) deficient in adolescent females in the United States of America
    D. Deficiency in Vitamin D has not been linked to increases in the risk of autoimmune diseases and nonskeletal chronic diseases like diabetes
    E. It is commonly found in foods that are eaten in United States of America and can replace lack of sun exposure

149. You are the team physician for the Paralympic wheelchair basketball team. One of the new players comes to you asking about "boosting" that he heard another team talking about. Which of the following describes a form of "boosting"?

    A. Wearing tight leg straps to increase sympathetic tone
    B. Taking 10 grams of carbohydrates every 30 minutes during exercise
    C. Emptying his bladder and bowels before each workout
    D. Using caffeine in excess to boost the metabolism

150. Which of the following symptoms or findings is most suggestive of ankylosing spondylitis in a patient with two-year history of back pain?

    A. Prominent morning back stiffness
    B. Presence of HLA-B27
    C. Recurrent sciatic pain
    D. Symmetric peripheral arthropathy
    E. Presence of rheumatoid factor

151. Which of the following is an example of a modifiable internal risk factor for musculoskeletal injury?

    A. A snow-covered natural grass field
    B. An athlete's gender
    C. An athlete's prior history of musculoskeletal injury
    D. An athlete's joint range of motion

152. A 35-year-old high-level female marathoner presents to your office with complaint of four to six weeks of left heel pain. She reports that her pain started gradually while increasing her mileage in preparation to run the Boston Marathon. She notes that she recently started using new running shoes about six to eight weeks ago. Training includes both indoor and outdoor surfaces. She also notes in her history that she is a paralegal who wear high heels to work at least four days a week. She locates most of her pain to the posterior ankle and denies any subsequent numbness or tingling. She has increased pain with walking uphill or upstairs. On physical examination, there is soft tissue swelling of the distal portion and attachment of the Achilles tendon. There is severe tenderness to palpation of this swelling as well as pain with both plantar and dorsiflexion. The patient has significant pain with toe-raising. X-rays of the left ankle show a retrocalcaneal exostosis. Which of the following is the most appropriate diagnosis?

    A. Posterior impingement-type syndrome
    B. Sever's disease
    C. Tarsal tunnel syndrome
    D. Haglund's syndrome

153. A college fullback is struck on the anteromedial knee. He has difficulty walking but is able to bear weight. He is unable to continue playing in the game, and you are asked to evaluate his knee in the training room after the game. The player reports that his knee is sore laterally, that he has mild swelling, and that he feels that his foot his weak. The most likely diagnosis is which of the following?

    A. Lateral collateral ligament injury
    B. Isolated popliteus strain
    C. Lateral meniscus injury
    D. Posterolateral corner injury
    E. Anterior cruciate ligament tear

154. A 50-year-old left-hand-dominant female patient with a history of diabetes had an insidious onset of left shoulder pain that has been progressively worsening over three months. She can no longer comb her hair and wash her back with the left arm. She has no neck pain, paresthesias, or radiating pain. Pain is deep in her shoulder and worsens with any motion. There are no mechanical symptoms. Active and passive range of motion is limited in both flexion and external rotation. Plain films radiographs were normal. Which of the following is the next step?

    A. An MRI is needed with intra-articular gadolinium to evaluate for a labral tear
    B. This condition often will resolve on its own in the next few months
    C. Anti-inflammatory medications shorten the overall length of the symptoms by altering the pathophysiologic process
    D. This condition is much more common among diabetics
    E. Scapular strengthening should be the focus of rehabilitation for this problem

155. Which of the following statements is true for epidemiology of collegiate women's soccer injuries?

    A. Rate of injury is higher in practices compared to games
    B. Concussion is the most common injury in both games and practices
    C. The majority of game injuries involve non-contact mechanisms
    D. The majority of practice injuries involve non-contact mechanisms
    E. ACL injury is the most common injury in both games and practices

156. A seven-year-old female soccer player presents to your office with pain in her left knee. The pain began during a soccer practice, and she was unable to walk after onset. On examination, she is acutely tender on the inferior aspect of her patella. She is unable to perform a straight-leg raise. Which of the following is the most likely diagnosis in this patient?

A. Traction apophysitis of the tibial tubercle (Osgood-Schlatter's disease)
B. Traction apophysitis of the distal patellar pole (Sindig-Larsen-Johansson disease)
C. Patellofemoral dysfunction
D. Patellar sleeve fracture
E. "Growing pains"

157. A high school freshman with office-spirometry-confirmed exercise-induced asthma comes into the office, complaining of shortness of breath 10 minutes after she starts running in gym class. She feels as if she cannot get air into her lungs. She is using her albuterol inhaler 30 minutes prior to gym class. She uses the albuterol again when the shortness of breath starts, but has no response. Gym class is the only time that she gets short of breath. The shortness of breath started two weeks ago when she had an asthma attack in gym class after forgetting her albuterol inhaler that day. Which of the following is the appropriate treatment of the shortness of breath?

A. Repeat the office spirometry testing with an exercise challenge; continue the albuterol as needed for shortness of breath and 30 minutes prior to gym class; reassess in one week
B. Refer the patient to a pulmonologist for pulmonary function tests; add a long-acting bronchodilator and corticosteroid combination for better control of her asthma; continue the albuterol 30 minutes prior to gym class; reassess in one week
C. Continue albuterol 30 minutes prior to gym class; teach the patient relaxation and slowed breathing techniques for when the attack happens; reassure her that her asthma is controlled with the albuterol; reassess in one week
D. Repeat the office spirometry with an exercise challenge; add a long-acting broncholdilator, and continue albuterol 30 minutes prior to gym class and as needed for shortness of breath; reassess in one week

158. The sport with highest overall number of catastrophic cervical spine injuries is which of the following?

    A. Ice hockey
    B. Gymnastics
    C. Equestrian sports
    D. Football
    E. Snowboarding

159. Which of the following are correct about testicular torsion?

    A. Prehn's sign is a reliable way of distinguishing testicular torsion from epididymitis
    B. A painless swollen testicle is common as an early finding
    C. Cremasteric reflex is absent on affected side
    D. Radionuclide imaging is the imaging modality of choice

160. If the lateral tubercle of the posterior talus ossifies separately, which of the following bones is formed?

    A. Fabella
    B. Os vesalianum
    C. Os trigonum
    D. Os calcis

161. The current American College of Sports Medicine (ACSM) and Centers for Disease Control and Prevention (CDC) guidelines for adult physical activity are which of the following?

    A. 20 minutes of physical activity at 80% to 90% of maximal heart rate most days of the week
    B. 30 minutes of low-intensity physical activity three days per week
    C. 30 minutes or more of moderate-intensity, physical activity on most if not all days of the week
    D. 20 to 50 minutes of vigorous-intensity physical activity on all days of the week

162. You see a high school football player in the training room for an injury, which occurred yesterday morning. He says his dog bit him on the arm. On exam, there is a 4 cm long laceration. The wound is fairly deep but you see no injury to bone, muscle, or tendon. There is minimal erythema or swelling. He believes he had a tetanus shot within the last five years. The best initial management to prevent infection is which of the following?

    A. Suture the wound
    B. Use a cyanoacrylate tissue adhesive to close the wound
    C. Irrigate and debride
    D. Give a Td booster

163. A collegiate gymnast has a chronic history of biceps femoris muscle strain in his left leg, which has precluded him from participating in three consecutive meets. He is concerned because the league meet is four weeks away, and he wants to be healthy for that event. Which of the following statements is true regarding the most effective timing for stretching?

    A. It is most effective during the warm-up phase of the exercise regimen
    B. It is most effective during the workout phase of the exercise regimen
    C. It is most effective during the cool-down phase of the exercise regimen
    D. Stretching is most effective between workouts

164. With regard to the Good Samaritan laws and being a team physician, one should understand which of the following?

    A. Good Samaritan laws exist throughout all 50 states and will protect the physician covering any event
    B. Good Samaritan laws apply only if receiving nominal financial compensation
    C. No matter what the Good Samaritan laws are in your area, it is best to clearly define responsibility and level of coverage in written form
    D. Compensation for event coverage is based on absolute dollar amounts
    E. Documentation of medical care is not required if the physician is acting solely as a Good Samaritan

165. You are consulted on a female track athlete with a known seizure disorder. Her favorite events are in the middle distances, and she has never had a seizure training or in competition. She has not had a seizure in three years and has not changed medications. The school is concerned about whether she should be allowed to compete due to her medical condition. Refraining from which of the following sports is most appropriate for this patient?

    A. Track
    B. Cycling
    C. Singles ice skating
    D. Football
    E. Gymnastic uneven parallel bars

166. A 72-year-old physically active man presents to your clinic for a regular check-up. He enjoys golf, walking, light jogs, and tennis. He is generally healthy, he states "I want to stay that way," and he seeks your expertise about exercise in the older person. Your advice for him is which of the following?

    A. Strength trained older athletes maintain muscle fiber type distribution similar to their younger counterparts
    B. Maximum heart rate declines with age and aerobic training does not slow its decline
    C. VO_2max declines with age, and aerobic training does not slow its decline
    D. Masters athletes who already participate in high intensity training programs can maintain that intensity for at least a decade
    E. Weight training in older athletes does not result in muscle hypertrophy

167. A 22-year-old vegetarian female runner presents with increasing fatigue over the past three to four months. She denies changes in her exercise routine, but has noted that her times have increased over that period and that her recovery times have increased as well. On examination, you notice pale conjunctivae. Her laboratory studies reveal a microcytic, hypochromic anemia. Which of the following is the most likely underlying etiology for her anemia?

    A. Foot strike hemolysis
    B. Vitamin B12 deficiency
    C. Folate deficiency
    D. Iron deficiency anemia
    E. G6PD deficiency

168. An 18-year-old soccer player presents to the training room with left elbow and forearm pain, with swelling and obvious deformity. While running during practice, she was accidentally pushed by another player and sustained a FOOSH (fall on outstretched hand) injury. Her neurovascular exam is intact. Fluoroscopy in the training room reveals a fracture of the proximal third of the ulna with dislocation of the radial head. Which of the following is the correct diagnosis?

    A. Nightstick fracture
    B. Greenstick fracture
    C. Monteggia's fracture
    D. Galeazzi's fracture
    E. Rolando's fracture

169. A 22-year-old male football player suffers a hyperpronation injury of the right forearm and this results in a first-time dorsal-ulnar dislocation of the distal radioulnar joint (DRUJ). Radiographs rule out fracture and adequate closed reduction is achieved. How should this injury be managed?

    A. Thumb spica splint for two weeks
    B. Short arm cast for four weeks
    C. Long arm cast for six weeks
    D. Orthopedic referral for arthrodesis
    E. Ulnar gutter splint

170. A 36-year-old female athletic trainer comes in with a two-day history of severe low back pain. This started after she lifted a water cooler from the ground and felt a "pop" before a football game the previous day. She reports that the pain goes down to her buttocks and posterior thigh with any type of movement. The exam today is limited because of pain, although she is positive for straight leg raise, both sitting and supine. Plain films are negative. An MRI shows lumbar disc herniation. She wants to get back to working as soon as possible because of the upcoming games. Which of the following is the most appropriate next step to get her back to activity?

    A. Epidural steroid/analgesic injection
    B. Soft lumbar bracing and analgesics as needed, go back to regular activity
    C. Bed rest as needed with early mobilization and NSAIDs/analgesics, reevaluate
    D. Microsurgical discectomy
    E. Traction therapy

171. Which of the following is a criterion for x-ray, according to the Ottawa Ankle Rules or Ottawa Foot Rules?

    A. Pain over the talus
    B. Positive anterior drawer sign
    C. Positive Talar tilt test
    D. Inability to bear weight for four steps either immediately or in the emergency room
    E. Pain over the shaft of the fifth metatarsal

172. A 16-year-old high school linebacker misses his tackle and receives a knee to the right side of his helmet. He loses consciousness for a few seconds but then is able to get up by himself and walk toward the sideline. He complains of a headache and blurry vision. After an initial medical evaluation onsite using standard emergency management principles, he sits on the bench for the rest of the first half. During halftime, he is reevaluated and states that he has no more symptoms and would like to return to play. Your sideline evaluation at that time does not show any significant neurological deficiencies. According to the recent consensus guidelines from the Zurich conference in 2008, what is the minimum time frame that has to pass before he can return to the game unrestricted?

    A. Seven days with return to game play on the eighth day if he remains asymptomatic
    B. Five days with return to game play on the sixth day if he remains asymptomatic
    C. Three days with return to game play on the fourth day if he remains asymptomatic
    D. The next day if he is still asymptomatic
    E. Second half if he is still asymptomatic

173. You are covering a college football game and are called to the field to evaluate a running back that has remained on the ground after a fumble recovery. A number of players had piled on him, and he is lying on his back, complaining of severe pain at the right sternoclavicular joint. You note exquisite tenderness at the joint and a non-palpable medial head of the clavicle. There is evidence of jugular venous congestion on that side, and he is noted to have stridorous respirations. You diagnose a posterior dislocation of the clavicle. The next-most appropriate step in management would be which of the following?

    A. Ice to the area and a sling for the right arm
    B. Figure-of-eight splint and relocation in the emergency room at the end of the game
    C. Transport by ambulance to the nearest emergency room with cervical spine immobilization
    D. Attempt emergent sideline reduction of the dislocation because of vascular and airway compromise

174. A 22-year-old track athlete presents to you for a follow-up visit after a grade 2 ankle sprain. Which of the following modules should be added to her rehabilitation in the intermediate stage, after she successfully had early rehabilitation measures?

    A. Range of motion exercises
    B. Isometric strength training
    C. Isotonic strength training
    D. Proprioceptive training

175. A 16-year-old male patient presents for his preparticipation evaluation. He has no significant medical problems and a normal physical examination. Which of the following are currently recommended as part of his screen?

    A. Complete blood count
    B. Electrocardiogram
    C. Screening echocardiogram
    D. Urinalysis
    E. No additional testing is generally required

176. A 35-year-old female long-distance runner who is training for a marathon by running 50 to 70 miles per week presents with a one-month history of right anterior hip and groin pain. The pain develops after two miles of running and is alleviated by stopping. Her exam demonstrates right anterior groin tenderness to palpation over the pubic ramus and pain with hopping on the affected leg. Which of the following statements is correct in regards to the diagnosis of a pubic ramus stress fracture?

   A. Men are more susceptible to pubic rami stress fractures than women
   B. A positive radionuclide bone scan definitively confirms the diagnosis of a pubic ramus stress fracture
   C. A small avulsion fracture off the inferior pubic ramus is pathognomonic of a pubic ramus stress fracture
   D. Pubic rami stress fractures are caused by the adductor and gracilus muscles pulling on the lateral aspect of the pubic ramus
   E. "Flamingo view" plain radiographs are useful in the diagnosis of a pubic ramus stress fracture

177. You are approached by parents of one of your patients, a 17-year-old male with Down syndrome. They are interested in exploring the possibility of his participation in Special Olympics sporting activities. Which of the following are important considerations regarding Special Olympics participation?

   A. There are no special considerations for his participation, and he can be cleared after a routine preparticipation evaluation
   B. Because of the increased incidence of atlantoaxial instability in Down syndrome patients, he should have cervical spine radiographs prior to participating in sports activities
   C. Epidemiologic studies have shown increased incidence of injury in Down syndrome patients who participate in winter sports
   D. Eye problems are an unusual finding among Special Olympics participants
   E. Although there is an increased incidence of seizures among Special Olympics participants, no special precautions are taken around water sports venues

178. With respect to the normal gait cycle, which of the following statements is true?

    A. There is one step in each gait cycle
    B. The faster the walking speed, the more time one will have in the swing phase
    C. The stance to swing ratio is stable when moving from walking to running
    D. The gait cycle has one double-support phase
    E. Cadence is the number of steps over distance

179. Injection for a carpal tunnel syndrome is best done in which manner?

    A. At a site just ulnar to the palmaris longus tendon and at the proximal wrist crease
    B. At a site just radial to the palmaris longus tendon and at the proximal wrist crease
    C. Volar side of the forearm 4 cm proximal to the wrist crease between the tendons of the flexor carpi radialis and flexor carpi ulnaris
    D. Volar side of the forearm 4 cm proximal to the wrist crease between the tendon of the flexor carpi ulnaris and the palmaris longus tendon

180. Children are a population at risk for heat-related injuries because of which of the following?

    A. Children sweat more and thus are at increased risk for dehydration
    B. Children have a lower surface area to body mass ratio and consequently they dissipate heat less efficiently
    C. Children produce higher temperature elevations because they tend to generate more heat secondarily to higher percentage of adipose tissue
    D. Children have higher surface area to body mass ratio, which may cause higher absorption from ambient environment

181. The recurrence rate after a primary, traumatic glenohumeral dislocation in an athlete less than 20 years old with non-surgical management is which of the following?

    A. 10%
    B. Less than 30%
    C. 50%
    D. Greater than 60%

182. A 32-year-old male recreational squash player is seen in your sports medicine clinic for a one-week history of right volar wrist pain with associated numbness and tingling along the volar aspect of the radial half of the hand. He spends a significant amount of time working at a computer, using a mouse without a wrist pad, and takes a "smoke break" about every three hours. He recalls an injury involving a fall onto his outstretched right hand the day prior to the onset of symptoms. Your examination reveals nonspecific tenderness in multiple areas of the right wrist, and a positive Tinel's sign over an area that approximates the median nerve. The best next step in the management of this case would be which of the following?

    A. Recommend night wrist splints, occupational therapy, and ergonomic precautions such as the use of gel wrist pads at work
    B. Perform a corticosteroid injection into the carpal tunnel
    C. Obtain electrodiagnostic studies of the upper extremity, including a complete electromyogram and nerve conduction studies
    D. Obtain a complete set of point-of-care plain film radiographs including a clenched fist and carpal tunnel views
    E. Obtain a workup for metabolic causes for peripheral neuropathies

183. A 23-year-old cross-country runner is complaining of a generalized papular itchy rash that occurs only during exercise. You would recommend that he do which of the following?

    A. Use sunscreen with PABA (para-aminobenzoic acid) at least 20 minutes prior to exercise
    B. Use topical steroids on the rash during exercise
    C. Take a hot shower the night before a long run, or try an antihistamine tablet one hour prior to exercise
    D. Desensitize with PUVA (psoralen + UVA)

184. According to most recently published studies, there is general agreement that repetitive heading of a soccer ball can demonstrate which of the following?

    A. Evidence of lasting neurocognitive deficits in well-controlled studies
    B. Ball type and size not important in epidemiology of head injuries
    C. Protective headgear not helpful in reducing ball impact to the head
    D. No evidence of gender differences in contact type and incidence of injuries

185. Examples of appropriate activities to improve cardiorespiratory endurance include which of the following?

    A. Jogging and cycling
    B. Wind sprints and weight lifting
    C. Power lifting
    D. Handheld video games
    E. Pilates

186. At a local collegiate football game, a player on the sidelines presents to you after he felt an insect sting. He feels like his throat is tightening, and you notice that it is becoming increasingly difficult for him to breath. The drug of choice to be administered first to this patient would be which of the following?

    A. Diphenhydramine
    B. Epinephrine
    C. Ranitidine
    D. Loratadine
    E. Nebulized beta-2 agonist

187. A 17-year-old basketball player visits her school's training room complaining of a 10-day history of insidious onset right-sided chest pain that is constant but worse with adduction of the right shoulder. There was no antecedent trauma. She is otherwise well and denies any medical problems and takes no medications. On exam, the athlete is in no distress. Heart rate is 72 bpm, BP 110/84 mm Hg in the right arm, and respiratory rate 16 breaths/minute. Inspection of the chest reveals no abnormalities. Palpation of the chest elicits tenderness over the cartilaginous articulations of the second through fifth ribs. There is no warmth or swelling. Auscultation of the lungs and precordium are normal. The most likely diagnosis is which of the following?

    A. Costochondritis
    B. Epidemic myalgia
    C. Pulmonary catch syndrome
    D. Slipping rib syndrome
    E. Tietze's syndrome

188. A 12-year-old swimmer is evaluated at the poolside during a water polo match after kicking another player's foot. She has a gross deformity of the fourth toe, and the clinical exam suggests a fracture. She would like to continue competing in this event. As pertaining to fractures of the phalanges, you explain that if pain permits, she can buddy tape the injured toe to an adjacent toe and continue competing. Regarding fractures of the phalanges, which of the following is true?

A. Overall, most toe fractures require referral and specialist management
B. Referral is usually not recommended for first toe fracture-dislocations, displaced intra-articular fractures, and children with first-toe fractures involving the physis because they may require internal fixation
C. Circulatory compromise and open fractures do not warrant orthopedic referral
D. Children with nondisplaced Salter-Harris types I and II fractures do not warrant an orthopedic referral
E. Unstable, displaced fractures can be treated with splinting and a rigid-sole shoe to prevent joint movement

189. During coverage of a cross country ski meet, an athlete presents to the medical team after she finished the race. She is shivering and slow to respond to your questions. You suspect hypothermia and quickly determine her rectal temperature to be 91.4 degrees Fahrenheit (33 degrees Celsius). Which of the following warming strategies should be considered first?

A. Encouraging the athlete to move as much as possible to generate body heat
B. Administration of warmed IV fluids
C. Extracorporeal blood rewarming using cardiopulmonary bypass
D. Removal of all wet clothing followed by application of warm blankets

190. Correct fit of a road bicycle is critical for optimal performance and reduction of overuse injuries. Which of the following factors is most important when fitting a bike?

A. Forward/back saddle adjustment: This adjustment is made with the pedals at 3 and 9 o'clock or parallel to the ground, correct position is reached when the forward knee is in front of the corresponding pedal spindle/ball of the foot
B. Saddle height: When seated on the bike with one pedal at the 6 o'clock position, the seat height is adjusted so the knee is flexed < 30 degrees
C. The handlebar position should always be higher than the seat height when viewed from the side
D. Bicycle frame size should be as tall as possible (longer seat tube length), optimizing power output per stroke

191. The pathology on the radiograph shown is indicative of which of the following injuries?

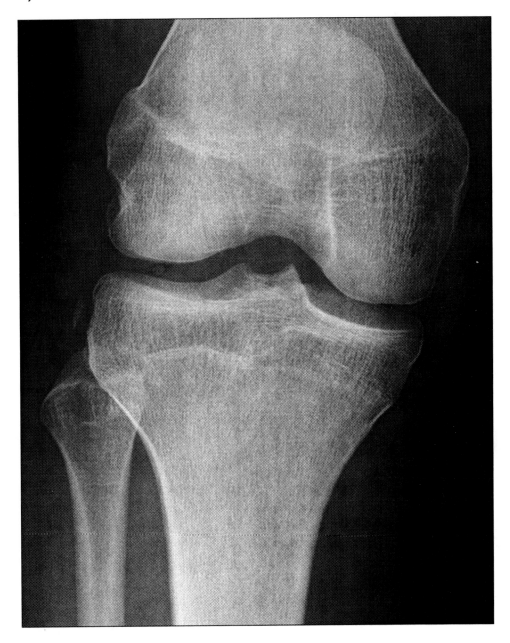

A. ACL tear
B. MCL tear
C. PCL tear
D. LCL tear

192. Identify which of the following dermatomes of the upper extremity is *not* appropriately matched with its corresponding nerve root supply?

    A. Lateral upper arm: C5
    B. Axilla: C7
    C. Lateral forearm: C6
    D. Medial upper arm: T1
    E. Medial forearm: C8

193. A 13-year-old softball player is struck in the right eye with a batted ball. Upon ophthalmological evaluation at the local emergency room, a fluid level is visible in the lower third of child's anterior chamber, and there is a slight drop in visual acuity when compared to the non-traumatized eye. The remainder of the eye exam is unremarkable. Therapy will be directed to avoid which of the following complications?

    A. Hemosiderin lens staining
    B. Rebleeding
    C. Further deterioration of visual acuity
    D. Clot formation in the anterior chamber
    E. Retinal hemorrhage

194. Which of the following is true of resistance training during childhood and adolescence?

    A. Strength gains are not lost during detraining
    B. Growth in height and weight of pre-adolescents can be influenced by resistance training
    C. Resistance training can result in increased strength without muscle hypertrophy or changes in body composition
    D. Resistance training is generally discouraged in children and adolescents due to safety concerns

195. Which of the following carpal bones is at highest risk for avascular necrosis?

    A. Trapezium
    B. Triquetrium
    C. Lunate
    D. Pisiform

196. After what time period does evaluation of microscopic hematuria after an intense run in an under-40-year-old warrant further investigation?

    A. 12 hours
    B. 24 hours
    C. 36 hours
    D. 48 hours
    E. 96 hours

197. A 42-year-old male is interested in beginning an exercise program. Which of the following is true regarding cardiovascular health and exercise?

    A. Arterial compliance increases with normal aging
    B. Aerobic exercise increases arterial compliance
    C. Resistance training increases arterial compliance
    D. Once resistance training is stopped, arterial resistance will increase

198. A 17-year-old male is playing a casual soccer game with his friends after school. He plants his right foot, and as he cuts sharply, he feels a pop on the outside of his ankle. He is not able to bear weight and has radiographs at the local urgent care facility that shows soft tissue swelling, closed physis, and a small fleck of bone lateral to the lateral malleolus at the level of the mortise. He is placed in a posterior splint, and he is seen in clinic two weeks later. The maneuver most likely to reproduce his symptoms is which of the following?

    A. Anterior drawer
    B. Syndesmosis squeeze
    C. Peroneal subluxation test
    D. Inversion stress test
    E. Passive dorsiflexion and external rotation of the foot

199. An athlete travels from sea level to a city at 3,000 m altitude in anticipation of a competition. Which of the following is a true physiological adaptation that occurs in this setting?

A. Mild hyperventilation induces respiratory alkalosis
B. Mild hypoxia increases stage 3 and stage 4 sleep
C. Decreased diuresis and increased plasma volume
D. Increased red blood cell mass in two to four days due to increased erythropoietin secretion
E. Pulmonary arterial vasodilation to increase PaO_2 (alveolar partial pressure of oxygen)

200. A 20-year-old female collegiate hockey player comes into your office with symptoms of fever, sore throat, and "swollen glands" in her neck for the last several days. In addition to collecting a throat swab for strep, of the following tests, which is the next best test to order at this time?

A. Epstein-Barr nuclear antigen
B. EBV IgG
C. EBV IgM
D. Heterophile antibody
E. Erythrocyte sedimentation rate (ESR)

3

Test 1
Answers, Critiques,
and References

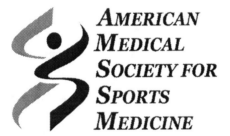

AMERICAN
MEDICAL
SOCIETY FOR
SPORTS
MEDICINE

Leading Sports Medicine into the Future

1. A 25-year-old presents to your office with popliteal artery entrapment syndrome (PAES). Which of the following is true about this condition from an anatomical, presenting signs, and diagnostic workup?

   A. It is more common under 30 years of age
   B. It occurs more commonly in females
   C. Pain at rest is pathognomonic for this disease
   D. Doppler studies show decreased velocity with knee flexion
   E. The popliteal artery derives from the deep femoral artery (profunda)

Correct Answer: A

Popliteal artery entrapment syndrome (PAES) causes calf pain during exercise due to compression of the popliteal artery by an abnormal relationship of the artery to the gastrocnemius and/or plantaris muscles. PAES is more common in those under 30 years of age (60%) and is more common in males (15:1, males:females). Unlike exertional compartment syndrome, symptoms are associated with intensity of exercise rather than volume. In addition, symptoms tend to resolve quickly after the conclusion of exercise until very late in the disease, when sclerosis of the artery creates a more chronic condition. Foot pulses tend to be normal at rest, but can decrease or disappear with dorsiflexion and plantarflexion of the foot. For this reason, diagnostic workup for the disorder includes Doppler ultrasonography or angiography in neutral position, dorsiflexion, and plantarflexion. Compartment pressures are usually normal or slightly elevated. Duplex ultrasound shows stenosis and increased velocity with flexion. This disorder is usually treated by cessation of causative activities followed by surgical release of the artery from the offending muscles. After surgical release, most patients can resume normal exercise.

The popliteal artery is a branch of the superficial femoral artery which distally gives off the anterior and posterior tibial arteries. Pain at rest is an ominous sign for more advanced disease of the popliteal artery, due to atherosclerosis, in a patient of much more advanced age than here.

1. Zetaruk M, Hyman J. Leg injuries. In: Frontera WR, Herring SA, Micheli LJ, Silver JK. Clinical Sports Medicine Medical Management and Rehabilitation. Philadelphia: Saunders Elsevier, 2007:451.

2. Wright L, Matchett W, Cruz C, James C, Culp W, Eidt J, et al. Popliteal artery disease: diagnosis and treatment. Radiographics 2004 Mar-Apr;24(2):467-479.

3. Shortell CK. Popliteal artery occlusive disease. Medscape. Accessed February 20, 2012 at http://emedicine.medscape.com/article/461910.

2. A 14-year-old boy nears the end of a five-minute-mile track race during an indoor track meet. He has sudden sharp pain over the left hip just proximal to the inguinal ligament. He has mild nausea and even one episode of emesis. In the office, his exam shows left low back tenderness and limited forward flexion at the waist without neurologic or radicular findings. He also has tenderness to direct and firm palpation over the left superior ilium along its anterior third. His physical exam also reveals no hernia, and the abdomen is benign. His plain radiographs and an abdominal CT in the emergency room are normal. MRI reveals a mild avulsion of the apophysis over the left superior ilium as well as some mild edema, indicating injury to the left quadratus lumborum. The plain film was read again showing the bony avulsion found on his MRI. Proper recommendations include which of the following?

    A. No running until radiologic healing is proven by plain x-ray
    B. Refer to orthopedic surgeon
    C. Conservative care, relative rest, return to running when pain has resolved and a full range of motion has returned
    D. Limit his passive hip flexion to allow healing
    E. Advise no further sprinting or racing on the track during this track and field season

Correct Answer: C

There are five apophyses near the hip. These secondary growth centers fuse by about age 25. Forceful or sudden traction at these sites can cause an apophysitis with pain and limitation of motion. Injury can also cause an avulsion of the apophysis itself. Treatment is conservative. There is no need to limit motion in general. Specific rehabilitation protocols have been described, and athletes have done well with them. Athletes may return to full activity with normal pain-free range of motion and normal strength. This teen had imaging evidence of two separate conditions on his MRI: an avulsion of the apophysis and an acute muscle strain. These conditions may be handled by primary care physicians. Surgery is generally not required. An MRI is usually not necessary to make the diagnosis but may be helpful to diagnose or rule out other pathology. Running the mile, bony injuries, and GI pathology can all cause nausea and vomiting.

1. DeLee JC, Drez D, Miller MD (eds). DeLee & Drez's Orthopaedic Sports Medicine. 2nd ed. Philadelphia: Saunders Elsevier, 2003:1475.
2. McKeag DB, Moeller JL. ACSM's Primary Care Sports Medicine. 2nd ed. Philadelphia: Lippincott Williams & Wilkins, 2007:447-461.
3. Esposito PW. Pelvis hip and thigh injuries. In: Mellion MB, Walsh WM, Madden C, Putukian M, Shelton GL (eds). Team Physician's Handbook. 3rd ed. Philadelphia: Hanley and Belfus, 2002:480-490.

3. When discussing an appropriate exercise prescription with your elderly patient, you include some of the general benefits that can be gained. Which of the following statements would you include in that discussion?

    A. Resistance training does not help maintain fat-free mass
    B. Benefits are only achievable at maximal intensity levels in the elderly
    C. Resistance training is a primary means for increasing $\dot{V}O_2$max
    D. Strength gains cannot be maintained with once weekly exercise
    E. Age-related decline can be attenuated with regular exercise

Correct Answer: E

Both aerobic and resistance training help to maintain the FFM (fat-free mass), so answer A is incorrect. Answer B is incorrect because various studies in multiple age groups, but especially in the elderly, show the benefits are witnessed at even minimal intensities. Answer C is also incorrect. Even though resistance training can help with strength, endurance, and maintaining one's fat free mass amongst other things, it is not a primary means for increasing $\dot{V}O_2$max. Answer D is incorrect. The recommended number of days per week of exercise is three to five or "most days" of the week. Maintaining the effects can be had with as little as one day per week for strength, and $\dot{V}O_2$max can be maintained with a two-thirds reduction in frequency and duration if intensity is unchanged. Answer E is correct as it has been shown that strength and flexibility declines are attenuated with regular exercise.

1. Pollock ML, Gaesser GA, Butcher JD, Despres JP, Dishman RK, Franklin BA, et al. American College of Sports Medicine position stand: the recommended quantity and quality of exercise for developing and maintaining cardiorespiratory and muscular fitness, and flexibility in healthy adults. Med Sci Sports Exer 1998 Jun;30(6):975-991.
2. Pescatello LS, DiPietro L. Physical activity in older adults: an overview of health benefits. Sports Med 1993 Jun;15(6):353-364.

4. A 12-year-old elite-level gymnast that is homeschooled presents to your office after three months of continued back and neck pain despite a thorough evaluation without findings and despite adequate radiologic and physical examination. After separating the child and parent, the child tells you that she just wants to spend time with her friends and she wants to go to the mall and be a normal 12-year-old. Which of the following is true?

   A. Elite-level gymnasts often present with back pain and should be pushed to "work through it" since she has a negative workup
   B. Burnout is common in elite-level child athletes as they often are subjected to excessive training loads during peak emotional and physical development times in pre-adolescence and adolescence
   C. Pressure from coaches and parents rarely leads to burnout in elite child athletes and only pushes them to work harder
   D. Respecting the child's request but not discussing it with the parent is best for the patient's recovery as the parent wants the child to continue training if the workup is negative
   E. A psychological consult is indicated as the athlete is obviously depressed

Correct Answer: B

Overtraining or "burnout" is the result of excessive training loads, psychological stress, or inadequate recovery. Back pain that has a negative workup (Answer A) needs to be evaluated for secondary concerns like psychological issues or overtraining. Burnout may occur in the elite child athlete when the limits of optimum adaptation and performance are exceeded. Clearly, excessive pain should not be a component of the training regimen. Elite-level athletes often have a large amount of pressure from coaches and parents (Answer C), and this will often lead to burnout if the child does not have the same goals as the parent or coach. Not discussing the child's concerns with the parent (Answer D) would be detrimental to the child's care; psychosocial concerns should be discussed with the parent in order to approach her back pain from a multifaceted direction. A psychological consult is not indicated at this time (Answer E), but if the child has depressive symptoms or is injuring herself for secondary gain, accessory consultation may be warranted.

1. Mountjoy M, Armstrong N, Bizzini L, Blimkie C, Evans J, Gerrard D, et al. IOC consensus statement: "training the elite child athlete." Br J Sports Med 2008 Mar;42(3):163-164.

5. A 50-year-old male complains of right medial knee pain for six months after an injury sustained while playing rugby. He was diagnosed with a medial meniscal injury four months ago, underwent surgical debridement, and has recovered uneventfully, but continues to have the same medial knee pain. Pain is deep aching/burning, often nocturnal, and radiates from the vastus medialis oblique region to the medial lower leg and dorsomedial ankle and foot. Pain is worsened by sitting a laptop computer on his lap for a prolonged time. There are no weaknesses or vascular changes noted on exam. He has no success with non-steroidal anti-inflammatory drugs or conservative therapies and pushes for further diagnostic testing. Your next step in making a diagnosis is which of the following?

A. MRI of the knee to evaluate the meniscus or other intra-articular pathology
B. Local nerve block at the adductor canal
C. Lumbar spine MRI to look for causes of lumbar radiculopathy
D. Repeat arthroscopy of the knee

Correct Answer: B

Saphenous neuritis or entrapment is an underrecognized cause of medial knee pain. Symptoms are purely sensory and follow the distribution of the saphenous nerve. On history the patient may report "lap sign" from pressure to the adductor canal, and on exam there may be a positive tinel's sign to this same area. Saphenous nerve entrapment often mimics medial meniscal injuries or is associated with them, and these patients will often report continued symptoms after the meniscal injury is treated. Initial treatment is with oral medicines or physical therapies. A local nerve block at the adductor canal can be both diagnostic and therapeutic. Electromyography and lumbar spine MRI may be needed to rule out other causes, but will not be diagnostic of saphenous neuritis.

1. Morganti CM, McFarland EG, Cosgarea AJ. Saphenous neuritis: A poorly understood cause of medial knee pain. J Am Acad Orthop Surg 2002 Mar-Apr;10(2):130-137.

6. A 20-year-old female cross country runner developed right thigh pain one week ago. She describes the pain as feeling like a pulled muscle. She has not had an injury but has recently added sprint workouts to her training regimen. She is on birth control pills but no other medication. She reports normal menses, a normal diet, and one previous stress fracture of her foot in high school. She has tenderness to palpation of the distal femur but no pain with firing the quadriceps muscle. She has pain with the single-leg hop test but not with the fulcrum test. She has normal knee and hip joint exams. AP and lateral views of the right femur are negative. Which diagnosis is most likely regarding her injury?

   A. Quadriceps muscle strain
   B. Adductor longus strain
   C. Patellofemoral pain
   D. Distal femoral stress fracture
   E. Quadriceps tendonopathy

Correct Answer: D

Stress fractures are very common in track athletes, but are at higher risk in female athletes that have increased training, poor dietary intake, amenorrhea, and osteoporosis. This athlete has recently increased her workout by adding sprints to her usual training program. A previous stress fracture is also a clue to questionable training methods and possible previous history of components of the female triad—disordered eating, altered menstrual function, and abnormalities in bone mineralization. These components are very important in diagnosing injury in female athletes. A quadriceps muscle strain is a possible etiology given the history, but she would have pain with firing of the quadriceps muscle and may have pain on the hop test. An adductor longus strain would present with muscular pain on adduction of the legs with no pain on the hop test. Patello-femoral pain would more commonly present with pain with long periods of sitting, poor quadriceps strength, and pain on change of leg positions. The single-leg hop test would not be positive. Quadriceps tendonopathy would also present with pain on palpation, possible pain on hop test, and the knee exam may be abnormal second to the tendonopathy distally. The fulcrum test applies the force of the arm of the examiner under the suspected fracture site with a bending force that reproduces the athlete's pain and is most commonly used to evaluate a femoral shaft stress fracture. The hop test on the affected leg also reproduces pain at the fracture site with femoral shaft stress fractures. Other tests that are used for diagnosing stress fractures clinically are the stork test (pars interarticularis stress fractures) and the tuning fork test for any fracture site. The tuning fork test has a high rate of false positives. X-rays are usually negative, and bone scan is nearly 100% sensitive but not specific. A triple phase technetium bone scan is usually positive in all phases with a stress fracture.

   1. Brukner P, Bennell K. Stress fractures in female athletes. Diagnosis, management and rehabilitation. Sports Med 1997 Dec;24(6):419-29.
   2. Bolin, DJ. Stress fractures. In: Mellion MB, Walsh WM, Madden C, Putukian M, Shelton GL (eds). Team Physician's Handbook. 3rd ed. Philadelphia: Hanley and Belfus, 2002:520-534.

7. Which pair of objective findings is most suggestive of increased intracranial pressure?

   A. Tachycardia, low blood pressure
   B. Bradycardia, elevated blood pressure
   C. Tachycardia, elevated blood pressure
   D. Bradycardia, low blood pressure

Correct Answer: B

Signs and symptoms that suggest a rise in intracranial pressure include headache, nausea, vomiting, ocular palsies, altered level of consciousness, and papilledema. If mass effect is present with resulting displacement of brain tissue, additional signs may include pupillary dilatation, abducens (sixth cranial nerve) palsies, and the Cushing's triad. The Cushing's triad involves an increased systolic blood pressure, a widened pulse pressure, bradycardia, and an abnormal respiratory pattern.

1. Smith ER, Amin-Hanjani S. Clinical manifestations of increased intracranial pressure. UpToDate. Accessed November 14, 2011 at www.uptodate.com/contents/evaluation-and-management-of-elevated-intracranial-pressure-in-adults.

8. In order to avoid overtraining, athletes can initiate training principles that include the use of microcycles, mesocycles, and macrocycles. Which of the following is the name for this type of training?

   A. Accommodation training
   B. Periodization training
   C. Progressive overload training
   D. Optimization training

Correct Answer: B

Periodization is a way to implement structural variation into a training program. In this form of training, one or more program variables are altered over time to maintain an optimum stimulus. Cycles of this training technique use differing amounts of rest and activity as well as intensity and duration of training to maximize performance.

1. Weir JP, Cramer JT. Principles of musculoskeletal exercise programming. In: Kaminsky, LA, Bonzheim KA, Garber CW, Glass SC, Hamm LF, Kohl HW, Mikesky A (eds). ACSM's Resource Manual for Guidelines for Exercise Testing and Prescription. 5th ed. Philadelphia: Lippincott Williams & Wilkins, 2005:355-356.

9. You are covering a weight lifting tournament, and the competitor misses the snatch (the olympic lift in which the athlete attempts to move a loaded barbell from the floor to an overhead postion in one fluid motion). You notice through your direct observation of the lift (and subsequent review of the videotape) that the loaded barbell (which weighed around 250 pounds) came down on the athlete's neck. The athlete was able to walk off the competition platform under his own power before you could reach the individual. Off the platform, the athlete complains of a sore neck and "nothing else." He denies radicular symptoms, limb weakness, headache, or parathesias. Your exam reveals normal peripheral neurological exam (deep tendon reflex, sensation, strength) but some paracervical muscle soreness and spinous process tenderness. Which of the following is the most likely diagnosis?

    A. C3-C4 cervical subluxation
    B. Rupture of the ligamentum flava
    C. Clay shoveler's fracture
    D. Paraspinal muscle strain
    E. Thoracic outlet syndrome

Correct Answer: C

Due to the ballistic nature of the lift and the weight of the loaded bar, one must consider all the above as possible diagnoses but must rule out the significant injuries first. The most serious are the subluxation and fracture. Thoracic outlet syndrome is a more chronic condition while the ligamnetum flava is virtually impossible to rupture. Cervical subluxation would present with limited range of motion and significant neurological findings, while clay shoveler's fracture would not. A simple radiograph would also confirm if either was present. The muscle energy involved in this maneuver would typically lead to an avulsion fracture of the seventh cervical vertebra posterior spinous process, also known as a clay shoveler's fracture.

1. Eiff MP, Hatch RL, Calmbach WL (eds). Spine fractures. Fracture Management in Primary Care. 2nd ed. Philadelphia: W.B. Saunders, 2003:220.

10. A 29-year-old hockey player complains of one day of eye pain. The pain began suddenly while he was sharpening his skates without using eye protection. Upon exam, his visual acuity is intact, as are extraocular movements. Seidel's test is negative. Inspection shows scleral erythema and a 0.5 mm brownish stain at 12 o'clock superior to the iris. In addition to standard management and removal of this corneal foreign body, which of the following steps must be taken?

A. Expansion of microbial coverage to include atypical organisms
B. Patching for one week to decrease spreading inflammation
C. Removal of products of iron oxidation from the cornea
D. Repair of corneal perforation in the operating room
E. Prolonged course of mydriatics

Correct Answer: C

The practitioner in this case has discovered a rust ring. This is the product of oxidation of iron materials that are embedded traumatically in the cornea. Not only must the iron shard be removed, but the rust ring must be removed to prevent vascularization degeneration of the cornea. There is no need presently to treat with expanded spectrum antibiotics. Patching is not necessary and may do harm. Seidel's test is negative, which rules out corneal perforation. Prolonged mydriatics have no further role in management of rust rings.

1. Jacobs DS. Corneal abrasions and corneal foreign bodies. UpToDate. Accessed November 14, 2011 at www.uptodate.com.

11. A 16-year-old male runner presents with a six-week history of worsening right-sided groin pain with activity. A femoral neck stress fracture is diagnosed by MRI. Conservative treatments are most appropriate initial management for which of the following types of this fracture?

   A. Superior neck fracture
   B. Tension-side fracture
   C. Compression-side fracture
   D. Displaced neck fracture

Correct Answer: C

Most femoral stress fractures respond adequately to a period of relative rest, attention to underlying biomechanical deficits, and a thorough assessment for any underlying nutritional, metabolic, or hormonal abnormalities, with treatments as indicated. However, both non-operative and operative care of stress fractures at the femoral neck can result in long-term morbidities such as osteonecrosis and arthritic changes at the femoral head. Surgical intervention should be determined on an individual case-by-case basis to decrease the risk of such complications, but is generally indicated for displaced fractures (Answer D), which have an increased rate of malunion and osteonecrosis, and tension-side fractures (Answer B), which have increased risk of nonunion and displacement. The superior cortex is the tension side of the femoral neck, making Answer A incorrect.

1. Harrast MA, Collono D. Stress fractures in runners. Clin Sports Med 2010 Jul;29(3):399-416.
2. Defranco MJ, Recht M, Schils J, Parker RD. Stress fractures of the femur in athletes. Clin Sports Med 2006 Jan;25(1):89-103, ix.

12. In which area would you not find a referred pain from sacroiliac joint dysfunction?

    A. Buttocks
    B. Hip joint
    C. Pubic symphysis
    D. Lower abdomen
    E. Lateral thigh

Correct Answer: B

In addition to the sacroiliac joint and the low back, pain can be felt in the locations in the question except the hip joint.

1. Isaac Z, Devine J. Sacroiliac joint dysfunction. In: Frontera W, Silver JR, Rizzo TD Jr (eds). Essentials of Physical Medicine and Rehabilitation. 2nd ed. Philadelphia: Saunders Elsevier 2001:267-270.
2. Joy EA, Cacintyre JG. Women in sports. In: Mellion MB, Walsh WM, Madden C, Putukian M, Shelton GL (eds). Team Physician's Handbook. 3rd ed. Philadelphia: Hanley and Belfus, 2002:91-93.

13. Which of the following is correct regarding the infrapatellar fat pad?

    A. The infrapatellar fat pad is located anterior to the patellar tendon
    B. Fat pad irritation is exacerbated by flexion of the knee
    C. Fad pad impingement is painful because it is a highly innervated structure
    D. Surgical excision is often necessary for definitive treatment of an irritated fat pad

Correct Answer: C

The infrapatellar fat pad is a highly innervated structure located at the inferior pole of the patella, posterior to the patellar tendon. Irritation or impingement can be caused by either a direct blow or due to hyperextension of the knee. People with fat pad irritation have exacerbation of the pain with extension of the leg (straight leg raises, prolonged standing). Treatment is often taping the knee either at the superior aspect of the patella to lever the inferior pole anteriorly or just distal to the fad pad to help support it.

1. McConnell J, Cook J. Anterior knee pain. In: Brukner P, Khan K (eds). Clinical Sports Medicine. 2nd ed. Sydney: McGraw-Hill, 2000:464-491.

14. Which of the following statements related to blood loss and anemia in athletes is false?

    A. Rupture of red blood cells occurs in the capillaries of the feet during endurance running events
    B. Hematuria in marathon runners lasts for several weeks after the marathon event
    C. Well-trained athletes with sickle cell trait perform similarly to athletes with normal hemoglobin at aerobic and anaerobic sports
    D. Iron deficiency anemia is the most common form of anemia found in athletes
    E. A drop in the hematocrit in well-trained endurance athletes can be a physiologic adaptation to exercise not requiring treatment

Correct Answer: B

"Sports anemia" has been considered an "innocent side effect of a healthy hobby." Answer E describes physiologic anemia in athletes, which is the increase in both blood volume and hematocrit with endurance training. It does not require treatment. True iron deficiency anemia in athletes is also an important issue. Iron deficiency causing anemia requires treatment. Studies show that this is the most common reason for anemia in athletes. There are many possible causes of iron deficiency anemia in the athletic population. Poor intake of iron-rich foods, menstrual losses, disordered eating in general, and a number of mechanical mechanisms of red cell destruction (capillaries in the feet and bladder motion during sports) can contribute. Low iron stores without anemia seems to affect performance as well, and iron supplementation in these athletes has become a common and successful protocol among college and elite endurance athletes, although the research evidence supporting this claim is running behind the observed benefits noted by team physicians and athletes. Studies show that athletes with sickle cell trait are more susceptible to exercise related collapse and should be informed of that risk. But they should not be disqualified from sports simply due to their sickle cell trait status. Trained athletes with sickle cell trait perform as well as trained athletes without sickle cell trait. Hematuria associated with endurance events should only last 48 hours or so. If hematuria persists in athletes, it should be addressed in a similar fashion as in the general adult population. Unexplained hematuria can result from a serious condition and should not be ignored.

1. Trojian TH, Heiman DL. In: McKeag DB, Moeller JL (eds). ACSM's Primary Care Sports Medicine. 2nd ed. Philadelphia: Lippincott Williams & Wilkins, 2007:261-269.
2. NATA consensus statement on sickle cell trait and the athlete. 2007. Accessed November 14, 2011 at www.nata.org/NR062107.

15. A 27-year-old female presents to your clinic, complaining of bilateral lower extremity pain that began about one month ago. She would like to run a marathon and has been training for the past three months. Initially, she felt a dull ache during the first mile of her run that she was able to run through. Gradually, the pain has increased, and she now feels it during and at the end of her run. She did try taking a week off and the pain completely subsided, but once she started running again, the pain returned. Her physical exam findings are remarkable for diffuse tenderness along the posterior medial aspect of the middle and distal tibia on both lower extremities. Her neurovascular exam is normal. You do not find focal or point tenderness and there are no abnormalities found on x-ray. You make the diagnosis of medial tibial stress syndrome (shin splints) and recommend which of the following treatments?

A. Relative rest to allow the patient to be pain free followed by a gradual increase in exercise intensity and duration on soft, level surfaces as long as she remains aymptomatic
B. Weight training avoiding cardiorespiratory fitness
C. Cam-walker-style boot for four to six weeks with the application of a bone-stimulator unit at night
D. A cool-down routine should be initiated emphasizing stretching before and after exercise

Correct Answer: A

The pathogenesis of this syndrome has not been clearly defined; however, excessive stress at the fascial insertion of the medial soleus or flexor digitorum longus muscles appears to be a likely source. Characteristic physical exam findings allow this syndrome to be diagnosed clinically. Stress fractures can be distinguished from MTSS (medial tibial stress syndrome) because they typically present with focal point tenderness and can be seen on x-ray. A bone scan could also be used to differentiate these two conditions. Exertional compartment syndrome would also be considered in this differential diagnosis; however, this condition is usually asymptomatic on exam. The onset of MTSS usually occurs after the initiation of a new running program with a rapid progression in intensity and duration. A reduction in both intensity and duration should alleviate the pain. It is generally recommended that these parameters may be increased approximately 10% per week so that the original training duration or distance is achieved in three to six weeks. Training may be increased more rapidly as long as the patient remains pain free; however, this increases the chance of reccurrence. Answer B is incorrect, as there is no evidence supporting weight training in the treatment of MTSS, although maintaining cardiorespiratory fitness will be important to the athlete and can often be achieved asymptomatically in other activities such as swimming or cycling. Answer C is incorrect. Immobilization is usually not required, unless briefly to allow pain-free activity but certainly not for four to six weeks. Answer D is incorrect. Heel cord stretching has been suggested to help prevent this injury; therefore, a warm-up routine including stretching may be recommended. A review of the literature failed to demonstrate a significant benefit. Ice massage can be helpful at reducing the patient's pain.

1. Kortebein PM, Kaufman KR, Basford JR, Stuart MJ. Medial tibial stress syndrome. Med Sci Sports Exer 2000 Mar;32(3 Suppl):S27-33.
2. Craig DI. MTSS: evidence-based prevention. Athl Train 2008 Apr-Jun;43(3):316-318.

16. Which of the following statements is true regarding cubital tunnel syndrome?

    A. MRI studies are often not helpful in the diagnosis of cubital tunnel syndrome
    B. Electromyogram (EMG) and nerve conduction studies are rarely helpful in the diagnosis of cubital tunnel syndrome
    C. Patients will usually complain of paresthesias in the thumb and index finger
    D. Patients may have weakness in thumb-index finger pinch (Froment's sign) in chronic cases
    E. In throwing athletes, the first-line treatment for cubital tunnel syndrome is ulnar collateral ligament reconstruction

Correct Answer: D

Cubital tunnel syndrome (a.k.a., ulnar nerve compression syndrome) is entrapment of the ulnar nerve at the elbow. Areas of entrapment include:
- The arcade of Struthers
- Hypertrophic medial head of triceps
- Spurs from the medial epicondyle and olecranon groove
- Anconeus epitrochlearis
- Cubital tunnel retinaculum (a.k.a., Osborne's ligament)
- Stenotic cubital tunnel
- The split of the humeral and ulnar heads of the flexor carpi ulnaris

It typically presents with paresthesias in the ulnar side of ring finger and in the small finger, but with no pain (Answer C is incorrect). Answer D is correct because the ulnar nerve innervates the adductor pollicis and deep head of the flexor pollicis brevis. Chronic ulnar neuropathy may lead to weakness in these muscles and decreased pinch strength (Froment's sign). Answer B is incorrect because an EMG/NCS usually shows slowing of the conduction velocity across the elbow and can be helpful in the diagnosis. Answer E is incorrect because relative rest is usually the initial treatment. Throwing athletes with recurrent episodes may need surgery. MRI can be helpful in the diagnosis of ulnar nerve entrapment at the ellbow with the finding of increased signal intensity better than nerve enlargement.

1. Mehlhoff TL, Bennett JB. Elbow injuries. In: Mellion MB, Walsh WM, Madden C, Putukian M, Shelton GL (eds). Team Physician's Handbook. 3rd ed. Philadelphia: Hanley and Belfus, 2002:424.
2. Verheyden JR, Palmer AK. Cubital tunnel syndrome. Medscape. Accessed November 15, 2011 at http://emedicine.medscape.com/article/1231663.
3. Keefe DT, Linter DM. Nerve injuries in the throwing elbow. Clin Sports Med 2004 Oct;23(4):729-742, xi.
4. Waldman SD. Atlas of Pain Management Injection Techniques. Philadelphia: W.B. Saunders, 2000:103-106.

17. Which of the following tests is recommended during a typical high school preparticipation physical?

    A. Echocardiogram
    B. Electrocardiogram
    C. Pulmonary function testing
    D. Urine drug screen
    E. Auscultation of the heart in standing and lying position

Correct Answer: E

Multiple studies have evaluated utility of screening tests in unselected populations. All of the above tests are useful in selected populations but are not as of yet recommended as screening tests in unselected populations. Auscultation of the heart in two positions is recommended by the working group on the preparticipation examination to evaluate for hypertrophic cardiomyopathy.

1. McKeag D, Moeller J. ACSM's Primary Care Sports Medicine. 2nd ed. Philadelphia: Lippincott Williams & Wilkins, 2007:62-73.

18. Which of the following cervical spine injuries are both considered stable non-emergent fractures?

    A. Flexion teardrop fracture and clay shoveler's fracture
    B. Hangman fracture and posterior neural arch fracture
    C. Simple wedge fracture and flexion teardrop fracture
    D. Posterior neural arch fracture and simple wedge fracture

Correct Answer: D

A flexion teardrop fracture occurs when flexion of the spine, along with vertical axial compression, causes a fracture of the anteroinferior aspect of the vertebral body. For this fragment to be produced, significant posterior ligamentous disruption must occur. Since the fragment displaces anteriorly, a significant degree of anterior ligamentous disruption exists. This injury involves disruption of all three columns, making this an extremely unstable fracture that frequently is associated with spinal cord injury. A clay shoveler fracture occurs with abrupt flexion of the neck combined with heavy upper body and lower neck muscular contraction. The fracture may also occur with direct blows to the spinous process. The fracture is located at the base of the spinous process. This fracture is considered stable since the injury involves only the spinous process and is not associated with neurological impairment. A hangman fracture results from a hyperextension injury that fractures both of the pedicles of C2. It is considered an unstable fracture; however, it seldom is associated with spinal injury, since the anteroposterior diameter of the spinal canal is greatest at this level, and the fractured pedicles allow decompression. The posterior neural arch fracture occurs when the head is hyperextended and the posterior neural arch of C1 is compressed between the occiput and the strong, prominent spinous process of C2, causing the weak posterior arch of C1 to fracture. The transverse ligament and the anterior arch of C1 are not involved, making this fracture stable. A simple wedge fracture occurs with a pure flexion injury. The nuchal ligament remains intact. There is no posterior disruption, making this a stable fracture. Answer D is the only pairing of two stable fractures in the choices given.

1. Davenport M. Cervical spine fractures in emergency medicine. Medscape. Accessed November 14, 2011 at http://emedicine.medscape.com/article/824380.

19. Which of the following statements is true regarding skin infection in athletes?

    A. Rifampin is the first line treatment for MRSA (methicillin-resistant staphylococcus aureus) infections
    B. Any skin wound that is suspicious for staphylococcus infection should be cultured
    C. The gold standard treatment of MRSA is appropriate oral antibiotics
    D. First line treatment of MRSA should be topical antibiotics
    E. Special cleaning of locker room, equipment and playing area is needed if MRSA is diagnosed in an athlete

Correct Answer: B

The best answer is B. Any wound that is suspicious for staphylococcus infection should be cultured. Suspicious features include: chief complaint of "spider bite" or a non-healing wound and "pus under pressure" on examination. Generally, CA-MRSA wounds are clinically indistinguishable from methicillin-sensitive s. aureus and streptococcal skin infections. Rifampin may be used in combination with other antibiotics for a synergistic effect, but should never be used alone. The gold standard treatment of CA-MRSA infections is incision and drainage. The transmission of MRSA is primarily skin-to-skin, not via fomites; thus, good hygiene is most critical.

1. Benjamin HJ, Nikore V, Takagishi J. Practical management: community-associated methicillin-resistant staphylococcus aureus (CA-MRSA): the latest sports epidemic. Clin J Sports Med 2007 Sep;17(5):393-397.

20. Which of the following factors has most contributed to the dramatic decrease in catastrophic cervical spine injuries since 1976?

    A. Improved preparticipation physical exam screening
    B. Mental conditioning prior to games
    C. Improvement in helmet design
    D. Banning of spear tackling or primarily striking with the crown of the head

Correct Answer: D

The dramatic decrease in catastrophic cervical spine injuries since 1976 is attributed to the banning of spearing in football. The other choices have had less definitive impact.

1. Torg JS. Cervical spine injuries. In: Garrick JG (ed). Orthopaedic Knowledge Update: Sports Medicine 3. Rosemont, IL: American Academy of Orthopaedic Surgeons, 2004:3-18.

21. A 33-year-old male who is preparing for his third half-marathon is determined to improve his time at this year's race, so he decided to change several areas of his training that he thought would improve his performance, increasing his overall mileage and hill running. Unfortunately, he developed substantial lateral knee pain. His physical exam demonstrates a positive Ober's test. He responded very well to stretching and strengthening exercises. What else on the history and physical would you have expected to discover before beginning treatment?

A. Normal lower extremity alignment
B. Strong abductor muscles
C. Less pain with hill running
D. Positive Noble's test
E. Abnormal radiographs

Correct Answer: D

He has iliotibial band syndrome (ITBS). Noble's test is pain elicited when the ITB is pressed against the femoral condyle near 30 degrees of flexion, and is commonly found in ITBS, so Answer D is the best answer. Answer E is incorrect because radiographs are typically normal, and are actually not indicated in clinically clear cases of ITBS. Answer C should read that the pain is worse with hill running, which is common at presentation due to increased eccentric contraction. An increase in mileage is frequently identified as well. Answer B is incorrect because the abductors of the hip which include the tensor fascia lata, gluteus medius and gluteus minimus are often found to be weak upon investigation. The adductor muscles may frequently be tight. Contributing intrinsic factors in the lower extremity alignment that can contribute to ITBS include: ankle pronation including pes planus, forefoot varus, metatarsus adductus, and tibial torsion. This alignment could be all normal, but Answer A is not the best answer to this question.

1. Fredericson M, Wolf C. Iliotibial band syndrome in runners: innovations in treatment. Sports Med 2005;35(5):451-459.
2. Ellis R, Hing W, Reid D. Iliotibial band friction syndrome: a systematic review. Man Ther 2007 Aug;12(3):200-208.

22. Pain originating from the facet joint complex is a common cause of back pain. The purpose of the facet joint in its protection of the lumbar intervertebral disk is best characterized as which of the following?

    A. Protection against axial rotation and loading
    B. Protection against shearing forces
    C. Protection against anterior translocation
    D. Protection against caudal translocation

Correct Answer: A

Facet joints of the cervical region of the spine are oriented primarily in the coronal plane to resist axial rotation and loading. The thoracic spine lays in an intermediate position and the lumbar spine transitions to a sagittal orientation to protect against rotatory forces. The lumbar facets can resist rotation while the coronal position of the cervical facets allows a great deal of rotation.

1. Berven S, Tay B, Colman W, Hu, S. The lumbar zygapophyseal (facet) joints: a role in the pathogenesis of spinal pain syndromes and degenerative spondylolisthesis. Semin Neurol 2002 Jun;22(2):187-196.
2. Benzel E. Biomechanics of Spine Stabilization. New York: American Association of Neurological Surgeons/Thieme, 2001:3.

23. An otherwise healthy 16-year-old male gymnast presents with a three-month history of non-radiating bilateral low back pain that worsens when he does back hand springs. On physical examination, his pain worsens with extension based maneuvers, and he has markedly decreased bilateral hamstring flexibility. There is no evidence of spondylolisthesis on plain x-rays. A bone scan with SPECT and a thin-slice CT confirm your diagnosis. Which of the following rehabilitation programs would you prescribe?

A. Extension-biased spinal stabilization and quadriceps flexibility exercises
B. Flexion-biased spinal stabilization and hamstring flexibility exercises
C. Extension-biased spinal stabilization and hamstring flexibility exercises
D. Plyometric exercise program
E. A rehabilitation program is not indicated for this condition

Correct Answer: B

This athlete's most likely diagnosis is lumbar spondylolysis, a stress fracture of the par interarticularis. The pars interarticularis is the region of the spinal lamina between the superior and inferior articulating processes. Spondylolysis often occurs due to repetitive hyperextension and axial rotation stresses on the lumbar spine. This problem is very common in gymnasts. Lumbar spondylolysis most commonly occurs at the L5 level. Bilateral spondylolysis is more common than unilateral spondyloyisis and can lead to spondylolisthesis (slippage of one vertebral body on another). On physical examination, the patient may have vertebral paraspinal muscle tenderness at the affected level, limited painful range of motion in both flexion and extension, and significant worsening of the low back pain with extension-based spine testing maneuvers. Up to 80% of patients with lumbar spondylolysis will have associated decreased hamstring flexibility. Initial treatment is conservative management including complete rest from the athlete's sport, a therapy program focusing on core strengthening, flexion-biased spinal stabilization and hamstring flexibility and possibly lumbar spine bracing. An extension-based therapy program may exacerbate the athlete's symptoms.

1. Micheli LJ, Curtis C. Stress fractures of the spine and sacrum. Clin Sports Med 2006 Jan;25(1):75-88, ix.
2. Bono CM. Low back pain in athletes. J Bone Joint Surg Am 2004 Feb;86-A(2):382-396.

24. Which of the following is correct about acute zygomatic complex fractures?

    A. Raccoon eyes are pathognomonic
    B. Unequal pupil levels
    C. They are the third-most common facial bone fractures related to sports injury
    D. Involves mandible and associated bony structures

Correct Answer: B

Fractures of the zygomatic bone (cheekbone) usually result from direct, blunt force. Due to the close association with the orbit, signs of orbital injury can exist: unilateral periorbital edema, ecchymosis, or emphysema; subconjunctival hemorrhage; diplopia, enopthalmos, step-offs of bone-limiting orbital movement also giving unequal pupils. You could also see paresthesias of the cheek, flatness of the cheek bone, and limited mandible movement. Radiographic views include Waters, submental vertex, and PA and lateral skull views. CT scan is useful when ocular trauma involvement is suspected. Treatment involves reduction of the fragments, often resulting in stable positioning. Involvement with ophthomologist is recommended if the orbit is involved. Protective headgear is worn for three to four months. Answer A is incorrect because raccoon eyes are often a delayed (two to three days) finding after trauma involving the subocciput and are bilateral. Echymosis after zygomatic fracture (and often orbital floor fracture) is nearly immediate and unilateral. Answer C is incorrect. Zygomatic fractures are the second-most common facial bone fracture in sports-related injuries (nasal fractures are first, mandibular are third). Answer D is incorrect. The zygoma is lateral to the maxilla and not directly connected to the mandible, which is the lower jaw bone. Complex facial fractures of the face have a classification system based on the location: I, II, and III.

1. Tu HK, Davis LF, Nique TA. Maxillofacial injuries. In: Mellion MB, Walsh WM, Madden C, Putukian M, Shelton GL (eds). Team Physician's Handbook. 3rd ed. Philadelphia: Hanley and Belfus, 2002:394-395.
2. Eiff MP, Hatch RL, Calmbach WL. Facial and skull fractures. Fracture Management for Primary Care. 2nd ed. Philadelphia: Saunders, 2003:361-369.

25. You are on vacation, scuba diving in the Carribean. Just after lunch, one of your morning dive partners complains to you he is having palpitations, a headache, nausea, and abdominal pain. You briefly take a look and notice he is very anxious, maybe wheezing and has a red macular balanching rash on the trunk. You quickly confirm he is a 35-year-old experienced male diver with a history of hypertension. He denies numbness and tingling in his hands and feet. He denies fevers or chills. He states during his week he participated in four recreational dives over two consecutive days. He reported dive times and depths well within the safety parameters set by PADI (Professional Association of Diving Instructors). He takes lisinopril 10 mg a day for hypertension and has been on it for seven years. He has no allergies. He did eat some locally caught fish: tuna, mahi mahi, and other reef fish at the lunch buffet. His vitals are stable with a blood pressure of 132/86. This patient is most likely suffering from which of the following?

A. Arterial gas embolism
B. Pulmonary barotrauma of ascent
C. Scombroid poisoning
D. Decompression illness
E. Ciguartera poisoning

Correct Answer: C

The correct answer is C, scombroid poisoning. The clues to this are: onset soon after eating dark flesh fish (probably at room temperature too long) within 10 to 30 minutes of ingestion. The symptoms are allergic in nature from histamine (converted from decarboxylation of histadine in fish). It is often the result of (usually darker flesh fish) spoiling and hence releasing histamine in the flesh (fresh caugh fish not chilled or frozen fish left a troom temperature too long). Initial symptoms consistent with allergic reaction (flushing, palpitations, headache, numness/tingling of mouth, abdominal pain, nausea diarrhea anxiety, wheezing). Severe symptoms can progress to hypertension or hyppotension, severe wheezing (especially in asthmatics), and tachycardia. They may have a macular blanching red rash on the trunk. Diagnosis is clinical. Treatment is supportive with H1 and H2 antihistamines and bronchodilators as needed.

The answer is not arterial gas embolism (AGE) or pulmonary barotrauma of ascent because 90% of symptoms occur within five minutes of surfacing. It is not decompression illness because the symptoms did not start within 10 to 60 minutes of surfacing. It is not ciguertera poisoning with onset of symptoms 1 to 14 days after eating tropical fish, reef fish, barracuda, or moray eel. Hot/cold reversal is a pathognomonic symptom of this condition.

1. Trojian TA. Environment. In: McKeag D, Moeller J. ACSM's Primary Care Sports Medicine. 2nd ed. Philadelphia: Lippincott Williams & Wilkins, 2007:286-287.
2. Marcus EN. Marine toxins. UpToDate. Accessed November 14, 2011 at www.uptodate.com.
3. Bove AA. Diving Medicine. 3rd ed. Philadelphia: W.B. Saunders, 1997.
4. Schilling CW. The Physician's Guide to Diving Medicine. New York: Plenum, 1984.
5. Plantz SH. Scombroid poisoning. Medscape. Accessed November 15, 2011 at www.emedicinehealth.com/wilderness_scombroid_poisoning/article_em.htm.

26. Which statement is true regarding exercise-induced anaphylaxis?

    A. Pre-treatment with antihistamines is effective to reduce the occurrence rate
    B. Pre-treatment with NSAIDs or aspirin is effective to reduce the occurrence rate
    C. A common trigger is running within a couple of hours after ingesting a meal
    D. Initial treatment is immediate administration of anti-histamines and steroids
    E. Reccurrence is rare so affected athletes can run alone with little risk

Correct Answer: C

Affected athletes should never run alone, as there are no proven measures to prevent an attack. Nonsteroidal antiinflammatory drugs and aspirin are common triggers for such an attack, and their use should be avoided before exercising. The initial step in management is always epinephrine—preferably IM. Treatment with antihistamines and steroids are needed, but epinephrine is the first line of treatment.

1. Brown DL, Haight DD, Brown LL. Alergic diseases in athletes. In: O'Connor F, Sallis RE, Wilder RP, St. Pierre P (eds). Sports Medicine: Just the Facts. New York: McGraw-Hill, 2005:226-227.
2. Brooks C, Kujawska A, Patel D. Cutaneous allergic reactions induced by sporting activities. Sports Med 2003;33(9):699-708.

27. A 16-year-old male football player presents to your office with acute onset of mid-thoracic back pain, which began immediately after being struck in the back during a football game the previous evening. On exam, you note an area of point tenderness immediately lateral to the midline in the mid-thoracic region of the athlete's back. Other than some moderate paravertebral muscle spasm, he has no other physical findings. Radiographic evaluation reveals a nondisplaced transverse process fracture. Which of the following are appropriate management options for this athlete?

A. Immediate immobilization on a back board and transfer to the hospital for neurosurgical evaluation
B. Referral for fitting of a clam-shell type back brace
C. Use of local ice, analgesics, and antiinflammatory medication, with return to activity as tolerated
D. MRI evaluation to assess spinal cord compromise
E. Disqualification from participation in collision sports for a minimum of six months

Correct Answer: C

Transverse process fractures typically occur in sports as a result of a collision, usually involving rotation or extension. Athletes can typically relate immediate onset of sharp pain associated with the collision. Because of the relationship between the transverse process and other nearby structures such as ribs and paravertebral muscles, transverse process fractures are considered stable injuries. As such, they require no further surgical intervention. Bracing is contraindicated in the management of these fractures, as it often adds to the patient's discomfort. The diagnosis of transverse process fracture is made through plain radiograph or CT, and additional imaging is not necessary. Because of the stable nature of the fracture, treatment is designed to decrease discomfort, and athletes can return to play when they are comfortable, often using a flak jacket for additional protection.

1. Dillon W, Eismont FJ, Kitchel S. Thoracolumbar injuries. In: DeLee JC, Drez D, Miller MD (eds). DeLee & Drez's Orthopaedic Sports Medicine. 3rd ed. Philadelphia: Saunders Elsevier, 2010:733-734.

28. Which of the following statements is true regarding preadolescents and well structured weight lifting programs?

    A. Strength training increases both muscle strength and hypertrophy in preadolescents
    B. Strength training increases muscle strength, but not hypertrophy in preadolescents
    C. Strength training is considered harmful to maturation, but beneficial to growth in preadolescents
    D. Strength training can have a negative impact on maturation and growth in preadolescents

Correct Answer: B

Preadolescent resistance training programs that include protocols with weights and resistance machines and have a low instructor to participant ratio can have significant improvement in strength without hypertrophy of muscle or deleterious effects on growth or maturation. Muscle hypertrophy is typically not seen until the hormonal effects of puberty begin.

1. Malina RM. Weight training in youth-growth, maturation, and safety: an evidence-based review. Clin J Sports Med 2006 Nov;16(6):478-487.

29. A 16-year-old male snowboarder had an accident during the Olympic competition. It was significant enough that it was decided to transport him to the hospital. En route, he complained of left shoulder pain, but remained hemodynamically stable during transport. At the hospital, his hemoglobin remained normal and stable throughout. CT scanning with contrast revealed a grade II splenic injury. Which of the following is correct regarding his initial evaluation, management, and disposition?

    A. The spleen is rarely injured during sport
    B. Non-operative management would be preferred
    C. Splenic rupture is of minor concern in this patient
    D. Ultrasound is the preferred method of imaging in stable patients
    E. He should be vaccinated immediately

Correct Answer: B

Answer A is not correct. The spleen is the most commonly injured abdominal organ in sports. Answer B is the best answer for several reasons. The predominant reasons include the fact that he is an adolescent who is hemodynamically stable. Preservation of the spleen is always preferable in the long term. And since his competitive season is likely over for a while after the Olympics, he would be an excellent candidate for non-operative management, which is the currently preferred method of management. Healing can take several months. Answer C is incorrect because delayed splenic rupture is the greatest concern after 48 hours in the non-operatively managed patient. Answer D is incorrect because CT scanning has been shown to be superior to US. If the patient is unstable, portable ultrasound would then be the preferable imaging method, but it is not pertinent in this scenario. Answer E is correct if the patient is thought to need an urgent splenectomy. There was no indication that emergent surgery was needed, and therefore E is not the best answer.

1. Brown RL, Irish MS. Observation of splenic trauma: when is a little too much? J Pediatric Surg 1999 Jul;34(7):1124-1126.
2. Rifat SF, Gilvydis RP. Blunt abdominal trauma in sports. Curr Sports Med Rep 2003 Apr;2(2):93-97.
3. Gravlee JR, Schwenk TL. Management choices for splenic injury in a collegiate football player. Curr Sports Med Rep 2003 Aug;2(4):211-212.

30. Which of the following exercise prescriptions should you advise against for an HIV-infected individual with mild to moderate symptoms or CD4 count < 200?

    A. Moderate exercise (40% to 60% $\dot{V}O_2$max)
    B. Weight training
    C. Intense exercise (> 75% $\dot{V}O_2$max)
    D. Three times per week

Correct Answer: C

Ullman reported an impaired ability to mobilize neutrophils and natural killer cells in response to one hour of exercise at 75% $\dot{V}O_2$max. Otherwise, moderate exercise has been shown to increase CD4 counts and CD4:CD8 ratios. It has also been shown to lower anxiety and tension levels in this population. Weight training may enhance muscle strength, bulk, and function in HIV+ individuals and may mitigate muscle wasting.

1. Neiman DC, Courneya KS. Immunologic conditions. In: Kaminsky LA, Bonzheim KA, Garber CW, Glass SC, Hamm LF, Kohl HW, et al (eds). ACSM's Resource Manual for Guidelines for Exercise Testing and Prescription. 5th ed. Philadelphia: Lippincott Williams & Wilkins, 2005:533-537.

31. During the second football practice of the day on day three of the college preseason football camp, an offensive lineman is found sitting on the ground, unwilling to stand up. He states his left calf is cramping and that he feels lightheaded and exhausted. You suspect possible exertional heat stroke. Which of the following statements about this condition is true?

   A. Axillary, oral, or a rectal temperature greater than 104 degrees Fahrenheit (40 degrees Celsius) establishes the diagnosis of exertional heat stroke
   B. This condition occurs randomly without warning and cannot be predicted
   C. Cold/ice water immersion is an effective way to treat exertional heat stroke
   D. There are two patterns of presentation: sodium depletion and water depletion

Correct Answer: C

Cold/ice water immersion has received much criticism from both medical professionals and industry that propose more superior cooling methods. Potential complications have been raised, including cardiovascular shock, hypothermia due to excessive cooling, inadequate access for other medical interventions, peripheral vasoconstriction, and shivering. While important to consider these issues, none of them have been proven as valid reasons not to utilize rapid cooling via cold/ice water immersion to treat exertional heat stroke. EHS is defined as a rectal temperature greater than 104 degrees Fahrenheit (40 degrees Celsius) accompanied by symptoms or signs of organ system failure, most frequently central nervous system dysfunction. Answer A is incorrect because temperature devices that assess a site on the outside of the body should not be used for the diagnosis of exertional heat stroke in an athlete who has been exercising in the heat as none have been proven to be accurate. Therefore, oral and axillary temperatures should not be used. Two viable options to establish core body temperature currently exist:

- Rectal thermometer: Unfortunately, an obvious drawback to rectal temperatures is the invasive nature and the lack of privacy to perform this technique on the athletic field.
- The ingestible thermistor is a second viable field measure. These devices transmit a signal that is obtained by a receiver that is held near the athlete. They provide a rapid assesment of core temperature, but they are expensive and must be ingested before the problem arises.

Answer B is incorrect because studies of exertional heat stroke have identified multiple risk factors that can allow health professionals to recognize predictable patterns allowing for primary prevention of this condition. Common risk factors include low physical fitness or physical effort unmatched to physical activity, underlying illness, improper acclimatization, heat load corresponding to green flag or above WBGT > 80.6 degrees Fahrenheit (27 degrees Celsius), training at hottest hours, dehydration, and sleep deprivation. Answer D is incorrect, as this describes two patterns that can cause exertional heat exhaustion, not stroke.

1. Casa DJ, Armstrong LE, Ganio MS, Yeargin SW. Exertional heat stroke in competitive athletes. Curr Sports Med Rep 2005 Dec;4(6):309-317.
2. Armstrong LE, Casa DJ, Millard-Stafford M, Moran DS, Pyne SW, Roberts WO. American College of Sports Medicine position stand. Exertional heat illness during training and competition. Med Sci Sports Exerc 2007 Mar;39(3):556-572.

32. You are evaluating an obtunded athlete who collapsed toward the end of a marathon. Physical exam is significant for a rectal temperature of 98.6 degrees Fahrenheit (37 degrees Celsius), BP 110/60, heart rate of 110, and diffusely increased muscle tone. What is the most likely diagnosis as you prepare to have your athlete transported?

A. Heat stroke
B. Myocardial infarction
C. Rhabdomyolysis
D. Exercise associated collapse

Correct Answer: C

Heat stroke is incorrect because it is an environmental injury associated with altered mental status and elevated core body temperature, usually above 103 degrees Fahrenheit (39.4 degrees Celsius). A myocardial infarction can occur during a strenuous event like a marathon but should be associated with hypotension to cause the mental status changes seen in this athlete. Rhabdomyolysis is the correct answer because the athlete is normotensive, normothermic, and has increased muscle tone expected with severe muscle injury. Exercise associated collapse is not correct because it occurs at the end of the event when the athlete stops. At this point, the muscles are no longer pumping the blood back to the heart, causing transient hypotension, resulting in collapse of the athlete.

1. Muldoon S, Deuster P, Voelkel M, Capacchione J, Bunger R. Exertional heat illness, exertional rhabdomyolysis, and malignant hyperthermia: is there a link? Curr Sports Med Rep 2008 Mar-Apr;7(2):74-80.

33. While treating a member of your university's women's cross country team for a fifth metatarsal stress fracture, you suspect she may have female athlete triad. Which of the following statements would help confirm the diagnosis of anorexia nervosa?

A. Binging and purging at least twice a week for three months
B. Menses every six to eight weeks in a postmenarchal female
C. Normal body image
D. A weight less than 85% of expected ideal body weight

Correct Answer: D

Female athlete triad includes disordered eating, amenorrhea, and osteoporosis. Disordered eating encompasses a variety of harmful behaviors, including anorexia nervosa and bulimia nervosa. Answer A is a diagnostic criterion for bulimia nervosa not anorexia nervosa. Secondary amenorrhea is defined as the three-month absence of menstrual bleeding in a women with previously regular menses. Therefore, Answer B is incorrect. Answer C is incorrect as patients with anorexia nervosa have a disturbance in the way in which one's body weight or shape is experienced. Other diagnostic criteria for anorexia nervosa include failure to maintain body weight at or above a minimally normal weight for age and height (i.e., body weight less than 85% of expected weight, either from weight loss or because the individual failed to gain weight during a period of growth); intense fear of gaining weight or becoming fat, even though underweight; and amenorrhea in post-menarchal females. Eating disorders are associated with ballet dancers, runners, wrestling, figure skating, and gymnasts.

1. Landry GL, Bernhardt DT. Gender-based pathologies: female athlete triad. Essentials of Primary Care Sports Medicine. Champaign, IL: Human Kinetics, 2003:75-89.

34. Which of the following statements is true regarding metacarpal fractures?

   A. Most metacarpal fractures in athletes will eventually need a surgical procedure in order to regain full function
   B. Fifth metacarpal fractures are called "boxer's" fractures because of their common occurrence in boxers
   C. Splints and casts for metacarpal fractures should immobilize the proximal interphalangeal (PIP), metacarpophalangeal (MCP), and the wrist joint
   D. Although up to 30 degrees of angulation is acceptable for a fifth metacarpal fracture and may be treated non-operatively, fractures with malrotation should be referred for surgical reduction
   E. Fractures of the hand should be treated with prolonged immobilization since early motion leads to significant risk of non-union and poor functional outcome

Correct Answer: D

Most metacarpal fractures can be treated non-operatively; exceptions include some intra-articular fractures, open fractures, unstable fractures (which usually include transverse and short oblique fractures), severely displaced fractures, and fractures with rotational deformities. "Boxer's" fractures almost never occur while boxing; instead, they typically occur from striking a solid object with a closed fist (a more typical fracture suffered while boxing is an index finger metacarpal fracture). When immobilizing the hand, the proximal interphalangeal joints should be allowed motion, while the MCP should be immobilized in 70 to 90 degrees of flexion. Only small amounts of fracture angulation (< 10 degrees) are acceptable for the relatively immobile second and third metacarpals; however, the more mobile fourth and fifth metacarpals can tolerate more angulation deformity (20 degrees and 30 degrees, respectively) before surgical reduction is needed. Malrotation is an indication for surgical treatment. Early motion is essential to good outcome for hand fractures. Delaying motion beyond three to four weeks increases the risk of arthrofibrosis and poor functional outcome.

   1. Dye TM. Metacarpal fractures. Medscape. Accessed February 15, 2012 at http://emedicine.medscape.com/article/1239721.

35. You are participating as a volunteer physician in a preparticipation physical examination night for incoming freshman athletes at a local college. The examinations are station-based and quite busy with four physicians to evaluate 80 athletes. You see a female cross country runner with a height of 5'6"; weight 100 pounds; pulse of 45 and respirations of 18. She says she has always been thin and her mother is also thin. Her last menstrual period was more than a year ago. She has been told that the lack of menses is of no concern since she is an athlete. Physical exam is unremarkable except for the very thin stature. You recommend which of the following?

A. Cleared for participation, but needs nutrition evaluation
B. Not cleared for participation until nutrition evaluation
C. Not cleared for participation until further evaluation by team physician and completion of nutrition evaluation
D. Order labs to include estradiol, LH, FSH, and TSH, and if normal, clear her for participation

Correct Answer: C

Amenorrhea and extreme low body weight are hallmarks for eating disorder. This athlete needs more evaluation than can be performed at a typical preparticipation examination. Further workup including a more detailed medical and menstrual history by the team physician and input from other experts such as a nutritionist would be needed before this athlete could be safely cleared for participation.

1. Nattiv A, Agostini R, Drinkwater B, Yeager K. The female athlete triad. Clin Sports Med 1994 Apr;13(2):405-418.

36. A 42-year-old laborer and distance runner presents to clinic with a painful click in his right hip. Pain is deep in the anterior groin. Exam shows pain with flexion combined with either internal or external rotation. Plain radiographs are normal. The test most sensitive in attempting to establish the diagnosis in this patient is which of the following?

   A. Ultrasound
   B. Computed tomography (CT)
   C. Magnetic resonance imaging (MRI)
   D. Bone SPECT scan
   E. Magnetic resonance imaging with intra-articular contrast and intra-articular local anesthetic (MRI arthrogram)

Correct Answer: E

In this series, clinical assessment accurately determined the existence of intra-articular abnormality but was poor at defining its nature. Magnetic resonance arthrography was much more sensitive than magnetic resonance imaging at detecting various lesions but had twice as many false-positive interpretations. Response to an intra-articular injection of anesthetic was a 90% reliable indicator of intra-articular abnormality.

   1. Byrd JWT, Jones KS. Diagnostic accuracy of clinical assessment, magnetic resonance imaging, magnetic resonance arthrography, and intra-articular injection in hip arthroscopy patients. Am J Sports Med 2004 Oct-Nov;32(7):1668-1674.

37. Which of the following is a known result of resistance training?

    A. In elderly patients, improved balance, mobility, and strength to perform ADLs
    B. Decrease in bone mass and in strength of connective tissue
    C. Decrease in lean body mass
    D. Large improvement in cardiorespiratory fitness
    E. Decrease in glucose tolerance and lipid profiles when resistance is a component of circuit training

Correct Answer: A

Studies have shown that strength training in the elderly can improve balance, mobility, and strength to perform ADLs. Weight-bearing exercise can increase bone mass and density as well as increasing lean body mass. Glucose tolerance and lipid profiles also improve with regular activity. There is only slight improvement in cardiorespiratory fitness when resistance training is a part of circuit training.

   1. Williams MA, Haskell WL, Ades PA, Amsterdam EA, Bittner V, Franklin BA, et al. Resistance exercise in individuals with and without cardiovascular disease: 2007 update: a scientific statement from the American Heart Association Council on Clinical Cardiology and Council on Nutrition, Physical Activity, and Metabolism. Circulation 2007 Jul;116(5):572-584.

38. A 67-year-old woman presents to your clinic with a persistent foot drop after sustaining a fibular head fracture two years ago. What type of orthotic would you prescribe?

    A. Metatarsal bar
    B. Ankle foot orthosis (AFO)
    C. UCBL (University of California-Berkeley Lab) shoe insert
    D. Thumb spica splint
    E. Hinged knee brace

Correct Answer: B

This patient's foot drop is most likely due to a common peroneal nerve injury associated with her fibular head fracture. Because of her loss of ankle dorsiflexion strength and ankle eversion strength, an ankle-foot orthosis (AFO) is the best option for her. A metatarsal bar will help relieve pressure off of the metatarsal heads of her foot but will not address her foot drop. A University of California-Berkeley Laboratory (UCBL) shoe insert can help with conditions such as pes planus but not foot drop. Using a hinged knee brace does not address the patient's underlying ankle weakness. Splinting the patient's thumb will not help her foot drop.

   1. Hennessey WJ, Johnson EW. Lower limb orthoses. In: Braddom RL (ed). Physical Medicine and Rehabilitation. Philadelphia: W.B. Saunders Company, 2000:326-352.

39. Which of the following is not felt to improve physical performance or considered an ergogenic aid?

   A. Caffeine
   B. Creatine
   C. Anabolic steroids
   D. Alcohol

Correct Answer: D

Caffeine can improve or increase work and power via increased mobilization of free fatty acids, thus sparing glycogen and prolonging endurance. Caffeine also directly affects muscle contraction by potentiating calcium release from the muscle. Creatine is felt to increase the intramuscular concentration of phosphocreatine and, therefore, enhance anaerobic power, speed recovery from high-intensity exercise, enhance muscular strength, and increase lean body mass. Anabolic steroids are well known to improve performance. Acute ingestion of alcohol has deleterious effects on psychomotor skills such as reaction time, hand-eye coordination, and balance. It does not improve muscular work capacity and may actually decrease performance level and affect or impair temperature regulation during exercise in a cold environment.

   1. Green GA, Frankel DZ, Puffer JC. Drugs and doping in athletes. In: Madden CC, Putukian M, Young CC, McCarty EC (eds). Netter's Sports Medicine. Philadelphia: Saunders, 2010:171-183.

40. De Quervain's tenosynovitis involves which of the following tendon sheaths?

   A. Extensor digitorum profundus and extensor pollicis
   B. Flexor pllicis longus and abductor pollicis longus
   C. Flexor pollicis longus and abductor pollicis brevis
   D. Extensor pollicis brevis and abductor pollicis longus

Correct Answer: D

De Quervain's results from swellng or stenosis of the sheath around the extensor pollicis brevis and the abductor pollicis longus; therefore, Answer D is correct. This can be deduced from recalling the motion of the Finkelstein test, which would stretch the extensor and abductor tendons of the thumb.

   1. Ingari JV. The adult wrist. In: DeLee JC, Drez D, Miller MD (eds). DeLee & Drez's Orthopaedic Sports Medicine. 3rd ed. Philadelphia: Saunders, 2010:1355-1366.

41. The anterior tibialis is the main dorsiflexor of the ankle,. It originates on the anterolateral tibia and interosseus membrane and inserts on which of the following?

    A. Medial cuneiform and base of first metatarsal
    B. All three cuneiform bones, and the base of the second metatarsal
    C. Navicular bone
    D. Anterior talus

Correct Answer: A

The anterior tibialis muscle is the largest muscle in the anterior leg and the main occupant of the anterior compartment. In addition to dorsiflexing the ankle, the muscle also adducts and inverts the foot. The tendon crosses the anterior to the ankle joint just medial to the midline, then sweeps across the dorsum of the foot medially to insert on the plantar surface of the medial cuneiform and base of the first metatarsal. The muscle is innervated by the L4 nerve root contained in the deep peroneal nerve. Rupture of this tendon can occur and is typically seen in individuals over age 45 after a forceful plantarflexion of the foot.

1. Baer GS, Keens, JS. Tendon injuries of the foot and ankle. In: DeLee JC, Drez D, Miller MD (eds). DeLee & Drez's Orthopaedic Sports Medicine. 3rd ed. Philadelphia: Saunders, 2010:1975-1976.

42. Which of the following statements regarding sickle cell trait athletes is true?

    A. Sickle cell trait, in contrast to sickle cell disease, has little to no mortality in athletes
    B. Any cramping, struggling, or collapse in a sickle-trait athlete must be considered sickling—a medical emergency—until proven otherwise
    C. The symptoms of exertional sickling and heat illness (heat stroke or heat cramping) are not distinguishable
    D. Acclimation to intense training, increased hydration, and increased rest afford no protection to sickling in athletes

Correct Answer: B

Sickle cell trait is common and generally benign, but in athletes it can be fatal if appropriate steps are not taken to prevent and treat its sequelae. There have been several deaths caused by exertional sickling in college football players and numerous more in military recruits. During strenuous activity, sickling is promoted by displacement of oxygen from hemoglobin S by lactic acidosis and high tissue temperatures, by increased concentration of hemoglobin S through dehydration, and by decrease in blood oxygen due to muscle demand. These sickled red blood cells get jammed in blood vessels and cause collapse from ischemic rhabdomyolysis. Cardiac arrhythmias and acute renal failure, known complications of rhabdomyolysis, can cause death. The symptoms and signs of sickling are unique and can easily be distinguished from those of heat illness. Heat cramping may have early warning signs such as twitching or twinges in tired muscles, whereas sickling hits suddenly without warning. Heat cramping pain is the severe pain of sustained, full contraction of muscles, whereas sickling pain is a milder, ischemic pain from muscles working on diminished blood supply. Heat cramping athletes "hobble to a halt" as their fully contracted muscles no long work, whereas sickling athletes "slump to a stop" as their legs become weak and can no longer hold them up. The heat cramping athlete is often yelling in pain as his muscles are rock hard in full contraction, whereas the sickling athlete lies fairly still, saying his legs won't hold him up. The muscles look and feel normal. Major heat cramping can take hours to resolve, even if resting in a cool place and being treated with stretching, massage, and IV fluids. A sickling athlete feels normal after about 15 minutes of sitting in a cold tub, drinking fluids, and receiving supplemental oxygen. Sickling risk is increased by anything that increases the difficulty of the exercise, for example, hot weather, dehydration, high altitude, or asthma. Strategies that emphasize acclimation to conditioning and lifting regimens, modifying drills to allow for adequate rest between repeated sprints, good hydration, and athlete recognition of mild signs can decrease sickling in sickle cell trait athletes.

1. Eichner ER. Sickle cell trait and athletes: three clinical concerns. Curr Sports Med Rep. 2007 Jun;6(3):134-135.
2. Eichner ER. Sickle cell trait and the athlete. Gatorade Sports Science Institute. Sports Science Exchange 2006. Accessed February 15, 2012 at www.gssiweb.com/Article_Detail.aspx?articleID=724.

43. Which of the following is the only immunization currently required by law for entrance into specific countries?

    A. Yellow fever
    B. Malaria
    C. E. coli
    D. Rotavirus

Correct Answer: A

Immunization for yellow fever is the only immunization required by law and only for entrance into specific countries. Yellow fever causes a severe hepatitis. Note: Cholera or other immunizations may be required by some countries.

> 1. Centers for Disease Control and Prevention. Cetron MS, Marfin AA, Julian KG. Yellow fever vaccine. Recommendations of the Advisory Committee on Immunization Practices (ACIP), MMWR Recomm Rep 2002;51(RR-17):1-11.

44. Which of the following is a property of slow twitch (type I) muscle fibers?

    A. Low mitochondrial density
    B. Rely on anaerobic metabolism
    C. Higher rate of force production
    D. Major storage fuel is triglycerides

Correct Answer: D

Slow twitch, or type I fibers, are more efficient at using oxygen to generate ATP and they have higher mitochondrial densities and capillary to volume ratios. Their major storage fuel is triglycerides. This allows them to utilize ATP more slowly. They are known to fire more slowly than their fast twitch, type II, counterparts. This type of muscle fiber is important in endurance-type events such as distance running or cycling. Type II fibers, or fast twitch fibers, are broken down into type IIa and type IIx in humans. They are more reliant on anaerobic metabolism to create fuel through the use of glycogen and creatine phosphate. These fibers are utilized in short bursts such as with sprinting and weight lifting.

> 1. Caiozzo VJ, Rourke B. The muscular system: structural and functional plasticity. In: Tipton, CM (ed). ACSM's Advanced Exercise Physiology. Philadelphia: Lippincott Williams & Wilkins, 2006:112-143.

45. A 17-year-old football player tackles an opposing player and sustains a flexion injury of his neck. He falls to the ground. The ambulance is summoned, and he is boarded and taken to the hospital. He is found to have an injury to the anterior spinal cord of his neck. Which of the following clinical findings match this lesion?

   A. Loss of motor function and position sense on the same side of the body as the lesion and loss of pain and sensation on the opposite side of the body as the lesion
   B. Bilateral lower extremity paralysis that is greater than the upper extremity paralysis; bilateral loss of pain and temperature sensation; vibratory and proprioception is intact
   C. Weakness in both upper extremities that is more severe than the weakness in both lower extremities; sacral function is spared
   D. After the period of spinal shock has resolved, the patient has no motor or sensory activity below the level of the lesion

Correct Answer: B

Answer A is incorrect as it describes a Brown-Séquard lesion. Only one side of the cord is affected, and there is loss of motor function and position sense on the same side with pain and sensation on the opposite side. This is a fairly rare lesion but has the best prognosis as far as patient recovery. Answer B is correct. Anterior cord lesion often happens after a flexion injury and unfortunately has a poor prognosis. Lower extremities are usually affected with paralysis greater than the upper extremities. Temperature sensation, vibratory sensation, and proprioception are intact. Answer C describes a central cord lesion. This type of lesion most often happens with the hyperextension, not a hyperflexion injury, and can happen in elderly people with spondylosis who falls. Answer D is also incorrect and describes complete severing of the spinal cord. There is loss of both motor and sensory function below the level of the lesion. The bulbocavernosus reflex must be present to confirm that the spinal shock period is over.

1. Thompson JC. Netter's Concise Atlas of Orthopaedic Anatomy. Teterboro, NJ: Icon Learning Systems, 2002:39-43.
2. Arce D, Sass P, Abul-Khoudoud H. Recognizing spinal cord emergencies. Am Fam Phys 2001 Aug;74(4):631-638.

46. A 20-year-old male soccer player presents with four months of right groin pain. It is described as a deep ache just to the side of his pubic bone and radiates down the medial thigh when he plays soccer. He also reports some paresthesias along the medial thigh after exercise and difficulty with jumping. On exam, he is weak on hip adduction and tender with stretching his adductors. You decide to order an EMG, which shows a denervation pattern of the adductor longus and brevis consistent with entrapment of which of the following nerves?

A. Obturator nerve
B. Ilioinguinal nerve
C. Superior gluteal nerve
D. Inferior gluteal nerve

Correct Answer: A

This is a classic presentation of obturator nerve entrapment. It has been found most commonly in males who play soccer or Australian rules football. EMG (electromyography) is the test of choice for diagnosis. It is believed that a chronic adductor tendonopathy leads to fibrosis and fascial adhesions, which eventually entrap the nerve. Conservative measures have not been found to be effective and surgery remains the preferred treatment.

1. Brukner P, Bradshaw C, McCrory P. Obturator neuropathy: a cause of exercise-related groin pain. Phys Sportsmed 1999 May;27(5):62-73.
2. Bradshaw C, McCrory P, Bell S, Brukner P. Obturator nerve entrapment. A cause of groin pain in athletes. Am J Sports Med 1997 May-Jun;25(3):402-408.
3. Morelli V, Smith V. Groin injuries in athletes. Am Fam Physician 2001 Oct 15;64(8):1405-1414.

47. You have been asked to coordinate preparticipation physical exams for a college with approximately 300 Division II athletes. You have the aid of some local physicians, physical therapist and athletic trainers. You elect for station-based exams. Which of the following choices is a disadvantage of station-based preparticipation physical examinations?

    A. Examinations can be limited and brief due to time constraints
    B. Many examinations can be performed in a short period of time
    C. Compared to office-base exams, it is the most cost-effective method
    D. Communication among the sports medicine team is readily available

Correct Answer: A

One disadvantage of station-based examinations is that a large number of athletes that are to be evaluated in a given time period may compel an evaluator to obtain a suboptimal history and a more superficial evaluation. Taking a more detailed history or exam may not be performed because of the perceived rush to get through a large number of athletes. If parents are not available, questions regarding family history may not be known by the athlete. However, a team approach with other providers' help allows a larger number of athletes to be examined in a shorter period of time. A station-based approach has been shown to be more cost-effective. A great opportunity for greater communication within the sports medicine team is present with a sports medicine "team" present.

1. Seto CK. The preparticipation physical examination: an update. Clin Sports Med 2011 Jul;30(3):491-501.
2. Bernhardt D, Roberts WO. Preparticipation Physical Evaluation. 4th ed. American Academy of Pediatrics, 2010:11-17.

48. The most common mechanism of injury to the carotid artery in blunt cerebrovascular injuries is due to which of the following?

    A. Direct laceration from a sharp object
    B. Hyperextension injury to the neck
    C. Flexion injury to the neck
    D. Direct blow to the neck
    E. Laceration secondary to fracture of sphenoid or petrous bones

Correct Answer: B

There are three fundamental mechanisms of injury to the carotid artery in blunt cerebrovascular injuries. The most common is hyperextension (with contralateral rotation of the head) injury to the neck, causing stretching of the carotid followed by direct blow to the neck and laceration of the artery by adjacent fractures involving the sphenoid or petrous bones. Additionally, vertebral artery injuries are usually combinations of direct injury due to fracture of vertebrae involving the transverse foramen and hyperextension injury due to the tethering of the vertebral artery within the lateral mass of the cervical spine. Both of these injuries result in potential intimal tears, leading to nidus for platelet aggregation and either emboli or occlusion. It is recommended that during a potential lucent period (silent period) without symptoms—anywhere from 10 to 72 hours—that diagnostic studies be performed to determine if damaged and extent and then treat with anticoagulants or antiplatelet treatment. Currently, until the sensitivity and specificity of MRA and CTA improves, a four-vessel arteriography is recommended.

1. Cothren CC, Moore EE. Blunt cererbrovascular injuries. Clinics (Sao Paolo) 2005;60(6):489-496.

49. A 30-year-old male with T6 paraplegia presents to the office with a desire to begin a wheel exercise program. He has been gaining weight due to a lack of activity since the injury several years ago. He wants your advice on how to safely begin an exercise program. Along with advising proper equipment, carrying water, and avoiding hot or humid days, you also advise which of the following?

    A. Wear tight leg straps to increase sympathetic tone
    B. Take 10 grams of carbohydrates every 30 minutes during exercise
    C. Empty bladder and bowels before each workout
    D. Have cervical x-rays to rule out atlantoaxial instability

Correct Answer: C

Answer C refers to prevention of autonomic dysreflexia, a medical emergency. Autonomic dyreflexia is caused by increased sympathetic input from the splanchnic nerves, caused by noxious stimuli. The majority of cases are caused by a distended bladder (90%) or bowel (9%). Prevention includes bowel and bladder maintenance, and skin care. Answer A is incorrect as this can induce autonomic dysreflexia, (a practice known as "boosting"), and is illegal in paralympics sports. Answer B is a recommendation for a type 1 diabetic. Answer D is a recommendation for a patient with Down syndrome.

1. Richter KJ, McCann PD, Bruno PJ. In: Scuderi GR, McCann PD (eds). Sports Medicine: A Comprehensive Approach. 2nd ed. Philadelphia: Mosby, 2005:725-737.
2. Klenk C, Gebke K. Practice management: common medical problems in disabled athletes. Clin J Sport Med 2007 Jan;17(1):55-60.

50. A baseball player was hit in the upper thigh by a line drive, and he complains of swelling and pain immediately. You note a large hematoma present in the location of the injury. You begin your evaluation by palpating the borders of the femoral triangle. Which of the following structures does not form a border of the triangle?

    A. Medial border of the adductor brevis
    B. Inguinal ligament
    C. Medial border of the adductor longus
    D. Medial border of the sartorius

Correct Answer: A

Several important structures lie in the femoral triangle, including the femoral artery, vein, and nerve. It is also the location of compression for tamponade of the femoral artery to the leg where the femoral artery lies over the head of the femur. While the brevis does run in parallel to the adductor longus, it lies deep to the adductor magnus and therefore does not form a border of the triangle.

1. Netter FH. Atlas of Human Anatomy. 5th ed. Philadelphia: Saunders Elsevier, 2011:Plate 480.
2. Hollinshead HW, Rosse C. Textbook of Anatomy. 5th ed. New York: J.B. Lippincott Company, 1985.

51. You are seeing a new patient for a preparticipation exam, and this athlete would like to be cleared to scuba dive. Which of the following statements is true regarding SCUBA diving participation?

    A. An athlete with a well-controlled seizure disorder who is on a stable dose of medication and has been seizure-free for six months is safe to be cleared

    B. An athlete with a previous spontaneous pneumothorax can be cleared for shallow dives only

    C. An athlete with sickle cell trait has no more risk of hypoxia than the average diver and is safe to be cleared

    D. An athlete with myringotomy tubes in place for three months is safe to be cleared

    E. An athlete with an active otitis media if treated with antibiotics is safe to be cleared

Correct Answer: C

Anti-epileptic medication is an absolute contraindication to scuba even with ideal seizure control since seizure activity underwater is lethal. A previous spontaneous pneumothorax is an absolute contraindication to scuba, and it is important to remember that the greatest change in water pressure occurs in the first 10 feet. The risk of pneumothorax is actually highest at shallow depths. Alveolar rupture while breathing compressed air can occur in depths as shallow as four feet. If an athlete with sickle cell trait were to lose his source of oxygen while diving (out of air, drowning, equipment failure, etc.), then the cells would sickle. However, the low-oxygen tensions necessary to produce this phenomenon would have caused brain damage long before the red cells were involved. The person with sickle cell trait then is not at any greater risk from hypoxia (oxygen deficiency in body tissues) than the ordinary diver and is qualified for diving (if trained and physically fit otherwise). Myringotomy tubes allow water to enter the middle ear, and this can induce cold water calorics, causing potentially lethal nausea, vomiting, and vertigo. Otitis media prevents normal eustachian tube function, which in turn prevents normal middle ear ventilation. Normal eustachian tube function allows the equalization of air pressure between the middle ear and the external water pressure. Without this ability, the tympanic membrane is at increased risk of rupture.

1. Divers Alert Network: frequently asked questions. Accessed November 14, 2011 at www.diversalertnetwork.org/medical.
2. Morris GA. Scuba diving. In: Madden CC, Putukian M, Young CC, McCarty EC (eds). Netter's Sports Medicine. Philadelphia: Saunders, 2010:539-545.
3. Scubadoc's diving medicine. Accessed February 15, 2012 at www.scuba-doc.com/ftnss.htm.

52. A 37-year-old male who is otherwise healthy, but minimally active physically, has signed up as a charity runner for a local marathon in August. He has been training well per Jeff Galloway's training program for first-time marathoners. He comes to see you in June before the race with concerns about hydration for prevention of heat injury. Which of the following recommendations is appropriate for fluid hydration during endurance events?

A. Drink at each water stop along the race course
B. Drink ad lib based on thirst
C. Drink an adequate amount of fluids to keep urine output pale
D. Alternate water and glucose-electrolyte solution according to a pre-planned schedule

Correct Answer: B

Per a recent position statement on fluid replacement recommendations during marathon running, adequate hydration is very important for peak performance with exercise as well heat stress management. Numerous recent case reports of exertional hyponatremia (EH) during endurance events and in particular marathons have prompted changes in recommendations for hydration during these events. Most episodes of hyponatremia area associated with fluid overload or overconsumption and, therefore, many races are even decreasing the number of water stops as well, publishing many education flyers on hydration recommendations. The old adage that "When you are thirsty you are behind in fluid requirements" has fueled this misconception. Drinking fluids ad lib has been demonstrated to be the best protection for fluid overload.

1. Noakes T. Fluid replacement during marathon running. Position statement. Clin J Sports Med 2003 Sep;13(5):309-318.
2. Jeff Galloway's training program for first-time marathon runners is available at www.jeffgalloway.com/training/marathon.html.

53. Which component of the deep posterior compartment of the lower leg assists with plantar flexion of the foot?

    A. Tibialis posterior
    B. Flexor digitorum longus
    C. Soleus
    D. Tibialis anterior

Correct Answer: A

The deep posterior compartment contains the tibialis posterior (TP), flexor digitorum longus (FDL), and flexor hallucis longus (FHL) and can be remembered by the mnemonic "Tom, Dick, and Harry." The tibialis posterior inverts the foot and assists with plantar flexion. When the TP is weak or injured, a patient may have difficulty with performing a single-heel raise and may demonstrate a "too many toes" sign during inspection from behind. The soleus is part of the superficial posterior compartment. The tibialis anterior is part of the anterior compartment.

1. Thompson JC. Netter's Concise Orthopaedic Anatomy. 2nd ed. Philadelphia: Saunders Elsevier, 2010:319.

54. A 15-year-old wrestler presents to the clinic with localized swelling and tenderness in the helix of the right ear. The swelling developed after a day long wrestling tournament. Which of the following statements is incorrect?

    A. The injury is caused by repeated rubbing or by absorbing repetitive blows
    B. If not treated initially, the ear will develop a deformed cauliflower-like appearance
    C. Suturing a sterile button through the ear is an acceptable treatment
    D. Repeated aspirations should be avoided
    E. Sports commonly associated with this injury are wrestling, rugby, and soccer

Correct Answer: D

An auricular hematoma is caused by repeated rubbing or blows to the ear. Wrestling, boxing, and rugby are sports that commonly produce this injury. A hematoma develops in the helix, causing the skin to separate from the perichondrium. Initial treatment consists of the application of cold compresses. Any hemorrhage between the perichondrium and the skin should be aspirated under sterile conditions, and a compressive dressing should be applied to prevent reaccumulation of the hematoma. Multiple techniques have been described to apply the compressive dressing, including collodion casts, plaster of paris, and suturing a sterile button to the ear to hold the skin to the perichondrium. The ear should be checked again in 24 hours. Any reaccumulation of fluid should be reaspirated. If not treated, the ear can develop a classic deformed cauliflower-like appearance caused by chronic scarring within several weeks.

1. Grindel SH. Head and neck. In: McKeag DM, Moeller JL (eds). ACSM's Primary Care Sports Medicine. 2nd ed. Philadelphia: Lippincott Williams & Wilkins, 2007:334-335.

55. On average, $\dot{V}O_2$max is lower in postpubertal females when compared to postpubertal males. Which of the following statements is true concerning reasons for this difference?

    A. Females, on average, experience a relative decrease in body fat after puberty

    B. Females, on average, have increased cardiac output compared to males

    C. Females, on average, have larger muscle fiber area compared to males

    D. Females, on average, have lower blood hemoglobin content

Correct Answer: D

$\dot{V}O_2$max is an estimation the body's ability to utilize oxygen for energy; measured by the volume of oxygen per body weight per time (mL/kg/min). $\dot{V}O_2$max is dependent on the body's ability to deliver oxygen to muscle and extract oxygen for utilization in energy production. Females, on average, have about 10% lower blood hemoglobin content. This translates into 10% lower oxygen transport capacity and lower $\dot{V}O_2$max. The calculation is affected positively by an increase in lean body mass. Females, on average, experience a relative decrease in lean body mass after puberty due to an increase in body fat after puberty. Females, on average, have smaller hearts after puberty with resulting decreased cardiac output compared to males. This leads to lower maximal delivery of oxygen when compared to males. Females, on average, have smaller muscle fiber area compared to males, leading to decreased total extraction of oxygen for utilization.

1. Greydanus DE, Patel DR. The female athlete before and beyond puberty. In: Luckstead EF (ed). The Pediatric Clinics of North America. Philadelphia: W.B. Saunders, 2002;49(3):553-580.
2. Freedson P. Cardiovascular fitness. In: Costa DM, Guthrie SR (eds). Women and Sport: Interdisciplinary Perspectives. Champaign, IL: Human Kinetics, 1994:170-172.

56. Your patient, a 43-year-old male with long-standing type 2 diabetes mellitus, wishes to begin an exercise program. Which of the following are appropriate recommendations for this patient?

    A. There is limited information regarding the benefit of exercise in type 2 diabetes
    B. There is little risk of hypoglycemia in exercising diabetic patients
    C. Patients with proliferative retinopathy are at no greater risk than those with normal funduscopic findings
    D. Hypoglycemia is more likely to occur during morning exercise
    E. The patient should undergo exercise electrocardiography before beginning an exercise program

Correct Answer: E

Benefits of exercise in diabetic patients are well-documented, including increased insulin sensitivity, improved blood sugar control and enhanced sense of well-being. Although there are significant benefits from exercise, both type 1 and type 2 diabetics are at risk for hypoglycemic episodes during exercise. Patients with funduscopic evidence of proliferative retinopathy should avoid strenuous or jarring activity due to their increased risk of retinal hemorrhage. Due to diurnal variations in growth hormone, diabetics are more likely to have hypoglycemic episodes during evening exercise. Diabetes mellitus is considered to be an independent risk factor for coronary artery disease. Because of this, all diabetic patients over the age of 40 should undergo stress cardiac evaluation before beginning an exercise program.

1. White RD, Cardone D, Berg K. The athlete with diabetes. In: Madden CC, Putukian M, Young CC, McCarty EC (eds). Netter's Sports Medicine. Philadelphia: Saunders, 2010:223-228.

57. Which of the following does not cause delayed onset muscle soreness (DOMS)?

    A. Lactic acid accumulation in muscle tissues
    B. Structural damage to muscle fibers
    C. Eccentric exercise
    D. Swelling on a cellular level, which may activate and sensitize afferent nerve endings around damaged muscle fibers
    E. Training at an intensity greater than customary

Correct Answer: A

Delayed onset muscle soreness (DOMS) describes pain 24 to 72 hours after unaccustomed exercise. It usually resolves in several days to a week after onset. Previously, lactic acid accumulation at the muscle site was thought to cause DOMS, but it is now known that lactic acid is rapidly cleared and is not present at the time of DOMS. Studies have demonstrated that eccentric activities produce more muscle damage and more DOMS than concentric activities and this damage has been shown to involve structural damage to muscle banding patterns including disruption of sarcomere Z lines. Prostaglandin-induced swelling has been demonstrated to sensitize afferent nerve fibers of muscle connective tissue, which transmit sensation of dull pain to the central nervous system.

    1. Clarkson, PM. Muscle soreness: cause, consequence, and cure—Joseph B. Wolfe memorial lecture. American College of Sports Medicine 54th Annual Meeting: New Orleans, LA. May 30, 2007.
    2. Sellwood KL, Brukner P, Williams D, Nicol A, Hinman R. Ice-water immersion and delayed-onset muscle soreness: a randomized controlled trial. Br J Sports Med 2007 Jun;41(6):392-397.

58. Which of the following is the main arterial blood supply to the anterior cruciate ligament in the knee?

    A. Posterior tibial artery
    B. Superior medial genicular artery
    C. Anterior tibial artery
    D. Middle genicular artery

Correct Answer: D

The main blood supply of the anterior cruciate ligament is the middle genicular artery after it leaves the popliteal artery. The major innervation is the posterior articular nerve.

    1. Dienst M, Burks RT, Greis PE. Anatomy and biomechanics of the anterior cruciate ligament. Orthop Clin North Am 2002 Oct;33(4):605-620.

59. A Segond fracture is pathognomonic for which ligamentous injury?

    A. Medial collateral ligament
    B. Lateral collateral ligament
    C. Anterior cruciate ligament
    D. Posterior cruciate ligament

Correct Answer: C

A Segond fracture is a vertical avulsion fracture of the lateral tibial condyle, where the lateral capsular ligament attaches. It occurs with anterior cruciate ligament injuries.

1. Evaluation of ACL tear. Wheeless' Textbook of Orthopaedics. Accessed February 15, 2012 at www.wheelessonline.com/ortho/evaluation_of_acl_tear.
2. Segond fracture. Radiopaedia.org. Accessed February 15, 2012 at http://radiopaedia.org/articles/segond-fracture.
3. Levandowshi R, Cohen P. Knee injuries. In: Birrer RB, O'Connor FG (eds). Sports Medicine for the Primary Care Physician. 3rd ed. New York: CRC Press, 2004:633-634.

60. A 17-year-old football player exits the game after a play due to severe right shoulder pain. Pain symptoms are completely resolved by the time he is examined on the sideline, but he describes the pain as primarily over the lateral shoulder with some radiation to the posterior arm and lateral forearm. Examination reveals no deformity or tenderness to palpation of the shoulder. He has slight weakness to the deltoid, supraspinatus and infraspinatus muscles. He has normal muscle strength on shoulder shrug, biceps, triceps, grip strength, and wrist pronation, supination, flexion, and extension. He has mild sensory changes to the lateral shoulder but normal sensation over the arm, forearm, and hand. The most likely location for the injury is which of the following?

A. Radial nerve
B. Posterior cord
C. Upper trunk
D. Lower subscapular nerve
E. Lateral cord

Correct Answer: C

A stinger is defined as a stretch-type injury to the brachial plexus caused by forceful downward distraction of the shoulder while the neck side bends to the opposite side. Symptoms resolve in less than one minute. A radial nerve injury would cause sensory problems in the posterior arm and forearm and lateral aspect of the arm. The posterior cord would cause sensory problems over the lateral arm and motor problems to the subscapularis, teres major, deltoid, teres minor, and latissimus dorsi. Upper trunk injury would cause sensory changes to the shoulder joint and weakness to the supraspinatus, infraspinatus, and subclavius muscles. The lower subscapular nerve would innervate the subscapularis and teres minor but have no sensory innervation. Lateral cord injury would cause weakness to the pectoralis major and minor and no sensation changes.

1. Brachial plexus. Wheeless' Textbook of Orthopaedics. Accessed February 15, 2012 at www.wheelessonline.com/ortho/brachial_plexus.

61. During a preparticipation examination on one of your female high school cross country athletes, she admits to two episodes of fainting that occurred during last season's racing. Further questioning of both her and her parents reveals that these episodes occurred after she crossed the finish line, never during actual running, and are not associated with any other symptoms. She has no post-episode confusion and recovers quickly with minimal assistance. No significant cardiac history exists in her or her family. She has never had any workup for this before, and you are only able to do one test beyond a thorough history and physical examination, both of which are normal. The most helpful test at this point would be?

A. 12-lead ECG
B. Echocardiogram
C. Tilt table test
D. 24-hour event monitor

Correct Answer: A

Any athlete found to experience syncope related to exertion should have an electrocardiogram (ECG) before being cleared to return to sport. In post-exertion syncope, the most common cause is neurocardiogenic syncope related to postural hypotension. This is easily treated with simple measures such as laying the athlete in the head down/leg up position. In a young person with no other risk factors, this situation can be easily diagnosed by a thorough history and physical examination along with an ECG. Conditions such as HCM, prolonged QT interval, heart block, and pre-excitation syndromes such as Wolff-Parkinson-White may have characteristic findings indicating an arrythmogenic or structural cause of the event. If the ECG is normal and the history and examination highly suggest neurocardiogenic syncope, no further testing is needed. On the other hand, syncope occurring during active exercise has a greater likelihood of having structural or arrythmogenic causes and warrants complete cardiac evaluation.

1. McAward KJ, Moriarity JM. Exertional syncope and presyncope faint signs of underlying problems. Phys Sport Med 2005 Nov;33(11):7-20.

62. Two nights after a rapid ascent from sea level to an elevation of 3,500 m (11,500 feet), a non-acclimatized climber is experiencing symptoms of headache, dry cough, decreased exercise performance, tachypnea, and tachycardia at rest. In addition to descent, what is the most appropriate treatment for this climber?

    A. Dexamethasone
    B. High-flow oxygen
    C. Ibuprofen
    D. Furosemide
    E. IV fluids

Correct Answer: B

This climber is experiencing symptoms of high altitude pulmonary edema (HAPE). Early detection and treatment of HAPE decreases the mortality rate. HAPE usually occurs within two to four days of ascent above 2,500 m (8,200 feet). The incidence depends on rate of ascent, final altitude reached, and individual susceptibility. Symptoms may include persistent dry cough, decreased exercise tolerance, fatigue, central and peripheral cyanosis, tachycardia, and tachypnea at rest. Other symptoms (present in 50% of cases) of acute mountain sickness include headache, GI disturbance, insomnia, and dizziness. Pink or bloody sputum and respiratory distress occur late in the illness. Primary treatment of HAPE consists of descent and supplemental high-flow oxygen. Breathing supplemental oxygen can reduce pulmonary artery pressure 30% to 50% and increases arterial oxygen pressure, which can help reverse the effects of HAPE. Medications, if necessary, should be used as second-line treatment for HAPE because descent and oxygen are often definitive treatment. Dexamethasone is a treatment for high-altitude cerebral edema (HACE), and thus far has shown little to no benefit in treating HAPE. Ibuprofen may be used as an analgesic to help relieve the climber's headache; however, it will not treat the symptoms associated with HAPE. Furosemide has not consistently shown to be effective and has fallen out of favor as a treatment for HAPE. IV fluids are not indicated for HAPE. Of note, nifedipine (not listed as a choice) has been shown to decrease pulmonary vascular resistance and should be considered as adjunctive therapy if necessary. Nifedipine may also be used as prophylaxis. Studies have also shown phosphodiesterase inhibitors (tadalafil and sildenafil) and salmeterol (not listed as choices) to be beneficial in preventing HAPE.

1. Hackett PH, Roach RC. High-altitude illness. N Engl J Med 2001 Jul 12;345(2):107-114.
2. Committee to Advise on Tropical Medicine and Travel (CATMAT). Statement on high-altitude illnesses. Can Commun Dis Rep 2007 Apr 1;33(ACS-5):1-20.

63. When treating patients with osteoarthritis, what therapy program has been shown to be most effective in improving Western Ontario MacMaster (WOMAC) scores?

    A. Home exercise program to improve compliance
    B. Water therapy in a group setting
    C. Formal physical therapy for at least four weeks
    D. Supervised physical therapy followed by a home exercise program

Correct Answer: D

Both supervised physical therapy and a home exercise program improve function and pain scores, but the combination of the two is most effective in improving WOMAC scores.

1. Deyle GD, Allison SC, Matekel RL, Ryder MG, Stang JM, Gohdes DD, et al. Physical therapy treatment effectiveness for osteoarthritis of the knee: a randomized comparison of supervised clinical exercise and manual therapy procedures versus a home exercise program. Phys Ther 2005 Dec;85(12):1301-1317.

64. What is the most common cause of airway obstruction in an unconscious athlete?

    A. Mouthguard
    B. Tongue
    C. Swelling from anaphylaxis
    D. Inhaled foreign body

Correct Answer: B

The tongue is the one answer that would be present in all athletes. A mouthguard would be present only in contact sports. Anaphylaxis is a valid answer, but it is not the most common cause. Foreign body is also a valid option, but the inhalation of foreign bodies is not that common.

1. Weiss EA. Wilderness 911: A Step-by-Step Guide for Medical Emergencies and Improvised Care in the Back Country. Seattle: The Mountaineers Books, 1998.
2. American Heart Association. American Heart Association 2005 guidelines for cardiopulmonary resuscitation and emergency cardiac care. Circ 2005;112:IV-1-IV-5.

65. After going up for a rebound and being poked in the eye by an opponent's finger, a high school basketball player complains of eye pain, blurred vision, and sensation of something stuck in her eye. Which intervention may increase pain while the abrasion heals?

    A. Patching
    B. Topical NSAIDs (diclofenac)
    C. Oral analgesics (acetaminophen with codeine)
    D. Erythromycin ointment
    E. Topical mydriatic agent (1% cyclopentolate)

Correct Answer: A

Answer A is correct because there is level A evidence demonstrating that patching does not aid in corneal re-epithelialization and may increase pain in one half of all patients (Kaiser & Pineda). Topical NSAIDs may delay healing but will decrease pain and speed return to work/sport (level B). Oral analgesics will help decrease pain levels and have no effect on healing rates. Many practitioners will choose to prophylactically prescribe topical antibiotic ointments. This is not, however, evidence based. Topical mydriatic agents are ineffective for corneal abrasions (level A) but may decrease the patient's pain.

1. Kaiser PK, Pineda R II. A study of topical nonsteroidal anti-inflammatory drops and no pressure patching in the treatment of corneal abrasions. Corneal Abrasion Patching Study Group. Ophthalmology 1997 Aug;104(8):1353-1359.

2. Arbour JD, Brunette I, Boisjoly HM, Shi, ZH, Dumas J, Guertin MC. Should we patch corneal erosions? Arch Ophthalmol 1997 Mar;115(3):313-317.

3. Carley F, Carley S. Towards evidence-based emergency medicine: best BETs from the Manchester Royal infirmary. Mydriatics in corneal abrasion. Emerg Med J 2001 Jul;18(4):273.

4. Kabat AG, Sowka JW. Corneal atlas, part III: from abrasions to burns, how to manage corneal injuries. Review of Optometry 1999. Accessed February 15, 2012 at http://cms.revoptom.com/archive/issue/ro101f5.htm.

5. Peate WF. Work-related eye injuries and illness. Am Fam Physician 2007 Apr 1;75(7):1017-1022.

66. Which of the following is not true regarding iron deficiency anemia (IDA) in athletes?

   A. Women are at higher risk of developing IDA than men
   B. In the initial stage of IDA, serum iron concentrations are low while the ferritin and hemoglobin levels are normal
   C. Footstrike hemolysis is a known cause of IDA
   D. Inadequate calorie consumption and menstrual losses are common causes in female athletes

Correct Answer: B

Iron deficient anemia (IDA) is the most common true anemia found in athletes. Athletes are often asymptomatic but may also have symptoms including weakness, palpitations, shortness of breath, and pica. Women are at a higher risk of developing IDA than men due to menstruation and inadequate dietary intake of iron. Causes of iron loss in athletes include gastrointestinal, genitourinary, sweat, and foot strike hemolysis. Gastrointestinal losses are of the greatest importance. Initial lab values in IDA reveal only a low serum ferritin level (Answer B is the correct answer because the statement is incorrect). As the anemia progresses, the serum iron and hemoglobin concentrations will also drop.

1. Robertson JA, Ray TR. Hematologic problems in athletes. In: Madden CC, Putukian M, Young CC, McCarty EC (eds). Netter's Sports Medicine. Philadelphia: Saunders, 2010:209-211.

67. An obese patient (BMI > 30) without other comorbidities presents to your office. To improve compliance, one strategy for the patient's exercise prescription could include which of the following?

    A. Incorporating high-impact aerobic activities
    B. Emphasizing exercising after their morning meal
    C. Strict cardiovascular prescription at 85% maximum HR for at least 30 minutes five times per week
    D. Increasing weight-bearing activities very rapidly to increase metabolism
    E. Starting with non-weight-bearing activities such as swimming and recumbent bike

Correct Answer: E

In 2006, 49 of 50 states had an obesity rate of > 20% of the population, according to the CDC. Exercise prescription remains extremely important for both the sports medicine specialist and the primary care provider for these patients. Guidelines are specific for a generalized exercise prescription. Cardiovascular exercise should take place at least five days per week with the patient maintaining 85% of their maximum predicted HR for at least 20 minutes. In addition, progressive resistance training should be performed two to three days per week. Subsequent data also exists for patient's with comorbidities. This specific case deals with an obese patient without other comorbidities. A provider should prescribe non-weight bearing activities at first to avoid the increase stress on the lower extremities. The compliance rate alone for obese patients is very poor secondary to either pain or discouragement. Thus, the patient should perform as much exercise as they can (not the firm 20 minutes as stated above) to increase compliance. In addition, the patient should exercise prior to the morning meal to help with digestion. The lower the impact of the exercise prescription, the higher the compliance.

1. American College of Sports Medicine. ACSM's Guidelines for Exercise Testing and Prescription. 7th ed. Philadelphia: Lippincott Williams & Wilkins, 2006:216-219.
2. Healthy weight. Centers for Disease Control and Prevention. Accessed November 14, 2011 at www.cdc.gov/healthyweight/physical_activity/index.html.

68. A 17-year-old female presents after injuring her right knee. She was landing from a rebound and felt her knee "pop." She developed immediate swelling in the right knee and was unable to continue playing. On exam, the knee has a large effusion with positive Lachman and anterior drawer tests. Which of the following is true regarding her diagnosis?

    A. ACL injuries are less common in female athletes
    B. Traditional surgical reconstruction of the ACL may be performed in children regardless of physeal status
    C. The ACL is the primary restraint to posterior translation of the tibia with respect to the femur
    D. A hemarthrosis would be expected with aspiration of the injured knee
    E. Findings on standard radiography are usually specific for ACL injury

Correct Answer: D

ACL injuries are more common in female athletes. Surgical technique for reconstruction would depend on the physeal state with traditional approaches used if physes are closed or nearly-closed. The ACL is the primary restraint to anterior translation of the tibia. A hemarthrosis is suggestive for ACL injury. Standard radiographs are often normal or nonspecific.

1. Walsh MD, McCarty EC, Madden CC. Knee injuries. In: Madden CC, Putukian M, Young CC, McCarty EC (eds). Netter's Sports Medicine. Philadelphia: Saunders, 2010:421-422.
2. Maguire J. Anterior cruciate ligament pathology. Medscape. Accessed November 14, 2011 at www.emedicine.medscape.com.

69. An avid 25-year-old male cyclist, cycling 120 miles per week, complains of left testicular pain and some perineal numbness for the past two months. He has never experienced this before and reports no recent change in his equipment, training intensity, or duration in the recent month. He reports his pain as 6 to 8 out of 10 and is relieved by standing or walking. He has discussed this with his cycling teammates, and they have advised he consider changing his seat set-up and brand to a split seat to relieve his symptoms. The likely cause of his symptoms is which of the following?

    A. Pudendal nerve compression
    B. Adductor tendinopathy
    C. Ischial periositis
    D. Scrotal ischemia
    E. Testicular torsion

Correct Answer: A

Perineal symptoms including numbness of the genitalia were reported in 50% to 91% of all cyclists and erectile dysfunction was reported in 13% to 24% of all cyclists. Causes are related to compression of blood flow, soft tissue, or nerve compression. The interaction between the bicycle seat (saddle) and the perineum is the culprit in all cases of perineal symptoms in cyclists. The interaction is dependent on the vertical (downward) and shear (backward) force of the perineum on the saddle, the weight of the rider, the height and angle between the saddle and the handlebars, the saddle tilt angle, and the shape of the saddle. The narrow saddle is associated with more reduction of perineal blood flow and, therefore, more symptoms. In extreme cases of perineal pain, pudendal nerve entrapment can be a source of this pain. Some cyclists with induced pudendal nerve pressure neuropathy gained relief from improvements in saddle position and riding techniques or fluoroscopic guided injections.

1. Ramsden CE, McDaniel MC, Harmon RL, Renney KM, Faure A. Pudendal nerve entrapment as a source of intractable perineal pain. Am J Phys Med Rehab 2003 Jun;82(6):479-484.

70. In the absence of direct physical trauma, the activities with the highest incidence of spontaneous pneumothorax include SCUBA diving and which of the following?

    A. Soccer
    B. Weight lifting
    C. Football
    D. Swimming

Correct Answer: B

Spontaneous pneumothorax occurs due to bleb rupture in sports involving changes in intrathoracic pressure, including weight lifting and SCUBA diving. Pneumothorax is rare in football or soccer and associated with trauma, usually rib fracture. It is unlikely in swimming.

1. Morris GA. Scuba diving. In: Madden CC, Putukian M, Young CC, McCarty EC (eds). Netter's Sports Medicine. Philadelphia: Saunders, 2010:539-545
2. Partridge RA, Coley A, Bowie R. Sports-related pneumothorax. Ann Emerg Med 1997 Oct;30(4):539-541.

71. Which of the following is not a criterion for x-ray, according to the Ottawa Ankle Rules or Ottawa Foot Rules?

    A. Pain over the navicular
    B. Positive anterior drawer sign
    C. Bone tenderness at the posterior edge of either malleolus
    D. Inability to bear weight for four steps, either immediately or in the emergency room
    E. Pain over the base of the fifth metatarsal

Correct Answer: B

According to the Ottawa Ankle Rules, ankle x-rays are required only in the following circumstances: the presence of bone tenderness at the posterior edge of the distal 6 cm or tip of either malleolus. The patient is unable to weight-bear for at least four steps immediately after injury and at the time of evaluation. Foot x-rays are also indicated where there is bone tenderness at the base of the fifth metatarsal or at the navicular. The patient is unable to weight-bear for at least four steps immediately after injury and at the time of evaluation. The Ottawa Ankle Rules have been found to have a sensitivity of almost 100%, but they are not designed to be used in cases where intoxication, head injuries, multiple trauma, or sensory deficits are present.

1. Steil IG, Greenberg GH, McKnight RD, Nair RC, McDowell I, Worthington JR, et al. A study to develop clinical decision rules for the use of radiography in acute ankle injuries. Ann Emerg Med 1992 Apr;21(4):384-390.
2. Bachman LM, Kolb E, Koller MT, Steurer, TerRiet G. Accuracy of Ottawa ankle rules to exclude fractures of the ankle and mid-foot: systematic review. BMJ 2003 Feb 22;326(7386):417.

72. One of the new athletes to your college lists on his health history that he takes methylphenidate (Ritalin) for his attention deficit, hyperactivity disorder (ADHD). Regarding intercollegiate athletes taking stimulant medications, which of the following is a true statement (select the best answer)?

    A. The NCAA does not ban methylphenidate (Ritalin, Concerta) or amphetamine (Adderral) because their common use for the treatment of ADHD
    B. A medical exemption must be applied for and granted by the NCAA prior to athletic participation when stimulant medications are used for medical reasons
    C. The NCAA does not require the institution maintain, in the student-athlete's on-campus medical record, a copy of the physician's signed prescription for dispensing the medication
    D. The NCAA requires the institution to maintain, in the student-athlete's on-campus medical record, documentation from the prescribing physician detailing medical history, diagnosis, verification of that diagnosis through standard assessment, and dosing
    E. The NCAA tests for only anabolic substances and not stimulant medications

Correct Answer: D

The NCAA requires the institution to maintain, in the student-athlete's on-campus medical record, documentation from the prescribing physician detailing medical history, diagnosis, verification of that diagnosis through standard assessment, and dosing information. Amphetamine and methylphenidate are banned substances by the NCAA and the U.S. Anti-Doping Agency (Olympic committee), and these substances are included in testing programs. The United States Olympic Committee allows a therapeutic use exemption for athletes on stimulant medications in competition. The NCAA provides for medical exemption of stimulant medications as long as the institution maintains documentation from the prescribing physician that the standard assessment to diagnose ADHD as been completed. This documentation would be requested by the NCAA if there is a positive sample.

1. NCAA banned drugs and medical exemptions policy guidelines regarding medical reporting for student-athletes with attention deficit hyperactivity disorder (ADHD) taking prescribed stimulants. Accessed November 14, 2011 at www.ncaa.org/wps/wcm/conn ect/00e85e004e0b8a619ae5fa1ad6fc8b25/ADHD_QA2009.pdf?MOD=AJPERES&CA CHEID=00e85e004e0b8a619ae5fa1ad6fc8b25.
2. U.S. Anti-Doping Agency Drug Reference Online. Accessed November 14, 2011 at www. usantidoping.org.

73. A 19-year-old female tennis player comes to you for her preparticipation examination. She denies any cardiac symptoms and has always kept up with her peers. There is no history of heart disease or early death in the family. Examination is unremarkable except for a systolic ejection murmur that increases with Valsalva and standing, and decreases with fist clenching and squatting. Which of the following is the most significant predictor of sudden cardiac death in this athlete?

A. Sudden death in her brother
B. Muscle fiber disarray on biopsy
C. Septal thickness of > 1.8 cm
D. Paroxysmal atrial fibrillation on Holter monitoring
E. Resting BP 120/75, and BP 95/70 after six minutes of exercise

Correct Answer: E

This athlete has physical findings concerning for hypertrophic cardiomyopathy. In an asymptomatic patient with hypertrophic cardiomyopathy, many potential predictors of sudden death have been described. The most widely recognized risk factors are: marked LVH (> 3 cm), resuscitation from sudden death, multiple sudden deaths in the kindred, and (perhaps) non-sustained VT. Biopsy is usually normal, but may show myofibrillar disarray. None of these have been shown to be prognostic. The only prognostic sign that has been consistently shown to be present is a drop in blood pressure with exercise. The answer here is, therefore, E.

1. Beckerman J, Wang P, Hlatky M. Cardiovascular screening of athletes. Clin J Sport Med 2004 May;14(3):127-133.
2. Maron BJ. Sudden death in young athletes. N Engl J Med 2003 Sep 11;349(11):1064-1075.
3. Pelliccia A, Maron BJ, De Luca R, Di Paolo FM, Spataro A, Culasso F. Remodeling of left ventricular hypertrophy in elite athletes after long-term deconditioning. Circulation 2002 Feb;105(8):944-949.

74. A 21-year-old female is brought to the medical tent near the finish line at your community's annual marathon after suddenly collapsing moments after completing the race. Her mental status is normal, and her temperature is 103.6 degrees Fahrenheit (38.9 degrees Celsius). She reports feeling slightly lightheaded and has difficulty standing up. Your intial treatment strategy should include which of the following?

    A. Provide the patient with walking assistance until she no longer feels it is difficult to stand or walk
    B. Place the patient in a supine position so that both her legs and pelvis are elevated
    C. Provide IV fluid replacement with 5% dextrose in half normal saline
    D. Provide IV fluid replacement with 5% dextrose in normal saline
    E. Provide active cooling with ice water tub immersion until her temperature drops below 104 degrees Fahrenheit (38.0 degrees Celsius)

Correct Answer: B

Exercise-associated collapse (EAC) occurs in athletes who participate in endurance events. The onset of symptoms and signs of postural hypotension occur when the participant suddenly stops exercising. By definition, it is an athlete that requires assistance after or during an endurance event that is not orthopedic or dermatologic.

Initially, one should not try to walk or assist the patient with ambulation, as this may lead to further injury of the athlete or possibly the provider (Answer A). Instead, patients should be instructed to lie with their pelvis and legs elevated in a head-down position. Most patients will respond to this simple maneuver with rapid abatement of their symptoms in just a few minutes. This will allow blood that has pooled in the dilated veins within the lower extremities to return to the central circulating blood volume (Answer B).

IV fluids (Answers C and D) are not recommended as part of the initial management of EAC in a patient with normal mental status. Oral fluids are the preferred method of fluid replacement in all mild and moderate cases if tolerated by the athlete.

A rectal temperature in addition to blood pressure and heart rate should be recorded. Hyperthermia defined as a body temperature > 103 degrees Fahrenheit (39.5 degrees Celsius) and hypothermia < 97 degrees Fahrenheit (36.1 degrees Celsius) should be be diagnosed and treated appropriately. This patient is normothermic (termperature between 97 degrees Fahrenheit and 103 degrees Fahrenheit) and should have her temperature monitored and maintained, not actively cooled (Answer E).

1. Divine J, Takagishi J. Exercise in the heat and heat illness. In: Madden CC, Putukian M, Young CC, McCarty EC (eds). Netter's Sports Medicine. Philadelphia: Saunders, 2010:142.
2. Asplund CA, O'Connor FG, Noakes TD. Exercise-associated collapse: an evidence-based review and primer for clinicians. Br J Sports Med 2011 Nov;45(14):1157-1162.

75. Which of the following statements is correct?

    A. Congenital sensorineural deafness is associated with long QT syndrome
    B. Albuterol should be encouraged in patients with suspected congenital prolonged QT interval
    C. Taking ciprofloxacin prolongs the QT interval
    D. Athletes with known prolonged QT can be cleared to run the 110 m hurdles, but not to run the 1,500 m in track and field

Correct Answer: A

Sudden cardiac death in young athletes is rare. Long QT syndrome is not the most common cause of sudden cardiac death, but there are important clinical issues related to long QT. Most deaf children and adults do not have long QT syndrome. There is an association with deafness, however. This is an inherited genetic association. Many common medications, including some stimulants, prolong the QT interval. This is particularly important for patients with a borderline QT interval or those currently using other medications where an altered QT interval is a potential side effect. Drug-drug interactions can affect the QT enough to lead to disaster. Albuterol has been shown to prolong the QT interval in addition to causing hypokalemia. Cardiac clearance for sprinters and hurdlers is essentially the same as cardiac clearance for middle distance runners. Sprinters may run many miles during a workout, and distance runners will sprint during their training and races. Ciprofloxacin has been linked to injury to soft tissues, including tendon rupture, but not to long QT syndrome.

1. Maron BJ, Zipes DP. 36th Bethesda Conference: Eligibility recommendations for competitive athletes with cardiovascular abnormalities. J Am Coll Cardiol 2005;45(8)1361-1362.
2. McKeag DB, Moeller JL. ACSM's Primary Care Sports Medicine. 2nd ed. Philadelphia: Lippincott Williams & Wilkins, 2007.
3. Maron BJ, Zipes DP. 36th Bethesda Conference. Introduction: Eligibility recommendations for competitive athletes with cardiovascular abnormalities—general considerations. J Am Coll Cardiol 2005;45(8):1318-1321.

76. Hypertension is the most common cardiovascular disease that the sports medicine physician will encounter. There are many aspects of both the patient and his chosen sporting activity to consider when selecting a pharmaceutical intervention in the management of the hypertensive athlete. Select the choice that represents the best antihypertensive for the given athlete?

   A. White female biathlete (cross country ski and riflery): metoprolol
   B. White male Olympic weight-lifter: hydrochlorothiazide
   C. Black female swimmer with a history of cholinergic urticaria: lisinopril
   D. White male lacrosse player: valsartan
   E. White female marathoner with a prior history of thyrotoxicosis-related atrial fibrillation: diltiazem

Correct Answer: D

Essential hypertension is by far the most common cardiovascular disease encountered by the sports medicine physician. In the management of the hypertensive athlete, several things must be considered including the severity of the hypertension (blood pressure classification), cardiovascular disease risk factors, comorbid conditions, and the athlete's chosen exercise or sporting activities. Aside from therapeutic lifestyle changes, the sports medicine physician may consider pharmaceutical intervention in the management of the hypertensive athlete. It is important to select the medications that would give the optimal therapeutic effect while minimizing adverse effects and adhering to any regulations set forth by the governing body of the athlete's particular sports. Beta-blockers, such as metoprolol, have a negative inotropic and chronotropic effect and would likely suppress the cardiovascular performance necessary for aerobic exercise. They may also offer an unfair advantage in long range riflery and are prohibited by most shooting sport governing bodies. Diuretics, such as hydrochlorothiazide, may mask the presence of androgenic steroids and are explicitly prohibited by the International Olympic Committee. Nondihydropyridine calcium channel blockers, such as diltiazem, also have negative inotropic and chronotropic effects, making them a suboptimal choice for endurance athletes. Angiotensin-converting enzyme (ACE) inhibitors (such as lisinopril) and angiotensin-receptor blockers (such as valsartan) are among the best tolerated by hypertensive athletes. However, their resulting increase of bradykinins may put the hypertensive athlete with a history of cholinergic urticaria at increased risk for exercise-induced anaphylaxis.

1. Chobanian AV, Bakris GL, Black HR, Cushman WC, Green LA, Izzo JL, et al. The seventh report of the Joint National Committee on prevention, detection, evaluation, and treatment of high blood pressure: the JNC 7 report. JAMA 2003 May 21;289(19):2560-2572.

2. Sachtleben T, Fields KB. Hypertension in the athlete. Curr Sports Med Rep 2003 Apr;2(2):79-83.

3. O'Connor FG, Meyering CD, Patel R, Oriscello RP. Hypertension, athletes, and the sports physician: Implications of JNC VII, the fourth report and the 36th Bethesda Conference Guidelines. Curr Sports Med Rep 2007 Apr;6(2):80-84.

77. In patients with chronic pulmonary disease, endurance training is often beneficial with improved pulmonary function and less symptoms. Which of the following is true regarding pulmonary rehabilitation?

    A. The American Thoracic Society (ATS) recommends a specific strength training program
    B. Successful rehabilitation requires optimal medical management, including pharmacotherapy
    C. Pulmonary rehabilitation resembles cardiac rehabilitation with similar applications
    D. In pulmonary rehabilitation, the patient is encouraged to exercise to maximal effect without relying on oxygen supplementation

Correct Answer: B

Successful pulmonary rehabilitation requires optimal medical management including: pharmacotherapy, oxygen supplementation, psychological support. The response to rehabilitation should translate into improved ADLs. The exercise program should be based on sound scientific evidence with an understanding of pulmonary response to exercise and pathophysiology of the pulmonary dysfunction. Hypoxemia should be recognized and treated with supplemental oxygen when needed which increases lung exercise capacity and improves life expectancy (Answer D). The ATS actually makes no specific recommendation on strength training due to the lack of good supporting literature (Answer A). Answer D is incorrect because there are significant differences in pulmonary and cardiac rehabilitation. Cardiac rehabilitation has more immediate, potentially life-threatening risks. Pulmonary rehabilitation is more complex due to: older age range, poorer baseline level of conditioning, and the complex nature of pathophysiology of chronic pulmonary disease.

1. Cooper CB. Exercise in chronic pulmonary disease: aerobic exercise prescription. Med Sci Sports Exerc 2001 July;33(7 Suppl):S671-S679.
2. Celli BR. Respiratory muscle training and resting in COPD. UpToDate. Accessed November 26, 2011 at www.uptodate.com/contents/respiratory-muscle-training-and-resting-in-copd.
3. Scherer TA, Spengler CM, Owassapian D, Imhof E, Boutellier U. Respiratory muscle endurance training in chronic obstructive pulmonary disease: impact on exercise capacity, dyspnea, and quality of life. Am J Respir Crit Care Med 2000 Nov;162(5):1709-1714.

78. Factors associated with increased risk of primary exertional headaches include which of the following?

    A. Exercise in cold weather
    B. Dehydration
    C. Intense exercise at sea level
    D. Age above 40 years
    E. Previous head trauma

Correct Answer: B

The best answer is B. Factors that increase the risk of exertional headache include hot weather, dehydration, and high altitude. Exertional headache can be related to intracranial bleeding, brain tumors, and myocardial infarction. Benign exertional headache occurs most frequently in women with an average age of 24 +/- 11 years. Typically, exertional headaches last from five minutes to 24 hours and are bilateral and throbbing.

1. Putukian M. Headaches in the athlete. In: Mellion MB, Walsh WM, Madden C, Putukian M, Shelton GL (eds). Team Physician's Handbook. 3rd ed. Philadelphia: Hanley and Belfus, 2002:299-311.
2. Cutrer FM, Swanson JW, Dashe JF. Primary exertional headache. UpToDate. Accessed February 7, 2012 at www.uptodate.com/contents/primary-exertional-headache.

79. A 16-year-old female soccer player receives a direct blow to the mouth from an opposing player's elbow. She immediately comes to the sideline and is noted to have bleeding from her mouth. In her hand, she is holding an intact, avulsed tooth. Which of the following management options will help to ensure the best outcome?

    A. Gently wipe away blood and tissue remnants from the tooth with sterile saline-moistened gauze, preserve in saline, and refer to dentist immediately
    B. Clean the tooth with sterile saline, protect it in dry sterile gauze, and follow up with dentist within eight hours
    C. Reimplantation of the avulsed tooth and immediate referral
    D. Preserve the tooth in milk and ensure follow-up with her dentist within eight hours
    E. Discard the tooth and salvage and stabilize the underlying tissue with a protective mouth guard

Correct Answer: C

Emergency sideline treatment of dental injuries aims to maintain the viability of the pulp, to prevent abnormal root resorption, and to restore function and aesthetics. Immediate care of an avulsed tooth is essential to a good outcome. Specifically, reimplantation within two hours is highly successful (Answer C) and should be followed up with urgent referral to a dentist or other specialized provider. The avulsed tooth must be handled carefully, and efforts should be taken to avoid contact with the exposed root and periodontal ligaments, so Answer A is incorrect. When reimplantation is not possible, the tooth should be preserved in the patient's buccal muscoa, sterile saline, milk, or other commercial medium such as Hanks' Balanced Salt Solution. Milk may preserve a viable tooth for up to four hours, so the follow-up period in Answer D is incorrect. Answer B is incorrect since the tooth should not be allowed to dry. The tooth should never be discarded (Answer E).

1. Echlin P, McKeag DB. Maxillofacial injuries in sport. Curr Sports Med Rep 2004 Feb;3(1):25-32.

80. During a masters race in mid-March, one of the runners collapses and dies shortly thereafter. While running a marathon, which of the following is the most common cause of sudden death in older athletes (> 35 years old)?

A. Hyponatremia
B. Neurocardiogenic syncope
C. Cerebral vascular accident
D. Poorly controlled diabetes mellitus
E. Coronary artery disease

Correct Answer: E

Most cases of SCD are related to undetected cardiovascular disease. In the younger population, SCD is often due to congenital heart defects, while in older athletes (35 years and older), the cause is more often related to coronary artery disease. Among older (> 35 years old) athletes, available estimates suggest that the frequency of sudden cardiac death is in the range of one in 15,000 joggers per year or one in 50,000 participants in marathon per year, with a marked predominance of deaths in men. Atherosclerotic coronary artery disease is the most common form of heart disease relevant to the masters population as a cause of nonfatal or fatal cardiovascular events. Men aged 40 and older and women aged 50 and older should also have an exercise stress test and receive education about cardiac risk factors and symptoms.

1. Franklin B, Fern A, Voytas J. Training principles for elite senior athletes. Curr Sports Med Rep 2004 Jun;3(3):173-179.

2. Noakes TD. Sudden death and exercise. In: Fahey TD (ed). Encyclopedia of Sports Medicine and Science. Nov 1998. Accessed November 26, 2011 at www.sportsci.org/encyc/suddendeath/suddendeath.html.

3. Maron BJ, Epstein SE, Roberts WC. Hypertrophic cardiomyopathy: a common cause of sudden death in the young competitive athlete. Eur Heart J 1983 Nov; 4(Suppl F):135-144.

4. Diseases and conditions. Cleveland Clinic. Accessed Feb 14, 2012 at http://my.clevelandclinic.org/heart/disorders/electric/scd.aspx.

81. A tight end receives a blow with a helmet to the right side of the chest wall while stretched out for a pass. He complains of right sided pleuritic chest pain and progressive dyspnea. On exam, you note contusion and a step-off of the rib. The right lung field is hyperresonant, and there are decreased breath sounds on the right. There is asymmetry in inspiration with the right chest wall not moving. Which of the following are the best indications for emergent, on-field, needle thoracostomy?

    A. Trachea deviated left and BP 124/82
    B. Trachea deviated left and BP 90/40
    C. Trachea midline and BP 162/94
    D. Trachea deviated right and BP 162/94
    E. Trachea deviated right and BP 90/40

Correct Answer: B

Tension pneumothorax is uncommon in sports, but it may occur with collision sports. It presents with progressive dyspnea, pleuritic chest pain, subcutaneous emphysema, hyperresonance and decreased or absent breath sounds on the affected side, deviation of the trachea away from the affected side, jugular venous distention, cyanosis, tachycardia, and ultimately hypotension. It has been shown that that the physical signs can be unreliable in making the clinical diagnosis. However, needle thoracocentesis can be life-saving, but also increases morbidity if preformed unnecessarily. The indications for needle thoracentesis are an appropriate mechanism of injury, the typical physical findings, respiratory distress, and hemodynamic instability (hypotension). Therefore, in this case, left tracheal deviation and BP 90/40 would indicate the need for emergent, on-field, needle thoracocentesis. The other answers do not fit with the clinical scenario of tension pneumothorax. Studies from trauma centers have shown the procedure may be beneficial, but has also been inappropriately used in cases when there was no respiratory or hemodynamic instability.

1. Blackwell T. Prehospital care of the adult trauma patient. UpToDate. Accessed November 14, 2011 at www.uptodate.com.
2. Rich BSE, Betteridge BB, Richards SE. Management of on-site emergencies. In: McKeag DB, Moeller JL (eds). ACSM's Primary Care Sports Medicine. 2nd ed. Philadelphia: Lippincott Williams & Wilkins, 2007:161.

82. An 18-year-old male baseball pitcher presents with a one-month history of fatigue and weakness in his throwing arm. His symptoms gradually worsen with increasing pitch counts and will resolve with rest. He reports normal sensation in his hands, but reports his right hand will feel cool after he has finished pitching. You suspect subclavian artery compression. Which of the following provocative maneuvers may recreate his symptoms if he has subclavian artery compression?

A. Roos stress test
B. Tinel's test at the wrist
C. Spurling's maneuver
D. Inability of the patient to make a circle with the index finger and thumb

Correct Answer: A

The correct answer is A: Roos stress test. The Roos stress test is performed with the patient holding his shoulders in abduction and external rotation of 90 degrees while maintaining elbow flexion at 90 degrees. The patient repeatedly opens and closes his hands for several minutes. Reproduction of symptoms or a sensation of heaviness and fatigue is consistent with the diagnosis of thoracic outlet syndrome. Additionally, the Adson maneuver consists of neck extension and turning of the head toward the shoulder being tested while that shoulder is abducted and extended. The subject inhales while the examiner palpates the ipsilateral radial pulse. Diminution or elimination of the pulse and reproduction of the paresthesias are positive test results, provided that they do not occur on the asymptomatic, contralateral side. The Wright test is performed with the subject's arm progressively hyperabducted and externally rotated while assessing for ipsilateral radial pulse diminution and reproduction of paresthesias. The thoracic outlet syndrome (TOS) can include a neurologic and/or a vascular component. Neurologic TOS is compression of the brachial plexus, whereas the vascular TOS is the result of compression of the subclavian blood vessels as they emerge from the thorax and enter the upper limb. The thoracic outlet is considered the space bounded by the first rib and clavicle below, the pectoral tendon and coracoid process above, and the anterior and middle scalene muscles medially and laterally. Narrowing of this outlet, putting compression on either the brachial plexus or the subclavian artery and its tributaries, may result in the syndrome. Answer B is incorrect, as this is used to test for carpal tunnel syndrome. Answer C is incorrect, this is used to test for cervical spine/cervical root disorder. Answer D is incorrect, this is classic finding in anterior interosseous syndrome (AIS).

1. Safran MR. Nerve injury about the shoulder in athletes, part 2: long thoracic nerve, spinal accessory nerve, burners/stingers, thoracic outlet syndrome. Am J Sports Med 2004 Jun;32(4):1063-1076.
2. Nuber GW, McCarthy WJ, Yao JS, Schafer MF, Suker JR. Arterial abnormalities of the shoulder in athletes. Am J Sports Med 1990 Sep-Oct;18:514-519.

83. A patient presents to your office unable to dorsiflex his great toe. Which of the following is true?

   A. The extensor hallucis longus, which inserts on base of the distal phalanx of the great toe, is the muscle responsible for extending the great toe
   B. The motor function for this is from L4 and L5
   C. The muscles that allow this action are all contained in the lateral compartment of the lower leg
   D. The muscles that allow this action are inervated by the tibialis anterior nerve

Correct Answer: A

The extensor hallus longus originates on the medial fibula in the interosseous membrane and it inserts onto the base of the distal phalanx of the great toe. It is inervated by the deep peroneal nerve, not the tibialis anterior nerve and it is inervated by L5, not L4. The muscles that act as extensors of the foot and toe are the anterior compartment of the lower extremity. The lateral compartment contains the proneous longus, proneous brevis, and the peroneal nerve.

   1. Thompson JC. Netter's Concise Atlas of Orthopaedic Anatomy. Philadelphia: Saunders, 2002:51.

84. When evaluating anterior knee pain, the defining characteristics of patellar tendinitis include which one of the following?

    A. There are findings on imaging that are "pathognomonic" for patellar tendinitis
    B. Surgery is more effective than rehabilitation
    C. Patellar tendinitis is common and rarely requires treatment
    D. Training errors are the most common cause

Correct Answer: D

Other than age range (teens to 40s), the most common identifiable risk factors are training errors, usually tight hamstrings and quadriceps. This is a clinical diagnosis; however, characteristics when imaged suggesting patello-femoral tendinitis include osteopenia at the distal pole of the patella and tractional osteophyte in proximal patellar tendon. Ultrasound, bone scan, and MRI identify change in the posterior proximal third of the tendon. Imaging is primarily useful to rule out more significant pathology within the knee or when considering surgery. Surgery is no better than conservative therapy. Surgical debridement of full-thickness abnormal tissue, then rehabilitation to eccentric training compared with rehabilitation to eccentric training alone showed no change in jump height, leg press strength, pain scores, or return to sports with or without pain. Common complications range from inability to return to sport at 6 and 12 months to rare tendon rupture. Treatment includes relative rest and rehabilitation.

1. Cook JL, Khan KM. What is the most appropriate treatment for patellar tendinopathy? Br J Sports Med 2001 Oct;35(5):291-294.
2. Bahr R, Fossan B, Løken S, Engebretsen L. Surgical treatment compared with eccentric training for patellar tendinopathy (Jumper's Knee). A randomized, controlled trial. J Bone Joint Surg Am 2006 Aug;88(8):1689-1698.
3. Witvrouw E, Bellemans J, Lysens R, Danneels L, Cambier D. Intrinsic risk factors for the development of patellar tendinitis in an athletic population. A two-year prospective study. Am J Sports Med 2001 Mar-Apr;29(2):190-195.

85. You accept responsibility to cover a local football game in a stadium. Which of the following choices is your top priority for this or any other athletic event?

    A. Investigate EMS coverage
    B. Confirm AED availability
    C. Coordinate the entire sports medicine team in advance
    D. Review the chain of command with covering physicians
    E. Require an ATC to be present

Correct Answer: C

Agreement to cover a team implies assumption of leadership and responsibility for all aspects of events—especially liability. The development of a comprehensive emergency action plan (EAP) is essential. Emergencies are rarely predictable; the response must be rapid and controlled. Specific priorities and elements of the EAP include awareness of the venue (access, AED locations); credentials, skills, and assignment of duties of medical team; coordination with EMS (duties vary by locale); and communication among team members.

> 1. Mellion MB, Walsh W. The team physician. In: Mellion MB, Walsh WM, Madden C, Putukian M, Shelton GL (eds). Team Physician's Handbook, 3rd ed. Philadelphia: Hanley and Belfus, 2002:1-11.

86. Of the following, which is not an appropriate indication for the use of a sugar tong splint?

    A. Colles' fracture
    B. Prevention of supination
    C. Elbow immobilization
    D. Prevention of pronation
    E. Scaphoid fracture

Correct Answer: E

A Colles' fracture can be treated with a sugar tong splint. Answer B, C, and D are correct because a sugar tong splint prevents all those movements. Answer E is the correct choice because a sugar tong splint cannot appropriately immobilize the thumb, which is required for a scaphoid fracture.

> 1. Eiff MP, Hatch RL, Calmbach WL (eds). Fracture Management in Primary Care. 2nd ed. Philadelphia: W.B. Saunders, 2003:101,120.

87. A day after being struck with a pitched ball on the ulnar aspect of the left wrist and hand, a professional baseball player develops "pins and needles" in the small and ulnar half of his ring fingers. He finds it extremely difficult to grab the bat to participate in batting practice. After x-rays demonstrate no acute abnormalities of the left wrist and hand, he is diagnosed with Guyon's canal syndrome. What two bones form Guyon's canal?

A. Pisiform and triquetrum
B. Pisiform and hamate
C. Hamate and lunate
D. Triquetrum and lunate

Correct Answer: B

Guyon's canal syndrome is entrapment of the ulnar nerve as it passes through a tunnel in the wrist called Guyon's canal. The canal is formed by the most lateral bones of the proximal and distal carpal rows—the pisiform and hamate, respectively—and the ligament that connects them. The ulnar nerve is accompanied by the ulnar artery as it passes through this canal. Symptoms can include a sensation of pins and needles in the small and ulnar half of the ring fingers, decreased sensation in the same distribution, as well as weakness of the small muscles of the palm and the muscle that pulls the thumb toward the palm.

1. McKeag D, Moeller J. ACSM's Primary Care Sports Medicine. 2nd ed. Philadelphia: Lippincott Williams & Wilkins, 2007:412-413.

88. An important aspect of the preparticipation physical exam is the blood pressure reading. Which of the following statements is true regarding blood pressure readings in children?

   A. The JNC 7 classification of hypertension in adults can be also be used for children under age 18
   B. Stimulant use is rarely a cause for blood pressure elevation in children under age 18
   C. One isolated elevation in a child's blood pressure greater than 95th percentile should fully restrict sports participation
   D. Blood pressure charts based on sex, age, and height percentile should be used for children under age 18

Correct Answer: D

In the PPE setting, blood pressure should be measured with an appropriately sized cuff, should be repeated after sitting quietly for five minutes if initially elevated, and if needed checked again after 10 to 15 minutes of supine rest. Percentile of elevated blood pressure in children under age 18 should be determined from charts for classification by age, sex, and height percentile. Athletes with elevated blood pressure should be questioned about stimulant use (caffiene, nicotine, ephedrine). Mild to moderate hypertension (> 95th percentile) does not necessarily preclude the athlete from sports participation, but may require modified clearance until further evaluation. Severe hypertension (> 99th percentile) would require temporary clearance restriction until further evaluation.

1. Bernhardt D, Roberts WO. Preparticipation Physical Evaluation. 4th ed.: American Academy of Pediatrics, 2010:44
2. National High Blood Pressure Education Program Working Group on High Blood Pressure in Children and Adolescents. The fourth report on the diagnosis, evaluation, and treatment of high blood pressure in children and adolescents. Pediatrics 2004 Aug;144(2 Suppl 4th Report):555-576.

89. Which of the following statements about fibula fractures is true?

    A. The best x-ray view to identify whether there is any widening between the talus and fibula is the AP view

    B. A proximal fibula fracture (Maisonneuve) occurs most commonly secondary to an inversion mechanism

    C. A proximal fibula fracture (Maisonneuve) is usually unstable and requires orthopedic surgical referral and intervention

    D. A proximal fibula fracture (Maisonneuve) is usually stable and can be treated in a non-weight bearing cast

    E. A proximal fibula fracture (Maisonneuve) occurs most commonly from a direct blow to the proximal fibula

Correct Answer: C

A proximal fibula fracture (Maisonneuve) results typically from an eversion mechanism. These eversion injuries often lead to medial ankle ligament injury as well as syndesmotic injury and are inherently unstable. The best way to evaluate for this instability is with a mortise view that shows the space between the talus and fibula, which is necessary to evaluate for widening. A standard AP view shows overlap between the talus and fibula, making it difficult to evaluate for widening of the mortise. The inherent instability seen with these fractures makes orthopedic referral necessary for surgical stabilization.

1. Fields KB. Fibula fractures. UpToDate. Accessed November 15, 2011 at www.uptodate.com.

2. Wolfe MW, Uhl TW, Mattacola CG, McCulsky LC. Management of ankle sprains. Am Fam Physician 2001 Jan 1;63(1):93-104.

90. A mother brings her 15-year-old son in for evaluation of curvature of the back noted by the athletic trainer at his school. He has no complaints about back pain and a normal neurological exam. After your evaluation, to include a scoliosis radiographic evaluation, you identify that he has dextroscoliosis with a Cobb angle of 15 degrees. His Risser classification is Risser 3. On further exam, his leg lengths are equal. Which of the following is an appropriate recommendation for follow-up evaluation?

   A. Follow up with evaluation in six months
   B. Refer for physical therapy
   C. Refer to a pediatric spine surgeon
   D. Order a lumbar MRI
   E. Only follow up as needed if symptomatic

Correct Answer: A

Scoliosis is a common adolescent diagnosis. Many of these adolescents are identified in school, during preparticipation physical exam or incidentally during evaluation of back or related complaints. Although most scoliosis does not progress or require anything more than observation, the adolescent growth spurt is a period when these curvatures can progress. Peak growth velocities typically occur during Tanner 2-3 in girls and Tanner 3-4 in boys. Generally, the peak growth velocity period is ages 12 to 14 in girls and 13 to 15 in boys. A more objective measure of growth is the Risser classification, observing the closure of the iliac apophysis. The iliac apophysis develops early in adolescence and can be observed as a radiolucent line over the iliac crest on a pelvic AP view. This apophysis fuses from lateral to medial such that Risser 0 is no observed fusion, Risser 1 is fusion of the lateral 25%, Risser 2 up to 50%, Risser 3 up to 75%, Risser 4 up to 100%, and Risser 5 complete fusion. When peak growth velocity has passed and curvature is equal or less than 30 degrees, the likelihood of progression is very low. Magnetic resonance imaging (MRI) should be obtained in patients with an onset of scoliosis before eight years of age, rapid curve progression of more than 1 degree per month, an unusual curve pattern such as left thoracic curve, neurologic deficit, or pain.

1. Greiner KA. Adolescent idiopathic scoliosis: radiographic decision making. Am Fam Physician 2002 May 1;65(9):1817-1822.
2. Weiss HR, Negrini S, Rigo M, Kotwicki T, Hawes MC, Grivas TB, et al. Indications for conservative management of scoliosis (guidelines). Scoliosis 2006 May 8;1:5.

91. In the majority of people, the median nerve courses between the two heads of which one of the following muscles in the forearm?

    A. Supinator
    B. Pronator teres
    C. Flexor carpi ulnaris
    D. Pronator quadratus

Correct Answer: B

The median nerve passes between the two heads of the pronator teres at the elbow. Entrapment at this area may lead to symptoms such as a dull, ache-like pain in the forearm, fatigue of the arm, and/or reduced sensation in the radial three-and-a-half digits. This condition is called pronator syndrome since this is the most common location of a median nerve entrapment at the elbow. The radial nerve passes between the two heads of the supinator, and this is an area of radial nerve entrapment about the elbow and forearm. The ulnar nerve passes through the ulnar and humeral heads of the flexor carpi ulnaris muscle after exiting the cubital tunnel. The pronator quadratus muscle is in the distal forearm and does not cause entrapment neuropathies.

1. Mackinnon SE, Novak CB. Compression neuropathies. In: Green A, Wolfe S, Hotchkiss R, Pederson W, Kozin S (eds). Green's Operative Hand Surgery. 6th ed. Philadelphia: Churchill Livingston, 2010:985-994.

92. A female volleyball player is in clinic for a preparticipation evaluation. Her history is negative except for frequent right ankle sprains. Her exam shows a positive anterior drawer and mild weakness of her peroneal muscles. In addition to having her do an ankle rehabilitation program, you recommend she use which of the following prophylactic devices to most effectively reduce her rate of recurrence?

    A. High top shoes
    B. Ankle brace
    C. Medial shoe wedge
    D. Ankle elastic wrap

Correct Answer: B

A shoe that is supportive that prevents heel inversion may reduce ankle sprains, but the height of the shoe has not been shown to reduce ankle sprains. Prophylactic use of a double-upright ankle brace reduced ankle sprains in female volleyball players in a recent AJSM article. A lateral shoe wedge can also be used to reduce ankle sprains by preventing the heel to invert. A medial shoe wedge may predispose to ankle sprains.

1. Pedowitz DJ, Reddy S, Parekh SG, Huffman GR, Sennett BJ. Prophylactic bracing decreases ankle injuries in collegiate female volleyball players. Am J Sports Med 2008 Feb;36(2):324-327.

93. The most common nerve injury in glenohumeral shoulder dislocations is which of the following?

   A. Suprascapular nerve
   B. Axillary nerve
   C. Long thoracic nerve
   D. Radial nerve
   E. Musculocutaneous nerve

Correct Answer: B

The suprascapular nerve innervates the supra and infra spinatus muscles; injury is produced by stretching or compression, not dislocation. The axillary nerve is the most common nerve injured by shoulder dislocation. The long thoracic nerve is usually injured by a direct blow or compression, which leads to paresis of the serratus anterior and scapular winging. The radial nerve can be compressed at multiple sites along its course, even at the high axillary location. It is not typically injured during shoulder dislocation. While injury to the musculocutaneous nerve due to dislocated shoulder is reported, it is uncommon; more common is compression with excessive resistive elbow extension such as in bench press or push-ups.

1. Hodge DK, Safran MR. Sideline management of common dislocations. Curr Sports Med Rep 2002 June;1(3):149-155.

94. A 34-year-old African-American Florida native is visiting her cousin in Colorado in early January. Temperatures are near record lows (−80 degrees Fahrenheit, −62 degrees Celsius). While her cousin is at work, she decides to go out snowshoeing with cotton socks and bindings that are a bit tight. After about five minutes, she notices numbness in her toes. She comes in to urgent care with white, cold, and firm toes. Further questioning reveals that she has smoked one pack of cigarettes per day since age 18. The definitive treatment is which of the following?

A. Vigorously rub the toes with warm hands to stimulate circulation
B. Warm the toes by immersion in a 104-degree Fahrenheit (40-degree Celsius) whirlpool
C. Immediately amputate the affecte d toes
D. Wrap the affected toes with warm blankets
E. Use a small heater to warm the toes

Correct Answer: B

This patient has frostbite. Warming in a 104-degree Fahrenheit whirlpool is the definitive treatment (Answer B). Rubbing the toes can cause tissue damage and more loss (Answer A). Surgery should be delayed 90 days to assess areas of revitilization and mummification (Answer C). While wrapping the toes is a passive way of rewarming, the definitive treatment is immersion in a 104-degree Fahrenheit whirlpool.

1. Seto CK, Way D, O'Connor N. Environmental illness in athletes. Clin Sports Med 2005 Jul;24(3):695-718.

95. Which of the following is true regarding children and sports activity?

    A. Preteen athletes most commonly injure lower limbs, whereas teenagers injure upper limbs
    B. Salter-Harris II fractures generally require surgical intervention
    C. Joint dislocations and ligamentous injuries are more common than buckle and other types of fractures
    D. Physes close on average at 14.5 years in girls and 16.5 years in boys
    E. Non-union fractures are common in the immature skeleton

Correct Answer: D

After physeal closing, injury patterns are similar to those in adults, but physes close at about 15 years of age in girls and 17 in boys. Preteens have injuries in the upper limbs (Answer A), including contusions, strains, and simple fractures, whereas teenagers more commonly injure the lower limbs—knee injury being the most common. Salter-Harris II fractures (Answer B) are the most common type of physeal fracture at the transphyseal location with extension into the epiphysis and exiting from the joint. These do not often require surgical intervention. Open epiphyses are three to five times weaker than the surrounding capsular and ligamentous tissues so fractures are more common than dislocations and ligamentous injuries (Answer C). Non-union is rare because the immature skeleton forms callous early and heals quickly. Non-unions are more common in adults than children.

1. Miner C, Berg K. Youth sports issues. In: Mellion MB, Walsh M, Madden C, Putukian M, Shelton G (eds). Team Physicians Handbook. 3rd ed. Philadelphia: Hanley and Belfus, 2002:61-67.

96. In order to improve athletic performance, endurance athletes may train at altitude. Which of the following is true about this technique?

    A. Sleeping and training at altitude provide the best performance improvement
    B. Altitude training only improves performance for athletes of lower fitness levels
    C. The altitude required to create benefit is 3,000 m (9,800 feet) or greater
    D. Athletes with iron-deficiency status can gain significant benefits from this training technique
    E. The training effect can persist for three weeks after returning to previous living altitude

Correct Answer: E

Altitude training can improve performance in athletes of various fitness levels if certain conditions are met. Living high and training low, optimal training elevation of 2,100 m to 2,500 m, and having the greatest and most sustained elevation of erythropoetin provided the best response, while those with low iron stores did not improve performance.

1. Mazzeo RS, Fulco CS. Physiological systems and their responses to conditions of hypoxia. In: ACSM's Advanced Exercise Physiology. Philadelphia: Lippincott Williams & Wilkins, 2006:576-579.
2. Levine BD, Stray-Gunderson J. High-altitude training and competition. In: Madden CC, Putukian M, Young CC, McCarty EC (eds). Netter's Sports Medicine. Philadelphia: Saunders, 2010:158-161.

97. A three-phase bone scan can aid in the diagnosis of complex regional pain syndrome. Which of the following diagnostic findings would be the most helpful?

   A. Focal increased activity on bone scan
   B. Diffuse increased activity with juxta-articular accentuation uptake on delayed images
   C. Normal bone scan in late stage of syndrome
   D. Focal changes on phases 1 and 2

Correct Answer: B

Increased uptake is seen in two-thirds of adult patients with complex regional pain syndrome. It is usually diffuse but can be seen on delayed images the best. Focal increased activity is not consistent with complex regional pain syndrome.

1. Wheeler AH. Complex regional pain syndrome. Medscape. Accessed February 15, 2012 at http://emedicine.medscape.com/article/1145318.
2. Peterson AR, Bernhardt DT. Complex regional pain syndrome. In: The 5-Minute Sports Medicine Consult. 2nd ed. Philadelphia: Lippincott Williams & Wilkins, 2011:91-93.

98. Which of the following statements is correct in regards to the diagnosis of a pubic ramus stress fracture?

    A. Female soldiers are more susceptible to pubic rami stress fractures than male soldiers
    B. Plain films are the imaging study of choice to diagnose pubic rami stress fractures
    C. The hop test is not helpful in the clinical diagnosis of a pubic ramus stress fracture
    D. Pubic rami stress fractures are caused by the abductor and sartorius muscles pulling on the lateral aspect of the pubic ramus
    E. "Flamingo view" plain radiographs are useful in the diagnosis of a pubic ramus stress fracture

Correct Answer: A

Pubic rami stress fractures are relatively rare—only 1.25% of all stress fractures. They are more commonly seen in military recruits and female runners. An increase in the incidence of pubic rami stress fractures corresponds to the increase in female participation in marathon running. Women are more susceptible to pubic rami stress fractures than men. The reason that women are more susceptible to pubic stress fractures is unknown, but may be related to the different anatomical configuration of the female pelvis or differences in gait. Although highly sensitive in the detection of stress fractures, radionuclide bone scintigraphy lacks specificity and provides poor anatomical detail. It has been reported to be falsely positive in as high as 32% of patients presenting with hip or groin pain. This is presumably due to high osteoblastic activity in the area because of high stress loads and constant remodeling. Periosteitis, adductor tendonitis, and avulsion fractures are other causes of a positive bones scan. An MRI has both sensitivity and specificity for detecting pubic rami stress fractures as well as those arising from the femoral neck, acetabulum, and sacrum. A fatigue fracture of traumatic etiology involving the bony attachment of the gracilis muscle to the pubic ramus is termed the "gracilis syndrome." This results in an avulsion fracture of the tendinous insertion of the gracilis muscle at the anterior edge of the inferior pubic ramus. Pubic rami stress fractures differ from other sites as being caused by a response to tensile forces rather than compressive forces. The tensile forces are produced by muscular forces of the adductor and gracilis muscles pulling on the lateral aspect of the pubic ramus and ischium during hip extension. Radiographic evaluation with plain films has shown limited usefulness in the diagnosis of pelvic and femoral neck stress fractures. Bony changes typically lag behind onset of symptoms by two to four weeks and 50% of patients who have stress fractures never exhibit changes on plain films. "Flamingo view" plain films are useful in diagnosing osteitis pubis. These views are performed anteroposteriorly with alternating unilateral lower extremity weight bearing. Instability of the pubic symphysis, which is characteristic of osteitis pubis, is suggested when the symphysis is widened more than 7 mm or when the top surfaces of the superior pubic rami move more than 2 mm.

1. Nelson EN, Kassarjian A, Palmer WE. MR imaging of sports-related groin pain. Magn Reson Imaging Clin N Am 2005 Nov;13(4):727-742.
2. Morelli V, Espinoza L. Groin injuries and groin pain in athletes: part 2. Prim Care 2005 Mar;32(1):185-200.
3. Wiley JJ. Traumatic osteitis pubis: the gracilis syndrome. Am J Sports Med 1983 Sep-Oct;11(5):360-363.

99. Concerning the prevalence of exercise-induced bronchoconstriction (EIB) in athletes, _____% of all asthmatics have airways hyperreactive to exercise, and _____% of cross country skiers are reported to have EIB?

A. 50% to 90% and 50%
B. 25% to 50% and 15%
C. > 90% and 25%
D. > 90% and < 10%

Correct Answer: A

Exercise is the most common trigger of bronchospasm in known asthmatics. 50% to 90% of asthmatics experience bronchoconstriction in response to exercise. Though unrecognized EIB may be a significant percentage of total cases, many high level athletes report this diagnosis. The prevalence is especially high in cold weather sports (18% to 26% in Winter Olympic athletes) and is reported as 50% in cross country skiers.

1. Parsons JP, Mastronarde JG. Exercise-induced bronchoconstriction in athletes. Chest 2005 Dec;128(6):3966-3974.

100. A thumb spica cast is the treatment of choice for which of the following fractures?

    A. Boxer's fracture
    B. Colles' fracture
    C. Scaphoid fracture
    D. Lisfranc fracture
    E. Hangman's fracture

Correct Answer: C

A boxer's fracture should be treated with a Gutter or Burkhalter-type splint. A Colle's fracture should be treated with a short arm cast with the wrist in neutral position or a long arm cast with the wrist in slight flexion and ulnar deviation, the forearm in neutral position, and the elbow at 90 degrees. A Lisfranc fracture should be referred immediately because anatomic reduction is essential. A hangman's fracture requires surgical stabilization.

1. Eiff MP, Hatch RL, Calmbach WL. Fracture Management for Primary Care. 2nd ed. Philadelphia: Saunders, 2003:76, 101, 120, 217, 343.

101. Skeletal muscles that function as a group to stabilize the scapula against the posterior thoracic wall during upper extremity overhead activities include which of the following?

    A. Levator scapulae, rhomboid major, rhomboid minor, and serratus anterior
    B. Supraspinatus, infraspinatus, subscapularis, and teres minor
    C. Thoracic paraspinals, trapezius, latissimus dorsi, and posterior intercostals
    D. Deltoid, triceps brachii, pectoralis major, and pectoralis minor

Correct Answer: A

Levator scapulae elevates the scapula. Serratus anterior protracts and laterally rotates the scapula. Rhomboid major and minor retract and elevate the scapula. These muscles work together to control the position of the scapula and stabilize it against the posterior thoracic wall, thus providing a stable base for the glenohumeral articulation during overhead activities involving the upper extremity. Answer B represents the rotator cuff muscles, which stabilize the humeral head in the shoulder joint. Answer C does not stabilize against the posterior thoracic wall as a group. Answer D has lateral stabilizers mentioned.

1. Interactive Shoulder—Sports Injuries Edition 2.0. Thorax and Arm. Available at www. anatomy.tv/home.aspx.
2. Brukner P, Khan K. Clinical Sports Medicine. 2nd ed. Roseville (NSW): McGraw-Hill Australia; 2000:69-75.
3. The shoulder girdle. SUNY Health Science Center. Accessed February 15, 2012 at www. upstate.edu/cdb/education/grossanat/limbs3.shtml.

102. A high school football player presents to your clinic with his parents. They seek information about nutrition and supplements for athletes. Which of the following statements is true regarding nutrition and high intensity exercise?

    A. Fat is broken down to glycogen during exercise
    B. With regard to training in a hot, humid environment, thirst is a sensitive and reliable indicator of dehydration and estimating fluid loss
    C. Due to the increased demand on an athlete's body, protein supplements are necessary in addition to a healthy diet
    D. An athlete's diet should consist of about 60% carbohydrates

Correct Answer: D

60% of an athlete's diet should consist of carbohydrates. It is the main energy source for the body. During exercise, fats are broken down to fatty acids, which are carried to muscles and converted to ATP. Because the thirst mechanism lags behind the body's need for fluid replacement, thirst is not a good initial indicator of dehydration. Fluids should be ingested before, during, and after exercise. Although athletes need more protein than non-athletes, athletes consume more calories and thus consume more dietary protein, fulfilling the daily protein requirements. Supplements are not needed.

1. Manore MM. Exercise and the Institute of Medicine recommendations for nutrition. Curr Sports Med Rep 2005 Aug;4(4):193-198.
2. Robins A. Nutritional recommendations for competing in the Ironman triathlon. Curr Sports Med Rep 2007 Jul;6(4):241-248.
3. Casa DJ. American College of Sports Medicine roundtable on hydration and physical activity: consensus statements. Curr Sports Med Rep 2005 Jun;4(3):115-127.

103. Which of the following is true of hypertrophic cardiomyopathy?

    A. Hypertrophic cardiomyopathy (HCM) is a genetic disorder with an autosomal recessive pattern of inheritance
    B. HCM is characterized by right ventricular wall thickness of > 5 mm
    C. The murmur associated with HCM is exacerbated by the Valsalva maneuver
    D. Most patients have detectible signs of HCM before sudden death
    E. The best initial test for diagnosis is cardiac CT

Correct Answer: C

HCM is autosomal dominant in familial inheritance, and it is characterized by right ventricular wall thickness of 15 mm. The upper limit of normal wall thickness is 12 mm, and the gray zone is 13 mm to 14 mm. Valsalva maneuvers and position changes to standing will increase the murmur. Occasionally, no murmur is present. Most patients have no presenting signs or symptoms before sudden death; therefore, a thorough family history is critical for a physician to obtain for optimal screening. ECG is the best initial screening test for suspicion of HCM. Echocardiography is the best initial test after an abnormal ECG, although cardiac MRI is also being used to help rule in HCM.

1. Corrado D, Drezner J, Basso C, Pelliccia A, Thiene G. Strategies for the prevention of sudden cardiac death during sports. Eur J Cardiovasc Prev Rehabil 2011 Apr;18(2):197-208.
2. Gersh BJ, Maron BJ, Bonow RO, Dearani JA, Fifer MA, Link MS, et al. American College of Cardiology Foundation/American Heart Association Task Force on Practice Guidelines; American Association for Thoracic Surgery; American Society of Echocardiography; American Society of Nuclear Cardiology; Heart Failure Society of America; Heart Rhythm Society; Society for Cardiovascular Angiography and Interventions; Society of Thoracic Surgeons. 2011 ACCF/AHA guideline for the diagnosis and treatment of hypertrophic cardiomyopathy: executive summary: a report of the American College of Cardiology Foundation/American Heart Association Task Force on Practice Guidelines. Circulation 2011 Dec 13;124(24):2761-2796.
3: Seto C. The preparticipation physical exam: an update. In: Miller MD (ed) Clinics in Sports Medicine. Philadelphia: Elsevier, 2011: 491-501.

104. In response to intense exercise, catecholamine release will occur. These hormones can lead to several effects in the athlete. Which of the following is due to alpha receptor effect?

    A. Vasoconstriction
    B. Cardiac acceleration
    C. Lipolysis
    D. Bronchodilatation
    E. Increased myocardial contractility

Correct Answer: A

Only vasoconstriction is an alpha receptor controlled mechanism in this setting. Cardiac acceleration, increased myocardial contractility, and lipolysis are beta-1 receptor effects (Answers B, C, and E). Bronchodilatation is a beta-2 effect (Answer D).

1. Alpha adrenergic receptor. Family Practice Notebook. Accessed February 17, 2012 at www.fpnotebook.com/neuro/pharm/AlphAdrnrgcRcptr.htm.

105. A 21-year-old senior female softball player presents to the clinic with left-sided abdominal pain. She says she first noticed the pain after hitting a double and sliding head-first into second base in last night's game. She was able to finish the inning, but felt like she had trouble taking a deep breath and removed herself from the game. Today, she says she is breathing okay, but still has pain with deep inspiration. She has pain with trunk rotation and bending, and bruising in the antero-lateral abdomen of the left side. She has bilateral breath sounds equal in nature, and she is tender to palpation along her ribs and the abdominal wall of the left side. A chest x-ray and vital signs are normal. Her pain has likely resulted from which of the following?

    A. Rib fracture
    B. Costochondritis
    C. Internal oblique strain
    D. Splenic hematoma

Correct Answer: C

The question addresses a common mechanism of tearing an abdominal wall muscle: the swinging of a bat. A rib fracture would be uncommon even with a head-first slide. Costochondritis typically does not have bruising, and has a more confined area of tenderness. A splenic hematoma is possible, but would more likely present from more severe trauma, be accompanied by hemodynamic changes, or have an associated history of mono-like symptoms.

1. Connell D, Jhamb A, James T. Side strain: a tear of internal oblique musculature. Am J Roentgenol 2003 Dec;181(6):1511-1517.
2. Stevens KJ, Crain JM, Akizuki KH, Beaulieu CF. Imaging and ultrasound-guided steroid injection of internal oblique muscle strains in baseball pitchers. Am J Sports Med 2010 Mar;38(3):581-585.

106. An afebrile patient with acute low back pain notices pain going down the posterior-lateral aspect of her right thigh and leg. It is noted on your exam that she has the following: (+) straight leg raise test, a slight sensory deficit over the lateral aspect of the right lateral foot, a diminished Achilles tendon reflex and weakness with plantar flexion of the great toe. It is also noted that it is hard for her to walk on her toes. Which nerve root is most likely affected?

    A. L3
    B. L4
    C. L5
    D. S1
    E. L2

Correct Answer: D

This question focuses on knowing nerve root innervation and the dermatomes of the lower extremity. The S1 nerve root supplies sensation to the lateral aspect of the foot, is responsible for the ankle reflex, and gives strength in plantar flexion.

1. Melanga GA. Lumbosacral radiculopathy. Medscape. Accessed February 17, 2012 at http://emedicine.medscape.com/article/95025.
2. Humphreys SC, Eck JC. Clinical evaluation and treatment options for herniated lumbar disc. Am Fam Physician 1999 Feb;59(3):575-582, 587-588.

107. A 16-year-old male long jumper lands awkwardly with his right knee hyperextended, collapsing in the pit. He experiences acute swelling of the right knee immediately. He has a past medical history of resolved bilateral jumper's knee and prominent tibial tubercles diagnosed two years ago. There is anterior deformity and swelling immediately distal to the patella. Which of the following statements is true regarding tibial tubercle apophyseal fracture?

A. Patients with type II and III fractures of the tibial tubercle are able to actively extend the knee against gravity several degrees

B. Negative Lachman testing immediately after injury eliminates rupture of the anterior cruciate ligament as a possibility

C. Fracture at the tibial apophysis can be comminuted, displaced, or involve the tibial articular surface

D. Osgood Schlatter's disease is not associated with tibial tubercle fracture

Correct Answer: C

Type II fractures involve the inferior pole of the patella and type III fractures include the anterior tibial epiphysis. They may also be Salter Harris III or V fractures, depending on extent of damage to the tibial articular surface and growth plate respectively. Type I injuries involve the apophysis alone. The remaining patellar tendon/apophyseal unit allows terminal extension against gravity. In types II and III, active terminal extension is no longer possible due to complete disruption of tubercle/patellar anchor. This mechanism of injury is compatible with severe injuries, including ACL rupture, collateral ligament, and meniscal injury. Tibial apophyseal fractures and ACL rupture both may exhibit acute massive hemarthrosis. Complete assessment of suspected pediatric tibial tubercle avulsion requires MRI. Osgood Schlatter's disease (OSD) may predispose to tibial tubercle fracture. Rosenberg demonstrated with imaging that OSD is caused by tendinopathy at the anterior ossification center of the tibial tubercle and not apophysitis. One theory notes an association of OSD to subsequent comminuted fractures.

1. Ramachandran M, Skaggs DL. Physeal injuries. In: Green NE, Swiontkowski MF.. Skeletal Trauma in Children. 4th ed. Philadelphia: Saunders Elsevier, 2009:19-40.

2. Rosenberg ZS, Kawerblum M, Cheung YY. Osgood-Schlatter lesion: fracture or tendinitis? Scintigraphic, CT, and MR imaging features. Radiology 1992 Dec;185(3):853-858.

3. Ogden JA, Tross RB, Murphy MJ. Fractures of the tibial tuberosity in adolescents. J Bone Joint Surg Am 1980 Mar;62(2):205-215.

108. Which of the following statements is true regarding stretching and flexibility?

   A. Stretching has been proven to decrease rates of muscle injuries
   B. Stretching is most beneficial if performed 30 minutes prior to exercise
   C. Ballistic stretching should be avoided by all individuals, as it predisposes to muscle injury
   D. Increasing muscle temperature with light cardiovascular exercise is as adequate as stretching to increase muscle flexibility prior to exercise

Correct Answer: D

There are no definitive studies to indicate that stretching reduces the rates of muscle injuries; however, there is also not enough evidence to discourage its use. The ACSM recommends that stretching be incorporated into the warm-up and cool-down phases of exercise. However, there is some evidence to suggest that stretching prior to exercise may compromise the force-producing capabilities of muscle and should be avoided prior to strength training. A stretching regimen may consist of static, ballistic, dynamic, or proprioceptive neuromuscular facilitation stretching. The type of program utilized depends on the experience and fitness of the individual as well as his existing flexibility and injury history. Ballistic stretching that involves bouncing movements which quickly exaggerate joint ROM may be more appropriate for a more experienced athlete with no prior injury history due to the theoretical risk of ballistic stretching predisposing an individual to injury. There is evidence to suggest that applying heat packs to a muscle or increasing core body temperature with light cardiovascular exercise is equivalent to stretching in increasing muscle flexibility.

   1. Weir JP, Cramer JT. Principles of musculoskeletal exercise programming. In: Kaminsky LA (ed). ACSM's Resource Manual for Guidelines for Exercise Testing and Prescription. 5th ed. Philadelphia: Lippincott Williams & Wilkins, 2006:350-365.
   2. Thacker SB, Gilchrist J, Stroup DF, Kimsey CD Jr. The impact of stretching on sports injury risk: a systematic review of the literature. Med Sci Sports Exerc 2004 Mar;36(3):371-378.

109. Lisfranc injuries involve a disruption in which of the following joints?

    A. Inter-phalangeal joint
    B. Metatarsal-phalangeal joint
    C. Tarsal-navicular joint
    D. Tarsal-metatarsal (T-MT) joint

Correct Answer: D

Unrecognized injuries to the tarsal-metatarsal joint (Lisfranc) may be debilitating and produce chronic pain; thus, it is important to recognize these injuries early. Comparison AP weight-bearing and oblique views are often helpful to help identify these injuries.

    1. Latterman C, Goldstein JL, Wukich DK, Lee S, Bach BR. Practical management of Lisfranc injuries in athletes. Clin J Sport Med 2007;17:311-315.
    2. Burroughs KE, Reimer CD, Fields KB. Lisfranc injury of the foot: a commonly missed diagnosis. Am Fam Physician 1998 Jul;58(1):118-124.

110. You are performing a preparticipation exam on one of your patients, who happens to be a student at the high school you cover. Of the following items, which one would require further evaluation?

    A. Mononucleosis three years ago
    B. Mildly enlarged liver
    C. Non-palpable spleen
    D. Small tattoo
    E. History of appendectomy

Correct Answer: B

Answers A, C, D, and E are frequently seen in the younger population. While noting the history of the appendectomy, no further workup is necessary. Remote history of mononucleosis that has resolved does not require reevaluation. Absence of splenomegaly is reassuring, and clearly does not need further inquiry. The small tattoo has no relevance to suitability for athletics, unless it is somehow related to the enlarged liver or other medical problem. Answer B, the finding of any enlargement in the liver via exam, warrants further evaluation, including a history of tattoos, of course, and is the best answer.

    1. Wappes JR (ed). Preparticipation Physical Evaluation. 3rd ed. Minneapolis: McGraw-Hill, 2005.
    2. Myers A, Sickles T. Preparticipation sports examination. Prim Care 1998 Mar;25(1):225-236.

111. Which of the following is a property of anabolic steroids?

    A. They increase the actions of glucocorticoids and help metabolize ingested proteins, converting a negative nitrogen balance into a positive one
    B. They give the athlete a state of euphoria and decreased fatigue that allows the athlete to train harder and longer
    C. Anabolic effects increase the number of muscles in the body for larger size and strength and better performance
    D. They may induce hypotension, lung tumors, and delayed closure of growth plates
    E. Androgenic effects will not increase or decrease libido along with other side effects like gynecomastia

Correct Answer: B

Anabolic steroids are testosterone derivatives with three main mechanisms of action. The anticatabolic effects reverse the actions of glucocorticoids and help metabolize ingested proteins, converting a negative nitrogen balance into a positive one. The anabolic effects directly induce skeletal muscle synthesis, but they do not increase the number of muscles in the body. When muscle synthesis is increased, athletes experience better strength and performance as well as larger mass of muscles. The "steroid rush" is a state of euphoria and decreased fatigue that allows the athlete to train harder and longer. A randomized double-blind study of 40 men examined the effects of supraphysiologic testosterone doses and compared placebo with or without weight training with testosterone doses with or without weight training. The subjects in the exercise plus testosterone group had a 9% increase in mass and 23% increase in strength compared with 3% and 9% in the exercise plus placebo group. These doses were comparable with the doses that many athletes who use steroids take. Adverse effects of steroids include: sexual side effects like decreased or increased libido, decreased sperm production, gynecomastia, and hirsutism; psychiatric effects like euphoria, aggression or personality disorders; and serious irreversible side effects including hypertension, severe tendon ruptures, liver tumors, psychosis, premature closure of growth plates, and irreversible hirsutism and voice changes in women. Most sports organizations have rules that ban the use of anabolic steroids for any reason.

1. Ahrendt D. Ergogenic aids: counseling the athlete. Am Fam Physician 2001 Mar;63(5):913-922.
2. Bhasin S, Storer TW, Berman N, Callegari C, Clevenger B, Phillips J, et al. The effects of supraphysiologic doses of testosterone on muscle size and strength in normal men. N Engl J Med 1996 Jul 4;335(1):1-7.

112. Which of the following best describes the correct effect of cryotherapy in treatment of injuries?

    A. Cryotherapy increases tissue metabolism
    B. Cryotherapy decreases the pain threshold
    C. Cryotherapy decreases pain post operatively
    D. Cryotherapy increases motor perfusion
    E. Cryotherapy increases nerve conduction

Correct Answer: C

Cryotherapy is frequently used in the management of athletic injuries. Cryotherapy leads to vasoconstriction. Cryotherapy decreases tissue metabolism, inflammatory response, motor perfusion, recovery time, and muscle spasm. Cryotherapy increases the pain threshold.

1. Mellion MB, Putukian M,. Physical therapy modalities. In Mellion MB, Putukian M, Madden CC. Sports Medicine Secrets. 3rd ed. Philadelphia: Hanley-Belfus, 2003:409-416.

2. Swenson C, Swärd L, Karlsson J. Cryotherapy in sports medicine. Scand J Med Sci Sports 1996 Aug;6(4):193-200.

3. MacAuley DC. Ice therapy: how good is the evidence? Int J Sports Med 2001 Jul;22(5):379-384.

4. Mayer JM, Mooney V, Matheson LN, Erasala GN, Verna JL, Udermann BE, et al. Continuous low-level heat wrap therapy for prevention and early phase treatment of delayed-onset muscle soreness of the low back: a randomised conrolled trial. Arch Phys Med Rehabil 2006 Oct; 87(10):1310-1317.

113. With a scaphoid fracture, non-union is a common complication. Which fracture location order shows the correct risk for non-union, from most likely to least likely?

    A. Proximal pole, distal pole, waist
    B. Waist, distal pole, proximal pole
    C. Proximal pole, waist, distal pole
    D. Distal pole, waist, proximal pole
    E. Waist, proximal pole, distal pole

Correct Answer: C

The blood supply to the scaphoid bone enters on one end only, resulting in a high rate of nonunion, malunion, and avascular necrosis following scaphoid fractures. Because these fractures do not always show up on the initial plain radiograph, a high index of suspicion is required in order to treat the patient effectively. A fall onto an outstretched arm may cause a variety of specific injuries from the proximal humeral head and the gleniod down to the wrist and hand. This mechanism is a common cause of fractures of the scaphoid. Snuffbox tenderness on the physical exam is an important finding and should not be overlooked, even when the injury appears otherwise benign. 70% of all carpal fractures involve the scaphoid due to the central stabilizing role it serves within the wrist. The blood supply enters distally. The more proximal fractures have the longest healing times and are most susceptible to nonunion and AVN.

1. McKeag DB, Moeller JL. ACSM's Primary Care Sports Medicine. 2nd ed. Philadelphia: Lippincott Williams & Wilkins, 2007.
2. DeLee JC, Drez D Jr, Miller MD (eds). DeLee & Drez's Orthopaedic Sports Medicine. 2nd ed. Philadelphia: Saunders Elsevier, 2003.
3. Boles C. Scaphoid fracture imaging. Medscape. Accessed December 11, 2011 at http://emedicine.medscape.com/article/397230-overview.

114. A storm is approaching during a high school football game you are covering. You notice what appears to be a lightning strike in the distance but still have clear skies overhead. The most correct evaluation of the situation is which of the following?

    A. Since the most severe storms are only dangerous in the spring, you decide the players, coaches, and others are safe
    B. You should watch for a funnel cloud, as that would present the most likely danger. You, therefore, will take action when the funnel cloud is spotted
    C. You know that with the clear skies overhead that immediate danger is unlikely and continue to watch for further changes in the weather
    D. You realize that lightning can strike in a large radius surrounding any storm and decide to take the next appropriate step

Correct Answer: D

Lightning is an obvious risk to any outdoor event, and its risk cannot be overstated. A team physician needs to have a plan in place to respond to approaching storms and other weather risks. The old adage that "it will pass" puts everyone as risk for injury and in the worst case, mass casualty and injuries.

1. Walsh KM, Hanley MJ, Graner SJ, Beam D, Bazluki J. A survey of lightning policy in selected Division I colleges. J Athl Train 1997 Jul;32(3):206-210.
2. Walsh KM, Bennett B, Cooper MA, Holle RL, Kithil R, López RE. National Athletic Trainers Association position statement: lightning safety for athletics and recreation. J Athl Train 2000 Oct;35(4):471-477.
3. Makdissi M, Brukner P. Recommendations for lightning protection. Sport. Med J Aust 2002 Jul 1;177(1):35-37. Comment in: Med J Aust 2002 Oct 21;177(8):463-464; author reply 464. Comment in: Med J Aust 2002 Oct 21;177(8):464.

115. A 45-year-old tennis player presents with six weeks of low back pain with radiation to the left big toe made worse with bending over to tie his shoes. He wants to do physical therapy, and you write a prescription for which of the following back programs to reduce his current symptoms of pain?

    A. McKenzie exercises
    B. Williams exercises
    C. Back school
    D. Lumbar traction

Correct Answer: A

This patient likely has a herniated disc with radicular symptoms to the foot. Flexion maneuvers make his symptoms worse, so Williams exercises will exacerbate his symptoms. Back schools in a recent review published in Annals of Internal Medicine showed no decrease in pain or recurrence of low back pain but improved short-term recovery and return to work. The same review, in addition to a Cochrane Review, found little evidence to support the use of lumbar traction to decrease pain. McKenzie exercises are hyperextension maneuvers that reduce symptoms associated with disc disease.

1. Eddy D, Congeni J, Loud K. A review of spine injuries and return to play. Clin J Sport Med 2005 Nov;15(6):453-458.
2. Standaert CJ, Herring SA. Expert opinion and controversies in musculoskeletal and sports medicine: core stabilization as a treatment for low back pain. Arch Phys Med Rehabil 2007 Dec;88(12):1734-1736.
3. Chou R, Huffman LH. Nonpharmacologic therapies for acute and chronic low back pain: a review of the evidence for an American Pain Society/American College of Physicians clinical practice guideline. Ann Intern Med 2007 Oct 2;147(7):492-504.
4. Clarke JA, Van Tulder MW, Blomberg SEI, De Vet HCW, Van der Heijden G, Brønfort G, et al. Traction for low-back pain with or without sciatica. Cochrane Database Syst Rev 2007 April 18;(2):CD003010.

116. A fit 58-year-old male with bright red rectal bleeding and known hemorrhoids presents to your office following a canoeing marathon. Which of the following options is appropriate?

    A. Treat his hemorrhoids conservatively, avoid constipation, and watch for further bleeding

    B. Ask to see him in the office for a rectal exam and guaiac assessment, and follow his case clinically if the guaiac test is negative

    C. Ask him to call the office if the bleeding recurs (no other assessment is needed)

    D. A colonoscopy should be recommended

Correct Answer: D

The athlete has experienced rectal bleeding. A negative guaiac at this point does not change the history of rectal bleeding in this adult. Rectal bleeding in adults may indicate cancer. Hemorrhoids are common. Sports can commonly exacerbate hemorrhoids. Given his age, it is important to carry a high index of suspicion for GI malignancy when evaluating GI bleeding. With a colonoscopy, you are able to either diagnose an important GI condition contributing to bleeding or allow the athlete to be reassured that he may continue his endurance activities. Exercise induced intestinal ischemia may also produce lower gastrointestinal bleeding. Endoscopy within one to two days is required to diagnose ischemia in these cases; otherwise, the visible mucosal changes diagnostic for this condition may resolve.

1. Pfenninger J. Common anorectal conditions: part I. Symptoms and complaints. Am Fam Physician 2001 Jun 15;63(12):2391-2398.
2. Natarajan B, Torres JL, Mellion MB. Gastrointestinal problems. In: Mellion M, Walsh WM, Madden C, Putukian M, Shelton GL (eds). Team Physician's Handbook. 3rd ed. Philadelphia: Hanley and Belfus, 2002:244-248.
3. McKeag DB, Moeller JL. ACSM's Primary Care Sports Medicine. 2nd ed. Philadelphia: Lippincott Williams & Wilkins, 2007.

117. An 18-year-old returns from a trip to Colorado with ankle pain and an antalgic gait. She was treated initially for a severe ankle sprain after eversion injury during snowboard lessons. Ankle radiographs reveal a lateral process fracture of the talus that is typical in snowboarding injuries, and a CT scan verifies the non-displaced position of the small fragment. Appropriate treatment consists of which of the following?

   A. Ankle rehabilitation and return to activity if the CT scan shows a Hawkin's sign
   B. Ankle splint, weight bearing as tolerated, and aggressive ankle rehabilitation
   C. Non-weight-bearing in a cast for four to six weeks followed by progressive weight bearing and ankle rehabilitation
   D. Walking cast for four to six weeks, then ankle rehabilitation
   E. Emergent orthopedic consultation because of tenuous blood supply to the talus

Correct Answer: C

A small non-displaced fracture of the lateral process may be appropriately treated with cast immobilization for four to six weeks. Since the lateral process supports 16% to 17% of the body's weight through the leg, early weight bearing risks displacement and surgical fixation. Any option with early weight bearing should be excluded. The Hawkin's sign appears six to nine weeks after trauma and is indicative of vascular viability. The presence of the subchondral radiolucent band of the talar dome is 100% sensitive, but only 57.7% specific to rule out avascular necrosis of the talus. The tenuous, retrograde blood supply of the talus is of greater concern with fractures of the talar neck.

1. DiGiovanni CW, Bernirschke SK, Hansen ST. Foot injuries. In Browner BD, Jupiter JB, Trfton PG, Levine AM (eds). Skeletal Trauma. 3rd ed, Philadelphia: Saunders, 2003:2400-2402.
2. Tezval M, Dumont C, Sturmer KM. Prognostic reliability of the Hawkins sign in fractures of the Talus. J Ortho Trauma 2007 Sep;21(8):538-543.
3. Von Knoch F, Reckord U, Von Knoch M, Sommer C. Fracture of the lateral process of the talus in snowboarders. J Bone Joint Surg Br 2007 Jun;89(6):772-777.

118. Which of the following statements are correct in the management of sports-related concussion?

    A. There are three classifications of concussion according to the Zurich 2008 Summary and Agreement Statement of the 3rd International Conference on Concussion in Sport
    B. Tonic posturing occurring with a sports-related concussion is generally benign and requires no further management beyond the standard treatment of the underlying concussive injury
    C. Loss of consciousness less than 30 seconds is a sign that would classify a concussion as complex
    D. A concussed athlete in high school and/or college may begin a return to play protocol when symptoms decrease from sideline evaluation

Correct Answer: B

According to the Zurich guidelines (2008) they agreed most concussions (80-90%) resolve in a short period of time, 7 to 10 days and they agreed to abandon the two classifications of concussion previously posted by the Prague 2004 guidelines. In such cases, apart from limiting playing or training while symptomatic, no further intervention is required during the period of recovery, and the athlete typically resumes sport without further problem.

A variety of acute motor phenomena, such as tonic posturing or convulsive movements, may accompany a concussion. Although dramatic, these clinical features are generally benign and require no specific management beyond the standard treatment of the underlying concussive injury. During this period of recovery in the first few days following an injury, it is important to emphasize to the athlete that physical *and* cognitive rest is required. Activities that require concentration and attention may exacerbate the symptoms and, as a result, delay recovery. The return to play following a concussion follows a stepwise process: complete rest, light aerobic exercise without resistance training (walking or stationary cycling), sport-specific exercise with progressive resistance training (skating or running), non-contact training drills, full contact training, and finally game play. With this stepwise progression, the athlete should continue to proceed to the next level if asymptomatic at the current level. If any post-concussion symptoms occur, the patient should drop back to the previous asymptomatic level and try to progress again after 24 hours. There is data suggesting at the high school and college level, there may be subtle neuropsychological deficits that are present but not apparent on same day of injury evaluation, hence the recommendation is not to allow same day retur to play if concussed in this age group.

1. McCrory P, Meeuwisse W, Johnston K, Dvorak J, Aubry M, Molloy M, et al. Consensus statement on concussion in sport. The 3rd International Conference on Concussion in Sport held in Zurich, November 2008. Clin J Sport Med 2009 May;19(3):185-200.

119. Which of the following is the most appropriate long-term treatment option for fibromyalgia?

    A. Aerobic exercise
    B. Lidocaine patches
    C. Cyclobenzaprine
    D. Ibuprofen
    E. Hydrocodone

Correct Answer: A

Several high-quality aerobic training studies reported significantly greater improvements in the exercise groups versus control groups in aerobic performance and improvements in pain. Aerobic exercise training has beneficial effects on physical capacity and FMS (fibromyalgia syndrome) symptoms. Strength training may also have benefits on some FMS symptoms. Further studies on muscle strengthening and flexibility are needed. Research on the long-term benefit of exercise for FMS is needed.

1. Busch AJ, Barber KA, Overend TJ, Peloso PM, Schachter CL. Exercise for treating fibromyalgia syndrome. Cochrane Database Syst Rev 2007 Oct 17;(4):CD003786.
2. Busch AJ, Schachter CL, Overend TJ, Peloso PM, Barber KA.. Exercise for fibromyalgia: a systematic review. J Rheumatol 2008 Jun; 35(6):1130-1144.
3. Busch AJ, Webber SC, Brachaniec M, Bidonde J, Bello-Haas VD, Danyliw AD, et al. Exercise therapy for fibromyalgia. Curr Pain Headache Rep 2011 Oct;15(5):358-367.

120. A 16-year-old female basketball player presents with five days of sore throat, fever, and fatigue. On exam, she has an exudative pharyngitis and posterior cervical lymphadenopathy. She has a playoff game scheduled for the weekend and wants to know if she can play. Which of the following tests is the most sensitive and could assist with the decision to allow the athlete to play?

    A. Heterophile antibody–latex agglutination (monospot)
    B. Viral capsid antigen IgM
    C. Viral capsid antigen IgG
    D. Complete blood count

Correct Answer: B

This athlete has the classic presentation for mononucleosis. Hoagland's criteria for the diagnosis of mononucleosis includes fever, pharyngitis, lymphadenopathy, and positive serologic markers. Mononucleosis commonly has a lymphocytosis of 50% or more and atypical lymphocytes of 10% or more. The CBC is less sensitive than either the heterophile or viral capsid antigen antibody tests. Up to 25% of heterophile antibody tests ordered in the first week of symptoms will be negative. By the second week, the false negative rate decreases to 5% to 10%, and by the third week of illness, it is down to 5%. If a more sensitive diagnostic test is needed, then a viral capsid antigen IgM can be ordered. It has a sensitivity of 97% (95% to 99%) and a specificity of 94% (89% to 99%). Antibodies to viral capsid antigen are produced slightly earlier than the heterophile antibody and are more specific for EBV infection. The viral capsid IgG antibody persists past the stage of acute infection and signals the development of immunity.

1. Ebell MH. Epstein-Barr virus infectious mononucleosis. Am Fam Physician 2004 Oct 1;70(7):1279-1287.
2. Epstein-Barr virus and infectious mononucleosis. Centers for Disease Control and Prevention. Accessed January 24, 2012 at www.cdc.gov/ncidod/diseases/ebv.htm.

121. You are one of several first responders on the scene of an unresponsive 17-year-old female with witnessed collapsed during basketball practice. CPR is begun, EMS activated, and the AED placed. Shock is advised. The next step should be which of the following?

    A. Three consecutive shocks followed by resumption of CPR
    B. One shock, then check pulse/rhythm and immediately reshock if advised
    C. One shock, then resume CPR for five cycles before rechecking rhythm
    D. Two rescue breaths and five cycles CPR before proceeding with shock

Correct Answer: C

The 2010 AHA adult guidelines for CPR and emergency cardiovascular care (ECC) in the case of a witnessed collapse recommend immediate CPR, EMS activation, and AED placement as soon as possible. If the AED advises to shock, shock once, and resume CPR immediately without checking the pulse or rhythm until five cycles CPR have been completed. Previous protocols have involved a sequence of three shocks, but this has been found to cause a delay of up to 37 seconds between delivery of shock and chest compressions and is, therefore, no longer recommended. A change in the 2010 AHA Guidelines for CPR and ECC is to recommend the initiation of compressions before ventilations. While no published human or animal evidence demonstrates that starting CPR with 30 compressions rather than two ventilations leads to improved outcomes, it is clear that blood flow depends on chest compressions.

1. Drezner JA, Courson RW, Roberts WO, Mosesso VN Jr, Link MS, Maron BJ. Inter-association task force recommendations on emergency preparedness and management of sudden cardiac arrest in high school and college athletic programs: a consensus statement. Clin J Sport Med 2007 Mar;17(2):87-103.
2. 2010 American Heart Association Guidelines for Cardiopulmonary Resuscitation and Emergency Cardiac Care published in Circulation. Accessed December 10, 2011 at http://circ.ahajournals.org/content/122/18_suppl_3.toc.

122. A 17-year-old male high school baseball pitcher presents to your sports medicine clinic for review of an MRI ordered by another physician. The pitcher has pain in his throwing shoulder. The MRI demonstrates bone marrow edema and cortical flattening suggestive of a Hill-Sachs lesion in the proximal humerus with subchondral sclerosis in the posterosuperior aspect of the glenoid. You would anticipate which of the following physical exam findings based on the imaging study?

   A. Visible atrophy of the supraspinatus and infraspinatus with muscular weakness on testing
   B. Posterior shoulder pain with passive abduction and external rotation of the affected shoulder
   C. Marked weakness of shoulder internal rotators
   D. Enlarged cervical and peri-clavicular lymph nodes

Correct Answer: B

The MRI findings of bone marrow edema and cortical flattening suggestive of a Hill-Sachs lesion in the proximal humerus with subchondral sclerosis in the posterosuperior aspect of the glenoid may be seen in patients with internal impingement of the shoulder. Internal impingement may be clinically assessed with the "relocation test of Jobe." In patients with internal impingement abducting and externally rotating the affected shoulder produces posterior shoulder pain. Posteriorly directed humeral head pressure, "relocation," with the patient's shoulder in abduction and external rotation relieves the pain. Atrophy of supraspinatus and infraspinatus would not be expected findings. Internal impingement is typically seen in overhead throwers who generally have increased strength of shoulder internal rotators. Lymph node enlargement is not seen with this condition.

1. Moosikasuwan JB, Miller TT, Dines DM. Imaging of the painful shoulder in throwing athletes. Clin Sports Med 2006 Jul;25(3):433-443.
2. Gialori EL, Major NM, Higgins LD. MRI of internal impingement of the shoulder. AJR Am J Roentgenol 2005 Oct;185(4):925-929.

123. A 19-year-old basketball player, exchange student from Italy, has an episode of unexplained syncope during practice. The patient adamantly denies any previous cardiac history and believes he was just dehydrated. He does admit, however, that a cousin died suddenly at age 20 of cardiac causes. An ECG is obtained. Which abnormality would be suggestive of arrythmogenic right ventricular dysplasia?

   A. Normal ECG
   B. T-wave inversion
   C. Prolonged QT interval
   D. Q waves with ectopy
   E. Pre-excitation

Correct Answer: B

Arrhythmogenic right ventricular cardiomyopathy (ARVC) is a rare cause of sudden cardiac death in the United States but ranks much higher in European studies. An ECG is an appropriate first step in a cardiac workup for this patient. Classic ECG findings include T-wave inversion V_1-V_3, left bundle branch block, and rarely an epsilon wave, which is pathognomonic for this disease. The other choices listed can be seen in other diseases such as HOCM, myocarditis, mitral valve prolapse, or supraventricular tachycardia, to name a few, but not typically seen with ARVC.

1. Basilico F. Cardiovascular disease in athletes. Am J Sports Med 1999 Jan-Feb;27(1):108-121.
2. Burke AP. Arrythmogenic right ventricular cardiomyopathy pathology. Medscape. Accessed December 10, 2011 at http://emedicine.medscape.com/article/2017949-overview.

124. A 15-year-old high school football player was hit on his blind side as he was running with the football. He landed on the side carrying the football, and the tackler landed on top of him. After needing assistance to the sideline, he became tachycardic, hypotensive, and there was a clear change in his mental status. He was transported to the nearest hospital where he was reevaluated. The patient is initially stabilized with IV hydration. However, the patient's pain is persistent. Which of the following testing types is going to take the longest to produce results?

A. CT abdomen and pelvis
B. Peritoneal lavage
C. MR abdomen
D. Plain films of abdomen and chest
E. Abdominal ultrasound

Correct Answer: C

In the acute setting, any testing needs to be quick, efficient, and provide information about the severity of injury. MR of the abdomen is not quick, and the other tests listed will help the clinician identify a possible need for surgery.

1. Feliciano DV, Rozycki GS. Evaluation of abdominal trauma. American College of Surgeons. Accessed January 24, 2012 at www.facs.org/trauma/publications/abdominal.pdf.
2. Walter KD. Radiographic evaluation of the patient with sport-related abdominal trauma. Curr Sports Med Rep. 2007 Apr;6(2):115-119.
3. Hoff WS, Holevar M, Nagy KK, Patterson L, Young JS, Arrillaga A, et al. Practice management guidelines for the evaluation of blunt abdominal trauma: East practice management guidelines work group. J Trauma 2002 Sep;53(3):602-615.

125. A 40-year-old male distance runner presents for a routine physical. As part of the physical, you obtain a urine sample, which shows 1+ protein on a dipstick test. Which of the following would support a diagnosis of exercise-induced proteinuria?

   A. Regular creatine supplementation
   B. A history of completing an intense speed training workout just prior to the physical
   C. A history of a 150-mile bike race two weeks prior to the physical
   D. A history of uncontrolled type 2 diabetes mellitus
   E. A 20-year history of distance running with over 40 marathons in the past 10 years

Correct Answer: B

Exercise-induced proteinuria is seen fairly commonly and is felt to be related to elevated levels of angiotensin converting enzyme during exercise. The proteinuria typically occurs 30 minutes after vigorous exercise and is related to changes in intraglomerular hemodynamics. Creatine supplementation has been shown to not be related to proteinuria in athletes. The proteinuria typically clears within two days. Exercise increases proteinuria in patients with diabetes, but it is felt to be an unmasking effect of underlying diabetic nephropathy and not exercise-induced proteinuria. Exercise-induced proteinuria does not increase or decrease with regular physical training.

   1. Saeed F, Naga Pavan Kumar Devaki P, Mahendrakar L, Holley JL. Exercise-induced proteinuria? J Fam Pract 2012 Jan;61(1):23-26.
   2. Poortmans JR, Francaux M. Long-term oral creatine supplementation does not impair renal function in healthy athletes. Med Sci Sports Exer 1999 Aug;31(8):1108-1110.

126. A college springboard diver, while entering the water, felt pain at medial aspect of right thumb. Position of thumb during entry was hyperextended and abducted. On exam, she had tenderness and mild swelling along the medial aspect of first MCP, but with solid end point. Which of the following is the most appropriate initial management of choice for this injury?

   A. Immediate surgery
   B. No necessary intervention
   C. Taping
   D. Short arm thumb spica splint with wrist in slight extension, thumb in abduction
   E. Short arm thumb spica splint with wrist in slight flexion, thumb in abduction

Correct Answer: D

Diagnosis: UCL injury grade 1 and 2. Management of nondisplaced avulsion fractures or type 1 and 2 UCL sprains without joint laxity is thumb spica (cast or spint) for three to six weeks with reevaluation every two weeks. The optimal positioning of the thumb spica is wrist in slight extension and the thumb in slight abduction. For this case, surgery is not indicated and taping is insufficient. The positioning listed for choices D and E are incorrect. Care should be taken to assess for Stener lesion.

1. Eiff M, Hatch R, Calmbach W. Fracture Management for Primary Care. 2nd ed. Philadelphia: Saunders, 2003:67-70.

2. Melone CP Jr, Beldner S, Basuk RS. Thumb colateral ligament injuries. An anataomic basis for treatment. Hand Clin 2000 Aug;16(3):345-357.

3. Foye PM. Skier's thumb. Medscape. Accessed February 15, 2012 at http://emedicine.medscape.com/article/98460.

127. A 55-year-old female is a regular participant in her aggressive aerobics class at the park district community center five days per week. She presents with subjective pain with motion over the most lateral portion of the proximal right femur for two to three weeks. Her right hip joint motion is smooth, without pain, and symmetric passively and actively when compared to the left hip. There is tenderness to palpation over the most lateral portion of the proximal right femur. She responds to treatment with a conservative program consisting of icing, deep tissue massage using a foam roller, over-the-counter analgesics, and an injection into the painful area. Which of the following is the proper diagnosis?

    A. Iliopectineal bursitis
    B. Ischial bursitis
    C. Greater trochanteric bursitis
    D. Pes anserine bursitis

Correct Answer: C

Greater trochanteric bursitis is diagnosed easily with a thorough physical exam. Intraarticular pathology can be considered less likely when the athlete demonstrates tenderness directly over the bursa and excellent pain-free motion in all directions about the hip joint. The conditions mentioned in Answer A through Answer D are differentiated by specific tenderness over the specific bursa. Knowledge of musculoskeletal anatomy is required to make the diagnosis and perform appropriate soft tissue injections. The benefits of corticosteroid injections, a longstanding accepted treatment, have been questioned in recent articles.

1. McKeag DB, Moeller JL. ACSM's Primary Care Sports Medicine. 2nd ed. Philadelphia: Lippincott Williams & Wilkins, 2007.
2. Cardone D. Diagnostic and therapeutic injection of the hip and knee. Am Fam Physician 2003 May 15;67(10):2147-2152.
3. Alvarez-Nemegyei J. Evidence-based soft tissue rheumatology: III: trochanteric bursitis. J Clin Rheumatol 2004 Jun;10(3):123-124.

128. A 23-year-old mountain bike racer flips over his handlebars and lands on the posterior superior portion of his right shoulder. Evaluation in the medical tent demonstrates significant weakness with resisted extension of the shoulder when tested at 90 degrees flexion, 30 degrees lateral to the coronal plane, and with hand pronated (empty can test) as well as an inability to initiate abduction of the involved arm. The patient also has weakness with resisted external rotation. There are no sensory deficits to light touch or pin prick over the shoulder, arm, thorax, or back. Which nerve has most likely been injured?

   A. Axillary nerve
   B. Subscapular nerve
   C. Suprascapular nerve
   D. Dorsal scapular nerve

Correct Answer: C

All of the nerves in the answer could be damaged in an injury as described; therefore, it is important to discern the specific nerve involved by muscle testing. The accident described could also cause damage to muscles of the shoulder joint and shoulder girdle innervated by the nerves listed. However, the description of the specific area of impact indicates that an injury to the muscles is less likely than direct injury to the suprascapular nerve or via a fracture in the suprascapular notch or via compression injury. Involvement of the supraspinatus and the infraspinatus suggests damage to the suprascapular nerve prior to the spinoglenoid notch. The absence of sensory findings also rules out the axillary nerve as well without specifically testing the deltoid. Weakness with external rotation and not internal rotation further clarifies that the subscapular nerve is not involved as there are no sensory components of this nerve.

   1. Reeser J. Suprascapular neuropathy. Medscape. Accessed December 11, 2011 at http:// emedicine.medscape.com/article/92672-overview.

129. A 13-year-old female with a history of Legg-Calve-Perthes disease as a child presents to your clinic with worsening chronic left hip and groin pain. She reports occasional catching or locking. On exam, she has pain with passive range of motion and reduced internal rotation and abduction. On MRI of the hip, you expect to find which of the following?

    A. Osteochondritis dissecans of the femoral head
    B. Labral tear
    C. Normal hip
    D. Arthritis

Correct Answer: A

Legg-Calve-Perthes disease is idiopathic avascular necrosis of the femoral head in young people. It presents at age four to eight and is more common in males. It typically is self-limited and undergoes resorption and collapse, followed by repair of the capital femoral epiphyses. The result is impaired development of the hip joint. Half of children who develop Legg-Calve-Perthes disease will develop osteoarthritis later in life. Additionally, some patients do not spontaneously resolve and develop an osteochondral fragment, which fails to unite with the rest of the femoral head.

1. Kocker M, Tucker R. Pediatric athlete hip disorders. Clin Sports Med 2006 Apr 1;25(2):241-253, viii.
2. Katz J, Siffert R. Osteochondritis dissecans in association with Legg-Calve-Perthes disease. Int Orthop 1979;3(3):189-195.

130. The use of a TENS (transcutaneous electric nerve stimulation) unit does which of the following?

   A. Results in increased dorsal horn cell activity
   B. Most likely relieves pain via endorphin release with high frequency, low intensity modalities
   C. Is relatively contraindicated for a patient with an implantable cardiac defibrillator (ICD)
   D. Has been proven to reduce fracture pain
   E. Results in local analgesia that is typically long-lasting (> one hour) after stimulation is stopped

Correct Answer: C

Cardiac pacemakers may be relatively resistant to TENS signals, but there is one published report of an ICD being triggered by use of a TENS unit. Other relative contraindications to using a TENS unit include local skin irritation and contact dermatitis. TENS results in decreased dorsal horn cell activity after stimulation. High frequency, low intensity stimulation most likely produces analgesia via the gate theory, whereas high intensity, lower frequency signals work by endorphin release. Hypoanalgesia may persist for up to five minutes after cessation of stimulation.

1. Alfano AP. Physical modalities in sports medicine. In: O'Connor FG, Wilder RP, St. Pierre P (eds). Sports Medicine: Just the Facts. New York: McGraw-Hill, 2005:405-412
2. Gemmell H, Hilland A. Immediate effect of electric point stimulation (TENS) in treating latent upper trapezius trigger points: a double blind randomised placebo-controlled trial. J Bodyw Mov Ther 2011 Jul;15(3):348-354.

131. A 27-year-old male complains of pain and numbness in his palm and fourth and fifth fingers after his recent karate tournament. There is a tender mass in his hypothenar area and an abnormal Allen's test. You suspect damage to which of the following structures?

    A. Thrombosis of ulnar artery
    B. Thrombosis of radial artery
    C. Thrombosis of median artery
    D. Thrombosis of common palmar digital artery

Correct Answer: A

Repetitive trauma to the hypothenar area can cause injury to the ulnar artery with subsequent construction, thickening, thrombosis, and possible aneurysm formation. Ulnar nerve symptoms may present concurrently due to compression.

1. Ignari JV, Hand and Wrist in In: DeLee JC, Drez D, Miller MD (eds). DeLee & Drez's Orthopaedic Sports Medicine. 3rd ed. Philadelphia: Saunders Elsevier, 2010.
2. Ulnar artery: thenar hand syndrome. Wheeless' Online. Accessed February 14, 2012 at www.wheelessonline.com/ortho/ulnar_artery_hypothenar_hand_syndrome
3. Netter FH. Atlas of Human Anatomy. 5th ed. Philadelphia: Saunders Elsevier, 2011:440-459.

132. A 16-year-old male high school athlete presents to the ER after being hit in the testicle by a racquetball in the groin during a competitive match with his father. Patient was unable to finish the competition because of nausea, vomiting, and difficulty walking due to pain. Examination revealed a tender and swollen right testicle and scrotal hematoma measuring 2 cm in diameter. A scrotal US with Doppler revealed a testicular parenchymal fracture and intact testicular blood flow. His parents are very concerned about the patient's future fertility since he is their only child. The most appropriate next step would be which of the following?

    A. Oral antibiotics
    B. Rest, pain control and ice packs on groin for 24 to 48 hours
    C. Urology consult for surgery to repair the testicular integrity
    D. Percutaneous drainage of the hematoma for pain control
    E. Scrotal MRI

Correct Answer: C

With the scrotal US showing a fracture and intact blood flow, it would not be recommended to treat this patient conservatively with rest, pain management, and ice packs to the groin. An MRI is usually reserved for equivocal findings on ultrasound, which is not the case in this situation with a definite fracture identified. Antibiotics are usually not indicated in blunt testicular trauma. Exploration and surgery are necessary to prevent anti-sperm antibodies, and this should be accomplished ASAP. Hematoma drainage is not needed for pain control.

1. Terlecki RP. Testicular trauma. Medscape. Accessed December 11, 2011 at http://emedicine.medscape.com/article/441362.
2. Kukadia AN, Ercole CJ, Gleich P, Hensleigh H, Pryor JL. Testicular trauma: potential impact on reproductive function. J Urol 1996 Nov;156(5):1643-1646.

133. The erector spinae and abdominal musculature stabilize the spine in a strength ratio of 1.3:1. The muscles you palpate in the erector spinae when the athlete has low back pain include?

    A. Iliocostalis, longissimus, spinalis
    B. Longissimus capitus, semispinalis capitis, splenius capitus
    C. Semispinalis thoracis, multifidus, rotatores thoracis
    D. Interspinalis lumborum, lateral intertransversi, quadratus lumborum

Correct Answer: A

An imbalance of the erector spinae and abdominal musculature contribute to the development of low back pain in the athlete. The erector spinae is made up of the iliocostalis, longissimus, and spinalis muscles. The longissimus capitus, semispinalis capitus, and splenius capitis are the deeper musculature of the neck. The semispinalis thoracis, multifidus, and rotatores thoracis are the deeper musculature of the thoracic spine. The interspinalis lumborum, lateral intertransversi, and quadratus lumborum are muscles deep to the erector spinae.

1. Netter FH. Atlas of Human Anatomy. 4th ed. Philadelphia: Saunders Elsevier, 2006.
2. Trainor TJ, Trainor MA. Etiology of low back pain in athletes. Curr Rep Sports Med 2004 Feb;3(1):41-46.

134. A high school senior kicker was involved in a calamitous play during a kickoff return. Upon rushing the field to examine him, you immediately noticed what initially appeared to be a fracture. Your exam showed this to be an anterior dislocation of the knee. Although difficult, you were able to successfully reduce and stabilize the joint. After the reduction, you reevaluated his knee on the sideline. Which of the following items would concern you the most during that exam?

A. The difficult reduction of his anterior dislocation
B. Gross multidirectional instability on exam
C. Non-progressive dorsiflexion weakness on neurologic exam
D. Difficulty obtaining palpable pulses from the foot

Correct Answer: D

Anterior dislocations account for 40% of the total cases, but the difficulty in reduction is not necessarily a major concern. Therefore, Answer A is incorrect. However, a non-reducible dislocation is an emergency to avoid prolonged traction on the neurovascular structures. Multidirectional instability on exam would certainly be devastating and concerning. In many instances, it can confirm a spontaneously reduced knee, but it is not a finding that requires emergent intervention, and therefore Answer B is incorrect. Answer C is not the best answer. Non-progression of weakness is reassuring that an impending compartment syndrome is not occurring, especially if there are no other findings. This is consistent with injury to the common peroneal nerve which occurs in just under 20% of knee dislocations. Answer D demonstrates the immediate potential for vascular insufficiency from a possible tear of the popliteal artery which can occur in 20% of dislocations. This is a potential emergency requiring immediate consultation because the risk of amputation is 86% if revascularization is delayed past six to eight hours.

1. Rihn J, Groff Y, Harner C. The acutely dislocated knee: evaluation and management. J Am Acad Orthop Surg 2004 Sep-Oct;12(5):334-346.
2. Robertson A, Nutton RW. Dislocation of the knee. J Bone Joint Surg Br 2006 Jun;88(6):706-711.

135. A 16-year-old male presents to your clinic for a preparticipation physical evaluation. His best corrected visual screen reveals < 20/40 vision in his right eye and 20/20 vision in his left eye. He states he lost vision in this eye after he was struck in the fourth grade by a baseball. The remainder of his history and physical are unremarkable. He should be excluded from participation in which of the following sports?

   A. Football
   B. Wrestling
   C. Ice hockey
   D. Lacrosse

Correct Answer: B

The athlete in this vignette is considered monocular as his best corrected visual acuity in the weaker eye is less than 20/40. Wrestling, boxing, and full-contact martial arts are contraindicated in monocular athletes because adequate eye protection is unavailable. Monocular athletes must wear sports eye protectors that meet ASTM racquet sports standards in all sports that carry risks of eye injury, for all games and practices. Face masks are required in hockey, football, and lacrosse. In addition to the face mask, sports goggles with polycarbonate lenses and frames should be worn. Monocular athletes should wear polycarbonate lenses and frames while playing basketball. Monocular baseball players should wear sports goggles at all times. While batting or running bases, the appropriate helmet with a polycarbonate face guard and sports goggles should be worn. The functionally monocular athlete should be evaluated by an ophthalmologist before being admitted to participation in a particular sport.

1. Rodriguez JO, Lavina AM. Prevention and treatment of common eye injuries in sports. Am Fam Physician 2003 Apr 1;67(7):1481-1488.
2. Mellion MB, Walsh WM, Madden C, Putukian M, Shelton GL (eds). Team Physician's Handbook. 3rd ed. Philadelphia: Hanley and Belfus, 2002.

136. Which of the following statements is true regarding Legg-Calve-Perthes disease?

    A. Legg-Calve-Perthes disease occurs most commonly in girls in the first decade of life
    B. Most patients with Legg-Calve-Perthes disease will have excruciating hip pain, which results in a unilateral limp
    C. The most common exam findings are of reduced internal rotation and abduction of the hip
    D. Long-term sequelae of untreated Legg-Calve-Perthes disease are rare
    E. With Legg-Calve-Perthes disease, an older child has a better prognosis than a younger child

Correct Answer: C

The most common exam findings are of reduced internal rotation and abduction of the hip. Legg-Calve-Perthes disease most commonly occurs in boys ages four to eight years old. There is a 3:1 ratio of boys to girls. The most common presentation is an insidious, unilateral, painless limp. Half of those with untreated Legg-Calve-Perthes disease develop osteoarthritis in the fifth decade of life. Younger children seem to have a better prognosis possibly because of the greater time for subsequent growth and remodeling. Treatment with non-operative versus operative options is controversial. In general, surgical intervention is recommended for the more severe disease.

1. Kocher MS, Tucker R. Pediatric athlete hip disorders. Clin Sports Med 2006 Apr:25(2):241-253, viii.
2. Cheng JC, Lam TP, Ng BK. Prognosis and prognostic factors of Legg-Calve-Perthes disease. J Pediatr Orthop 2011 Sep;31(2 Suppl):S147-151.

137. You are asked to be the physician for a local summer league junior softball tournament. Which of the following factors are true in relation to the risk for heat illness?

   A. Children's sweat rates are equal to adults and, therefore, are at no greater risk
   B. Children usually stop before they get too hot and, therefore, are at no greater risk than adults
   C. Children don't absorb fluids as readily as adults and, therefore, are at greater risk than adults
   D. Children have increased heat production per kilogram of body mass and are at greater risk than adults

Correct Answer: D

With more children playing multiple sports and multiple seasons, it is important to realize the differences between adults and children and how these differences put the children at risk. The tournaments in the summer put the players—and siblings who are present—at risk especially since many of the fields (baseball/softball, soccer, football) have little or no shade. Because many of these tournaments are played throughout the day on Saturday and Sunday, the mid-day heat can be a potentially dangerous factor to consider.

   1. Grubenhoff JA, Du Ford K, Roosevelt GE. Heat-related illness. Clin Pediatr Emerg Med 2007 Mar;8(1):59-64.
   2. Jardine DS. Heat illness and heat stroke. Pediatr Rev 2007 Jul 1;28(7):249-258.

138. The most effective treatment for a symptomatic dorsal carpal ganglia is which of the following?

    A. Nothing, as most ganglia resolve spontaneously and do not require treatment
    B. Aspiration with corticosteroid injection
    C. Aspiration without corticosteroid injection
    D. Surgery

Correct Answer: D

Ganglion cysts account for approximately 60% of soft tissue, tumor-like swelling affecting the hand and wrist. They usually develop spontaneously in adults 20 to 50 years of age. There is a female-to-male preponderance of 3:1. The dorsal wrist ganglion arises from the scapholunate joint and constitutes about 65% of ganglia of the wrist and hand. The volar wrist ganglion arises from the distal aspect of the radius and accounts for about 20% to 25% of ganglia. Flexor tendon sheath ganglia make up the remaining 10% to 15%. The cystic structures are found near or are attached to tendon sheaths and joint capsules. The cyst is filled with soft, gelatinous, sticky, and mucoid fluid.

Cysts are self evident, being soft and ballotable, and occur along the dorsal and volar aspects of the wrist. Most ganglia resolve spontaneously and do not require treatment. If the patient has symptoms, including pain or paresthesias, or is disturbed by the appearance, aspiration with or without injection of a corticosteroid is effective (no recurrence of the cyst) in 27% to 67% of patients. However, a recent randomized controlled trial between surgery and aspiration combined with methylprednisolone acetate injection plus wrist immobilization in the treatment of dorsal carpal ganglion showed the success by excision was 81.8% and by aspiration combined with methylprednisolone acetate injection plus wrist immobilization was 38.46%. The p-value was 0.047 by Fisher exact test. The present study has clearly shown that surgical excision gave a better success rate in the treatment of dorsal carpal ganglion.

1. Talia AF, Cardone DA. Diagnostic and therapeutic injection of the wrist and hand region. Am Fam Physician 2003 Feb 15;67(4):745-750.
2. Limpaphyayom N, Wilairatana V. Randomized controlled trial between surgery and aspiration combined with methylprednisolone acetate injection plus wrist immobilization in the treatment of dorsal carpal ganglion. J Med Assoc Thai 2004 Dec;87(12):1513-1517.

139. What is the role of calcium in muscle contraction?

A. Calcium binds troponin, moving tropomysin and allowing crossbridge linkages and contraction

B. Calcium binds troponin, allowing for release of ATP and therefore initiating contraction

C. Calcium binds tropomysin, moving troponin and allowing crossbridge linkages and contraction

D. Calcium binds tropomysin, allowing for release of ATP and therefore initiating contraction

Correct Answer: A

Muscle contraction is triggered by an electrical impulse involving acetylcholine release, which subsequently results in calcium release from the sacoplasmic reticulum. Once released, calcium binds troponin, which causes tropomysin to move and, therefore, allowing activation of cross linkages and contraction.

1. Deuster P, Keyser D. Basics in exercise physiology. In: O'Connor FG, Wilder RP, St. Pierre P (eds). Sports Medicine: Just the Facts. New York: McGraw-Hill, 2005:34-36.

140. You are performing the preparticipation physical examination for one of the new soccer recruits for the college. He is an 18-year-old male who had his first generalized tonic-clonic seizure eight months ago. He was appropriately evaluated; testing confirming the diagnosis of idiopathic epilepsy, and was started on valproic acid. He has tolerated the medication well and has been seizure free for seven months. He resumed his workouts but has not returned to competitive soccer before this time. With regard to his participation with the college soccer program, your recommendations and counseling would be which of the following (select the best answer)?

A. There is no known risk for increasing seizure frequency with contact or collision sports, and since his seizures are well controlled, he may be cleared to participate

B. Persons with history of seizure should not be active in strenuous activities, even if their seizures are well controlled as physical activity lowers the seizure potential and activity speeds clearance of anti-seizure medications

C. There is still a significant risk of seizure, so he should not participate in any contact or collision sports (in addition, he should not participate in sports such as archery, riflery, swimming, diving, and weight or power lifting)

D. Valproic acid is a banned substance by the NCAA. Although he is well controlled and is cleared to participate in soccer on this medication, an exception based on your request must be granted by the NCAA before he can participate with the team

E. Because he has been seizure-free for more than six months, you can recommend stopping the valproic acid today (as long as he is seizure-free with non-contact sport activities for the next two weeks, he can be released for full activity)

Correct Answer: A

There is no evidence that shows athletes with good seizure control increase the frequency of seizure with strenuous activity or contact or collision sports. Although the evaluation of good control is debatable and generally accepted as seizure free for three to six months, it is noted that during medication withdrawal, most seizures occurred in the first three months. Because of the risks of injury should a seizure occur, most practitioners will counsel athletes to always have a companion who is aware of the seizure history present with activities so that assistance may be obtained. If seizures were not well controlled, the limitations on contact and collision sport, as well as high-risk non-contact sports (listed in Answer C) should be followed as stated in the PPE monograph. Valproic acid is metabolized by the liver and the metabolite excreted in the urine. There is no information showing that activity increases metabolism. Valproic acid is not banned by the NCAA or U.S. Anti-Doping Agency. Most experts would not recommend withdrawal of anti-seizure medications until a patient is seizure-free for at least two years, and then medications should be tapered.

1. Matheson GO, Boyajian LA, Cardone D, Dexter W, Difiori J, Fields KB, et al. The Physician and Sports Medicine. Preparticipation Physical Evaluation. 3rd ed. Minneapolis, MN: McGraw-Hill, 2005.
2. NCAA Banned Drug List 2011-2012. Accessed January 21, 2012 at www.wm.edu/sportsmedicine/2011-12_Banned_Drugs_Educational.pdf.
3. U.S. Anti-Doping Agency Drug Reference Online. Accessed January 21, 2012 at www.globaldro.org/us-en/default.aspx.

141. After completing heat acclimation, which of the following changes would be a physiologic change in an athlete after exercising in a heat environment?

A. An increase in plasma aldosterone
B. A significant decrease in the percent dehydration during exercise
C. A right shift of the sweat osmolality
D. A significantly higher plasma lactate concentration

Correct Answer: C

After getting heat acclimatized, the concentration and total content of sodium in sweat as well as plasma aldosterone are significantly decreased during exercise. After getting heat acclimatized, the percent dehydration during exercise is significantly increased due to the increase in loss of free water. After getting heat acclimatized, the sweat osmolality and the sweat sodium ion concentration shift to the right. There is a significantly lower sweat sodium ion concentration for a given sweat rate following heat acclimation. These results suggest that heat acclimation increases the sodium ion reabsorption. After getting heat acclimatized, a significantly lower plasma lactate concentration can be found in post-exercise tests.

1. Buono MJ, Ball KD, Kolkhorst FW. Sodium ion concentration vs. sweat rate relationship in humans. J Appl Physiol 2007 Sep;103(3):990-994.
2. Saat M, Sirisinghe RG, Singh R, Tochihara Y. Effects of short-term exercise in the heat on thermoregulation, blood parameters, sweat secretion and sweat composition of tropic-dwelling subjects. J Physiol Anthropol Appl Human Sci 2005 Sep;24(5):541-549.
3. Kirby CR, Convertino VA. Plasma aldosterone and sweat sodium concentrations after exercise and heat acclimation. J Appl Physiol 1986 Sep;61(3):967-970.

142. In order to prevent exercise-induced bronchospasm during competition, athletes with documented asthma would benefit from which of the following treatments?

    A. Pre-medicate with beta-adrenergic agonist
    B. Pre-medicate with oral corticosteroids
    C. Pre-medicate with inhaled corticosteroids
    D. Pre-medicate with antihistamines
    E. Pre-medicate with nasal steroids

Correct Answer: A

The use of anti-asthma medications helps to control EIB in most asthmatics. For individuals with asthmatic symptoms associated only with exercise, the prophylactic use of a beta-2 agonist inhaler before exercise prevents EIB in most cases. Short-acting beta-agonists have the advantage of providing prevention and rescue therapy for EIB. Although long-acting beta-agonists provide a longer duration of EIB prophylaxis, they should not be used as a first-line treatment for EIB because of their slow onset of action. Pre-treatment with corticosteroids is not indicated. Inhaled corticosteroids may be needed for moderate persistent asthmatics for control but not an acute state as with exercise. Answers D and E both are control medications and may be part of the treatment for an asthmatic that also has allergic rhinitis. However, these are not the mainstay to prevent EIB.

1. Nichols AW. Exercise induced bronchospasm. In: Puffer JC (ed). 20 Common Problems in Sports Medicine. New York: McGraw-Hill, 2002:299-300.
2. Parsons J, McCamey K, Mastronarde J. Exercise-induced bronchospasm. In: DeLee JC, Drez D, Miller MD (eds). DeLee & Drez's Orthopaedic Sports Medicine. 3rd ed. Philadelphia: W.B. Saunders, 2010: Section E.

143. Which of the following structures is the primary static stabilizer for preventing lateral subluxation of the patella?

   A. Medial patellofemoral ligament
   B. Vastus medialis obliquus (VMO)
   C. Medial patellotibial ligament
   D. Superficial oblique retinaculum

Correct Answer: A

Investigations to determine the soft tissue restraints to lateral subluxation of the patella identified the patello-femoral ligament as the primary stabilizer. At 20 degrees of flexion, the PFL contributed 60% of the total restraining force, while the patello-meniscal ligament and lateral retinaculum contributed 13% and 10%, respectively. The medial patellotibial ligament and superficial fibers of the medial retinaculum were not found to be functionally important in preventing lateral subluxation.

   1. Bicos J, Fulkerson JP, Amis A. Current concepts review: the medial patellofemoral ligament. Am J Sports Med 2007 Mar;35(3):484-492.
   2. Burks RT, Desio SM, Bachus KN, Tyson L, Springer K. Biomechanical evaluation of lateral patellar dislocations. Am J Knee Surg 1998 Winter;11(1):24-31.
   3. Desio SM, Burks RT, Bachus KN. Soft tissue restraints to lateral patellar translation in the human knee. Am J Sports Med 1998 Jan-Feb;26(1):59-61.

144. A 26-year-old African-American female presents to the medical treatment tent you are staffing at a large cross country ski race in upper Wisconsin. She is complaining of painful edematous purple lesions on her face. She is in excellent health, an avid cross country runner from southern Illinois. She denies pregnancy or any medical problems. She does not seem to be in any acute distress. She and her friends have been taking "nips" out of a pocket flask containing Blackberry brandy. Which of the following is true?

A. She has classic pernio (or chilblain)
B. She should immediately stop the race and be transported to the main medical tent 10 km away via ambulance
C. She can go back out after applying protective UV cold barrier ointment on her face
D. She should quickly rewarm her face by sitting next to the propane gas warmer in the tent
E. It is best to warm her face slowly, using cool water and then slowly applying heated water to prevent further tissue damage

Correct Answer: A

The patient has classic pernio, or chilblain, which is characterized by localized inflammatory lesions that result from acute or repetitive exposure to cold. The lesions are edematous, often purple, and are most common in young women. It is one of the milder forms of a cold injury. First-degree frostbite is characterized by a central area of pallor and anesthesia of the skin surrounded by edema. A second-degree frostbite is recognized by blisters containing a clear milky fluid surrounded by edema and erythema. Third-degree frostbite differs from second-degree frostbite as the injury is deeper and blisters are hemorrhagic. Alcohol use predisposes cold injury. Risk factors include smoking, previous cold injury, and exposure of hands and arms to vibration. African-American women may be at increased risk of cold injury. This patient does not have any other physical signs that would require immediate transportation to the main medical tent. The best medical advice would be to simply stop the race at this point, and get her to a warm environment. In some areas, protective ointments applied to the face have been advocated, but this practice may actually increase the risk of a cold injury. The area should be warmed as soon as possible, and it is best to get the patient into a warm environment and remove wet clothing. Stoves or open fires used to rewarm frostbitten tissue are not recommended as the tissue is insensitive and thermal injury can occur. If necessary, it is best to rewarm the area in a water bath 104 to 108 degrees Fahrenheit (40 to 42 degrees Celsius), which feels warm, but not hot, to the patient.

1. Frostbite. UpToDate. Accessed May 2, 2008 at www.uptodate.com.
2. Petrone P, Kuncir EJ, Asensio JA. Surgical management and strategies in the treatment of hypothermia and cold injury. Emerg Med Clin North Am 2003 Nov;21(4):1165-1178.
3. Simon TD, Soep JB, Hollister JR. Pernio in pediatrics. Pediatrics 2005 Sep;116(3):e472-475.

145. A college football player sprains his ankle at the bottom of a pileup. When considering diagnosis of syndesmotic ankle sprain, which of the following is true?

    A. Imaging shows < 5 mm of clear space and > 10 mm of tibiofibular overlap
    B. One mechanism of injury is a blow to the back of the externally rotated ankle while prone
    C. Anterior drawer, talar tilt, and squeeze testing are negative
    D. If interosseous sprain is strongly suspected and distal fibular pain is present, the Ottawa Ankle Rules do not apply, as x-rays are not needed

Correct Answer: B

Forced external rotation of the talus during dorsiflexion stretches and tears the interosseous membrane by laterally distracting the distal fibula. Syndesmosis injury is confirmed by > 5 mm of clear space or < 10 mm of tibiofibular overlap (the opposite of Answer A). Anterior drawer and talar tilt may be negative, but squeeze testing along with external rotation of the foot at the ankle cause pain at the ankle. The Ottawa Ankle Rules may disclose fibular or other fracture which shouldn't be neglected. The syndesmotic widening > 5 mm would be detected, and surgery should be considered.

1. Edwards GS Jr, DeLee JC. Ankle diastasis without fracture. Foot Ankle 1984 May-Jun;4(6):305-312.
2. Xenos JS. The tibiofibular syndesmosis: evaluation of the ligamentous structures, methods of fixation, and radiographic assessment. J Bone Joint Surg 1995 Jun;77(6):847-856.
3. Gerber JP. Persistent disability associated with ankle sprains: a prospective examination of an athletic population. Foot Ankle Int 1998 Oct;19(10):653-660.
4. Dubin JC, Comeau D, McClelland RI, Dubin RA, Ferrel E. Lateral and syndesmotic ankle sprain injuries: a narrative literature review. J Chiropr Med 2011 Sep;10(3):204-219.
5. Molinari A, Stolley M, Amendola A. High ankle sprains (syndesmotic) in athletes: diagnostic challenges and review of the literature. Iowa Orthop J 2009;29:130-138.

146. Which of the following measurements of left ventricular wall thickness on 2D-echocardiogram at the end of diastole is considered left ventricular hypertrophy in a 70 kg male?

    A. > 6 mm
    B. > 9 mm
    C. > 12 mm
    D. > 15 mm

Correct Answer: D

Although the definition of LVH is based on various cut-offs for LV mass, the use of left ventricular wall thickness can be used for screening. The end diastolic left ventricle wall thickness in a normal individual is usually between 6 mm to 11 mm. The upper limit of normal for left ventricular thickness is 15 mm in men and 13 mm in women.

1. Pelliccia A. Maron B, Spataro A, Proschan MA, Spirito P. Upper limit of physiologic cardiac hypertrophy in highly trained elite athletes. N Engl J Med 1991 Jan;324(5):295-301.
2. Pluim BM, Zwinderman AH, Van der Laarse A, Van der Wall EE. The athlete's heart: a meta-analysis of cardiac structure and function. Circulation 2000 Jan 25;101(3):336-344.
3. Whyte GP, George K, Sharma S, Firoozi S, Stephens N, Senior R, et al. The upper limit of physiological cardiac hypertrophy in elite male and female athletes: the British experience. Eur J Appl Physiol 2004 Aug;92(4-5):592-597.

147. There are several different types of muscle stretching techniques. Using a partner to stretch the hamstring passively, then pushing against the partner by contracting the muscle isometrically, and then stretching farther in the same range of motion is an example of which of the following?

    A. Static stretching
    B. Dynamic stretching
    C. Ballistic stretching
    D. Proprioceptive neuromuscular facilitation

Correct Answer: D

This is an example of proprioceptive neuromuscular facilitation. Static stretching is performed by slowly moving into a stretched position and holding the stretch for 15 to 30 seconds. Dynamic stretching involves maximal joint motion secondary to muscle contraction. The athlete uses controlled swinging of a limb with gradually increasing distance speed and intensity without exceeding his range of motion. Ballistic stretching involves quick bouncing movements that use momentum to achieve greater range of motion. This form of stretching is not recommended.

1. McKeag DL, Moeller JL. ACSM's Primary Care Sports Medicine. 2nd ed. Philadelphia: Lippincott Williams & Wilkins, 2007:134-135.
2. Moore MA, Hutton RS. Electromyographic investigation of muscle stretching techniques. Med Sci Sports Exerc 1980;12(5):322-329.

148. A 21-year-old type 1 diabetic athlete begins training for a 50-mile bike ride with a partner. She uses an insulin pump and is experienced with running cross country in high school. During her first 30-mile ride, she experiences symptoms of hypoglycemia at 25 miles and almost falls before stopping. She is confused, and her blood sugar level is 40. Which of the following is the most appropriate immediate action?

A. Eat a banana or sports bar
B. Administration of glucagon by her partner
C. Drink a carbohydrate sports drink then quickly resume riding to reach a safe destination
D. Drink eight ounces of water to improve volume status

Correct Answer: B

Glucagon has the most rapid onset of action in a confused, uncooperative athlete. Hyperinsulinemia due to the pump is the cause. A reduction of infusion by 50% is needed for longer bouts of exercise. A solid carbohydrate food will be absorbed too slowly to prevent potential serious CNS complications in this emergency. Resumption of exercise without adjusting the continuous pump plus a carbohydrate bolus will result in progressive hypoglycemia and CNS decline. Dehydration may exist for various reasons, but carbohydrate fuel is absolute necessity in this situation.

1. Sonnenberg GE, Kemmer FW, Berger M. Exercise in type 1 diabetic patients treated with continuous subcutaneous insulin infusion. Prevention of exercise induced hypoglycemia. Diabetologia 1990 Nov;33(11):696-703.

149. A 17-year-old male presents to your office with a chief complaint of heel pain. If this patient has Sever's disease, which of the following items collected during the history and physical examination would you expect?

   A. Skeletal maturity
   B. Normal foot radiograph
   C. Pain worse in the morning
   D. Tight gastrocnemius-soleus muscle complex
   E. Normal foot alignment

Correct Answer: D

Sever's disease is also known as calcaneal apophysitis. It is thought to occur secondarily to the strong vertical shear forces along the apophysis before fusion has been completed. The apophysis appears around 7 to 9 years of age, and is fused around 17. The mean age for presentation is 10 to 12. Therefore, you would not expect a skeletally mature patient as in Answer A. Radiographs of the foot are not diagnostic of Sever's disease. They may show sclerosis and fragmentation, but these findings are found in asymptomatic patients as well. The primary usefulness of the radiograph is to eliminate other causes of heel pain. Hence, Answer B is not the best answer. The classic presentation includes tightness of the Achilles tendon. It also typically includes a history of overuse found in a new sporting activity or season. These activities are typically high impact sports such as track, soccer, or tennis and with hard surfaces. Improper footwear and malalignment of the foot is also found commonly. With this in mind, the best answer of the remaining choices is D.

1. Hendrix CL. Calcaneal apophysitis (Sever disease). Clin Podiatr Med Surg 2005 Jan;22(1):55-62, vi.
2. Micheli LJ, Ireland ML. Prevention and management of calcaneal apophysitis. J Pediatr Orthop 1987 Jan-Feb;7(1):34-38.
3. Ishikawa SN. Conditions of the Calcaneus in Skeletally Immature Patients. Foot Ankle Clin 2005 Sep;10(3):503-513, vi.
4. Scharfbillig RW, Jones S, Scutter S. Sever's disease: a prospective study of risk factors. J Am Podiatr Med Assoc 2011 Mar-Apr;101(2):133-145.

150. The "clunk test" evaluates shoulder pathology caused by which of the following?

    A. Impingement
    B. Tendinopathy
    C. Labral tears
    D. Sliding biceps tendon
    E. Instability

Correct Answer: C

Snapping shoulder syndrome may be related to an intraarticular or extraarticular pathological condition. The initial evaluation of a patient with snapping shoulder should include thorough examination for mild glenohumeral instability and labral defects, which can be evaluated by the "clunk" test. This test, as described by Andrews and Gillogly, is performed with the patient supine and the arm in full overhead abduction. One of the examiner's hands is placed posterior to the humeral head to apply anterior pressure while the other hand is placed at the level of the humeral condyles to provide rotation and axial loading. A "clunk" or grinding may indicate a Bankart lesion or a labral tear caused by instability.

1. Hegedus EJ, Goode A, Campbell S, Morin A, Tamaddoni M, Moorman CT III, et al. Physical examination tests of the shoulder: a systematic review with meta-analysis of individual tests. Br J Sports Med 2008 Feb;42(2):80-92.
2. Clunk test and other shoulder tests from chart: shoulder examination stress tests, University of Western Alabama. Accessed February 15, 2012 at http://at.uwa.edu/Special%20Tests/SpecialTests/UpperBody/shoulder%20Main%20Page.html.

151. Which of the following statements is true regarding proximal biceps tendon rupture?

   A. A complete rupture results in formation of "Popeye" deformity with a large bulge in the proximal arm
   B. Must be treated with surgery within two weeks of injury in order to preserve function
   C. The typical mechanism of injury is forceful extension against excessive resistance
   D. Plain x-rays should be obtained to rule out avulsion of the bony origin
   E. The weakness caused by proximal biceps tendon rupture is significantly less than the weakness caused by distal biceps tendon rupture

Correct Answer: E

The best answer is E. Typically, complete rupture of the distal biceps tendon results in greater weakness and less endurance compared to proximal ruptures. These distal ruptures are more likely to require a surgical repair A complete rupture of the proximal biceps tendon usually results in considerable pain, swelling, and ecchymosis in acute injury. A visible hump in the mid-portion of the upper arm, the "Popeye" deformity is caused by retraction of the biceps muscle belly distally. Patients, especially those who place lower demands on the shoulder, often can be treated non-operatively for proximal biceps tendon rupture. The typical mechanism of injury is forced flexion of the elbow against excessive resistance. Plain x-rays are usually normal and do not contribute to the diagnosis. The most common location of injury is a complete disruption of the long head of the biceps as it passes through the bicipital groove.

1. Hutton KS, Julin MJ. Shoulder injuries. In: Mellion MB, Walsh WM, Madden C, Putukian M, Shelton GL (eds). Team Physician's Handbook. 3rd ed. Philadelphia: Hanley and Belfus, 2002:397-418.
2. Branch GL. Biceps rupture. Medscape. Accessed December 12, 2011 at http://emedicine.medscape.com/article/327119-overview.

152. Which of the following statements is true regarding hip flexor injury?

    A. X-ray to rule out hip flexor origin avulsion is needed in adolescents with the possible diagnosis of hip flexor pain and tenderness over the ischial tuberosity
    B. A hop test with pain in the ipsilateral groin is indicative of a hip flexor strain
    C. Patients with large, palpable defects in the rectus femoris rarely need surgery
    D. Hip flexor strains are commonly accompanied by a tingling sensation in the anterior thigh because of irritation of the lateral femoral cutaneous nerve
    E. Significant weakness is usually seen on exam with most hip flexor strains

Correct Answer: C

The best answer is C. Isolated deformities of the rectus femoris usually cause little to no functional disability and rarely need surgical intervention. The most common site of avulsion of hip flexors is the rectus femoris at the anterior inferior iliac crest, not the ischial tuberosity, which is the origin of the hamstrings (a hip extensor). A positive hop test is suspicious for a femoral neck stress fracture. Meralgia paresthetica is a condition caused by irritation of the lateral femoral cutaneous nerve (often at the inguinal ligament). Meralgia paresthetica is not commonly associated with hip flexor strains. Because the hip flexors are very strong muscles, most strains do not cause significant weakness, but instead have pain (and perhaps subtle weakness) with resistance testing.

1. Rosenberg J. Hip tendonitis and bursitis. Medscape. Accessed December 12, 2011 at http://emedicine.com/sports/topic49.

153. An 800 m open water swim is part of a short-course triathlon with over 800 registered athletes. It will be held in a shallow, protected lake that is usually calm but has been notorious for sudden weather changes. The race was cancelled the prior year because of excessive wave chop and poor visibility, and a duathlon (bike and run race) was held in its place. Since that time, you have implemented some changes to improve safety in the case of any adverse events. Which of the following is an adequate safety measure for this race?

   A. Local volunteer swim club members will be on hand at the finish to deal with common minor conditions
   B. A "mass start" will begin the swim to assure the race finishes at an early time
   C. There will be one certified lifeguard for every 50 swimmers in this non-ocean race
   D. There will be large, highly visible buoys positioned 1000 m or so apart and secured in a manner that will limit their movement in the most severe wave conditions in that body of water
   E. A highly mobile, powered watercraft will be "on call" in the area to facilitate any emergency plan that is implemented

Correct Answer: C

USA Triathlon event-sanctioning guidelines suggest that this ratio be no lower than one lifeguard for every 50 athletes in non-ocean swims and one lifeguard for every 35 athletes in ocean swims. (Triathlon Canada guidelines recommend a minimum ratio of one lifeguard for every 25 swimmers.) "Wave" starts minimize the number of competitors in the water at any one time. The rescuers should ideally have lifeguard training and minimally first responder training. Several highly mobile watercraft should be on site to facilitate any emergency. Large, highly visible buoys every 100 m should be secured in a manner to limit movement in severe conditions.

1. Dallam GM, Jonas S, Miller TK. Medical considerations in triathlon competition: recommendations for triathlon organizers, competitors and coaches. Sports Med 2005;35(2):143-161.
2. Martinez JM, Laird R. Managing Triathlon competition. Curr Sports Med Rep 2003 Jun;2(3):142-146.

154. A 12-year-old girl with no previous hip problems suffers an injury immediately after landing in the sand pit following setting her personal record in the long jump. She now has pain and tenderness deep within the hip over the proximal and medial femur. There is pain with passive internal and external rotation of the involved hip and with active hip flexion. The examination of the other hip is normal. The most accurate diagnosis is avulsion of the apophysis over which of the following?

    A. Ischial tuberosity
    B. Anterior superior ischial spine
    C. Anterior inferior ischial spine
    D. Lesser trochanter
    E. Greater trochanter

Correct Answer: D

The most common sites of avulsion fractures of an apophysis near the hip in a skeletally immature athlete are the anterior superior iliac spine (sartorius), the ischium (hamstrings), the lesser trochanter (iliopsoas), the anterior inferior iliac spine (abdominal rectus), and iliac crest (abdominal muscles). These are injuries resulting from sudden mechanical force and from weakness at the secondary growth site. This type of maximal effort causing an injury in an adult would most often lead to a simple muscle strain, not a fracture of a mature bone. These injuries occur in running and jumping sports during a maximal effort. Avulsion of the apophysis over the greater trochanter is rare. Presentation of apophyseal fractures is acute. Common bursitis reactions in the same areas present gradually, often with an overuse history. Plain radiographs can demonstrate these apophyseal avulsion fractures.

1. DeLee JC, Drez D, Miller MD (eds). DeLee & Drez's Orthopaedic Sports Medicine. 2nd ed. Philadelphia: Saunders Elsevier, 2003.
2. McKeag DB, Moeller JL. ACSM's Primary Care Sports Medicine. 2nd ed. Philadelphia: Lippincott Williams & Wilkins, 2007.
3. Hecht S. Gymnastics injuries. In: Mellion M, Walsh W, Madden, C, Putukian M, Shelton G (eds). Team Physician's Handbook. 3rd ed. Philadelphia: Hanley and Belfus, 2002:673.

155. Which of the following is listed as a minor criterion of Marfan syndrome?

    A. Ectopia lentis
    B. Dilation of the ascending aorta
    C. Lumbosacral dural ectasia
    D. Scoliosis > 20 degrees
    E. High-arched palate

Correct Answer: E

Skeletal major criteria include scoliosis greater than 20 degrees: more than 60% of patients have scoliosis. Progression is most likely with curvature of more than 20 degrees in growing patients. A highly arched palate is a minor skeletal criterion. One of the major criterions for ocular findings includes ectopia lentis. About 50% of patients have lens dislocation. The dislocation is usually superior and temporal. This may present at birth or develop during childhood or adolescence. A major criterion for cardiovascular includes aortic root dilatation involving the sinuses of Valsalva. The prevalence of aortic dilatation in Marfan syndrome is 70% to 80%. It manifests at an early age and tends to be more common in men than women. A diastolic murmur over the aortic valve may be present. Only one major criterion is defined for dural findings: dural ectasia must be present and confirmed using CT or MRI. Dural ectasia most frequently occurs in the lumbosacral spine.

1. De Paepe A, Devereux RB, Dietz HC, Hennekam RC, Pyeritz RE. Revised diagnostic Criteria for the Marfan syndrome. Am J Med Genet 1996 Apr 24;62(4):417-426.
2. Chen H. Marfan syndrome. Emedicine. Accessed December 12, 2011 at http://emedicine.medscape.com/article/946315.

156. A 26-year-old female triathlete comes in to see you in consultation at your sports medicine clinic. She asks for your nutrition recommendations to complement her current training regimen. For optimal post-exercise recovery, you recommend that she take which of the following?

    A. Low glycemic index carbohydrates and protein (in a ratio of 3:1), and no fat within 30 minutes of completing her workouts
    B. High glycemic index carbohydrates and protein (in a ratio of 3:1), and some fat within 30 minutes of completing her workouts
    C. Low glycemic index carbohydrates and fat (in a ratio of 3:1) within 30 minutes of completing her workouts
    D. High glycemic index carbohydrates and fat (in a ratio of 3:1) within 30 minutes of completing her workouts
    E. Low glycemic index carbohydrates and protein (in a ratio of 3:1), and some fat within 30 minutes of completing her workouts

Correct Answer: B

The primary fuel source for exercising muscles during moderate to high intensity endurance events is glycogen. An adequate glycogen supply helps prevent "bonking" or "hitting the wall," and is, therefore, crucial in exercise performance. Optimal recovery in preparation for future exercise bouts is directly related to the ability to restore this glycogen supply. However, depleted glycogen stores are replenished slowly, involving multiple factors and a complex array of biochemical interactions. Dietary carbohydrates are converted to glucose and stored in skeletal muscles and the liver as glycogen. Following the completion of an endurance event, there is a window of time (up to 30 to 60 minutes after the event) during which glycogen stores are more readily increased from dietary carbohydrates. Additionally, high glycemic index carbohydrates evoke larger increases in serum glucose, which in turn facilitates glycogen repletion. Studies have also suggested that coingestion of protein (amino acids), and perhaps a small amount of fat, with carbohydrates may also facilitate glycogen repletion, as well as enhance muscle protein balance—a critical component to muscle recovery. While more research is needed, current recommendations for optimal recovery of muscle glycogen stores and protein balance include ingesting 1.0 to 1.5 g of carbohydrates per kg of body weight within 30 minutes of completing an endurance event lasting longer than one hour, and repeated every two hours for four to six hours. Protein replacement at a protein to carbohydrate ratio of 1:3 (or 1:4) after exercise is also probably helpful.

1. Zawadzki KM, Yaspelkis BB III, Ivy JL. Carbohydrate-protein complex increases the rate of muscle glycogen storage after exercise. J Appl Physiol 1992 May;72(5):1854-1859.
2. Rasmussen BB, Tipton KD, Miller SL, Wolf SE, Wolfe RR. An oral essential amino acid-carbohydrate supplement enhances muscle protein anabolism after resistance exercise. J Appl Physiol 2000 Feb;88(2):386-392.
3. DiMarco NM, Samuels M. Nutritional considerations. In: O'Connor FG, Wilder RP (eds). Textbook of Running Medicine. New York: McGraw-Hill, 2001:469-477.

157. Which of the following has been reported in association with creatine use in an otherwise healthy athlete?

   A. Muscle cramping
   B. Cardiac complications
   C. Weight loss
   D. Renal complications
   E. Constipation

Correct Answer: A

Muscle cramps, diarrhea, and weight gain have been reported in athletes using creatine. The potential also exists for elevation in uric acid levels, leading to gout-like symptoms. Long-term effects of supplemental creatine have yet to be established, and no serious side effects have been consistently documented from creatine supplementation.

1. Rodriguez NR, DiMarco NM, Langley S, American Dietetic Association, Dietetians of Canada, American College of Sports Medicine. Position of the American Dietetic Association, Dietitians of Canada, and the American College of Sports Medicine: Nutrition and athletic performance. J Am Diet Assoc. 2009 Mar;109(3):509-527.
2. Gualano B, Ugrinowitsch C, Novaes RB, Artioli GG, Shimizu MH, Seguro AC, et al. Effects of creatine supplementation on renal function: a randomized, double-blind, placebo-controlled clinical trial. Eur J Appl Physiol. 2008 May;103(1):33-40.
3. Lattavo A, Kopperud A, Rogers PD. Creatine and other supplements. Pediatr Clin N Am 2007 Aug;54(4):735-760, xi.

158. The number of disabled athletes competing in sports has substantially increased over the years. Athletes with spinal cord injury (SCI) often have difficulty regulating body temperature during training or competition in both warm and cold environments. These conditions necessitate understanding which of the following true statements?

   A. In cold weather, SCI athletes are predisposed to hypothermia from paralysis and decreased muscle mass below the level of the lesion and a reduced ability to generate body heat by shivering
   B. In warm weather, impairment of sweating and control of peripheral blood flow below the level of the lesion (decreased surface area for cooling via evaporation) decreases the risk of hyperthermia
   C. Proper clothing, hydration and avoidance of activities during extreme temperatures are not as important because decreased peripheral sensation allows increased exposure time without significant detriment
   D. Athletes participating in cold weather sports need not be concerned about inspecting extremities to avoid frostbite if properly dressed for the activity

Correct Answer: A

Impairment of sweating in a SCI athlete increases the risk of hyperthermia. Athletes with impaired sensation should frequently inspect extremities to avoid cold injury, like frostbite, even when properly dressed.

1. Dec KL. Challenged athletes. In: McKeag DB, Moeller JL (eds). ACSM's Primary Care Sports Medicine. 2nd ed. Lippincott Williams & Wilkins, 2007:294-303
2. Klenck C, Gebke K. Practical management: common medical problems in disabled athletes. Clin J Sports Med 2007 Jan;17(1):55-60.

159. A 42-year-old female runner presents to your office with a history of multiple joint pain that started after her return from a sprint distance triathlon in Michigan last week. Her diet, menses, and weight are unchanged. She runs about 15 to 20 miles a week, swims three miles per week and bikes 50 miles a week. She denies a fever but does feel flushed at times. No history of autoimmune condition in her family. Her vitals are normal and afebrile. She has a normal musculoskeletal exam outside of subjective joint soreness. Her skin exam shows an abdominal rash, which is 6 cm in diameter, appearing as an annular homogenous erythema with a central purpura. The test you would most likely order **first** is which of the following?

A. CBC
B. Lyme titre
C. ANA
D. Rheumatoid factor
E. Thyroid stimulating hormone

Correct Answer: B

Image is of erythema chronicum migrans, which is pathognomonic for Lyme disease. In addition, the patient traveled to a Lyme-endemic area.

1. Meyeroff J. Lyme Disease. Medscape. Accessed February 15, 2012 at http://emedicine.medscape.com/article/330178.
2. Lyme disease. Centers for Disease Control and Prevention. Accessed February 15, 2012 at www.cdc.gov/lyme.

160. The most common site from which nosebleeds arise is which of the following?

A. Sphenopalantine artery
B. Anterior ethmoidal artery
C. Kiesselbach's plexus
D. Posterior ethmoidal artery

Correct Answer: C

Kiesselbach's plexus, in the anterior nasal septum is the most prominent anastomosis of the internal and external carotid circulation in the nose and is the most common site for epistaxis.

1. Gifford TO, Orlandi RR. Epistaxis. Otolaryngol Clin North Am 2008 Jun;41(3):525-536, viii.
2. Nguyen Q. Epistaxis. Medscape. Accessed December 12, 2011 at http://emedicine.medscape.com/article/863220-overview#a0104.

161. A professional basketball player comes to you, his team physician, during the off-season to discuss his medical history in light of his contract renewal option. He is medically healthy except for seven documented concussions over the course of his eight-year career. He had one concussion that included brief loss of consciousness. In no instance was he held out of competition for longer than one week. Which of the following would be a true statement to consider when advising him medically about retirement?

 A. Assessment of each prior concussion, particularly severity, should not influence his decision
 B. There is a higher risk of concussion after sustaining more than two concussions in a seven-year period
 C. Subsequent concussions could possibly resolve faster than prior ones
 D. A recently performed, normal MRI would lessen concerns
 E. There is potential risk for neurocognitive deficits

Correct Answer: E

A normal MRI does not rule out neurologic damage from one or more concussions. Severity of prior concussions does seem to play a role in not only the absolute risk of a subsequent concussion, but also in the recovery time for each. One study showed a three-fold higher risk of concussion after sustaining more than three concussions in a seven-year span. There are further risks that aren't completely understood including second-impact syndrome (although there is ongoing debate questioning whether this is a distinct clinical entity) and neurocognitive dysfunction.

1. Guskiewicz KM, McCrea M, Marshall SW, Cantu RC, Randolph C, Barr W, et al. Cumulative effects of recurrent concussion in collegiate football players: the NCAA Concussion Study. JAMA 2003 Nov 19;290(19):2549-2555.
2. Guskiewicz KM, Weaver NL, Padua DA, Garrett WE Jr. Epidemiology of concussion in collegiate and high school football players. Am J Sports Med 2000 Sep-Oct;28(5):643-650.
3. Lovell MR, Iverson GL, Collins MW, McKeag D, Maroon JC. Does loss of consciousness predict neuropsychological decrements after concussion? Clin J Sport Med 1999 Oct;9(4):193-198.

162. A 23-year-old professional snowboarder falls while making a jump. He lies on the snow and does not get up. When ski patrol reaches him, he is conscious and complaining of back pain. He is boarded and collared and transported to the nearest hospital. He is neurologically intact. A plain film radiograph shows a compression fracture of T12. Which of the following is the appropriate next step in his course of treatment?

   A. Obtain a CT scan to further assess the fracture
   B. Place the patient in a TLSO brace and perform follow-up x-rays in two weeks
   C. Consult the neurosurgeon for surgical correction of the fracture
   D. Consult interventional radiology for kyphoplasty of the fracture

Correct Answer: A

Answer A is correct. Burst fractures can be misdiagnosed as mere compression fractures with plain film radiographs. A CT scan can give more diagnostic information than plain radiographs. Lamina and articular process fractures are typically missed on plain films. If the fracture is established to be stable, the patient can be placed in a TLSO brace and followed with x-rays. Answer B did not assess whether the fracture was stable or not before placing the patient in a TLSO brace. If the fracture is established to be unstable or the patient has neurologic deficits, the neurosurgeon should be consulted for surgical stabilization with or without decompression as needed. Answer C did not assess the stability of the fracture. In Answer D, the patient was not assessed further to diagnose the burst fracture and was treated as a compression fracture.

1. Boden BP, Jarvis CG. Spinal injuries in sports. Neurol Clin 2008 Feb;26(1):63-78, viii.
2. Wennberg, RA, Cohen HB, Walker SR. Neurologic injuries in hockey. Neurol Clin 2008 Feb;26(1):243-255, xi.
3. Slotkin, JR, Lu Y, Wood KB. Thoracolumbar spinal trauma in children. Neurosurg Clin N Am 2007 Oct;18(4):621-630.

163. A volleyball player presents with right shoulder pain after attempting to spike the ball in practice. The player is holding her arm in slight abduction and external rotation. The humeral head is palpated anteriorly. Before proceeding, it is important to first evaluate which of the following?

    A. Supraclavicular nerve by testing sensation over the clavicular area
    B. Axillary nerve by testing sensation over lateral aspect of the shoulder
    C. Radial nerve by testing sensation over inferolateral arm
    D. Medial cutaneous nerve by testing sensation over medial aspect of arm

Correct Answer: B

Axillary nerve injury is a known complication of anterior dislocations of the shoulder. Before proceeding with x-ray and/or reduction, it is important to document neurovascular status by specifically checking sensation over the superior lateral aspect of arm (i.e., over the deltoid).

1. Thompson, JC. Netter's Concise Atlas of Orthopaedic Anatomy. Teterboro, NJ: Icon Learning Systems, 2002:47.
2. Wilson, S. Shoulder dislocation in emergency medical clinical presentation. Medscape. Accessed December 12, 2011 at http://emedicine.medscape.com/article/823843-clinical#a0217.

164. A 17-year-old woman notes on her preparticipation physical that she has had regular menstrual periods over the past four years until the last 10 months. During the last 10 months, she has had no menstrual periods. Her history reveals no obvious causes for this other than her participation in cross country and track. Her physical exam is unremarkable. Which of the following statements is the best statement that reflects her condition?

   A. She is suffering from exercise-related amenorrhea and should be counseled about starting on calcitonin to prevent osteoporosis
   B. She is suffering from oligomenorrhea and should be counseled to gain weight so that her menstrual cycles return to normal
   C. She is normal for her age and should wait one year to see if her menstrual cycle returns to normal
   D. She is suffering from an eating disorder and should be counseled to seek a mental health consultation
   E. She is suffering from amenorrhea and should be counseled to have laboratory testing to determine the cause

Correct Answer: E

A history of amenorrhea is one of the easiest ways to detect the female athlete triad in its earliest stages. Evidence suggests that menstrual history may predict current bone density in female athletes. In a study of young female athletes, longer, more consistent patterns of amenorrhea were found to have a linear correlation with measures of bone density. Amenorrhea should not be discounted by the family physician as a benign consequence of athletic training. Thus, in this case, further workup is indicated.

1. Warren M. Amenorrhea and infertility associated with exercise. UpToDate. Accessed December 12, 2011 at www.uptodate.com.
2. Hobart JA, Smucker DS. The female athlete triad. Am Fam Physician 2000 Jun 1;61(11):3357-3364, 3367.
3. Drinkwater BL, Bruemner B, Chesnut CH III. Menstrual history as a determinant of current bone density in young athletes. JAMA 1990 Jan 26;263(4):545-548.

165. A 33-year-old female runner has increased her running regimen for an upcoming marathon. She has had only three menstrual periods in the last six months. Her pregnancy test is negative. The most likely etiology of her menstrual dysfunction is which of the following?

    A. Increased testosterone
    B. Increased LH
    C. Decreased GnRH
    D. Increased prolactin

Correct Answer: C

Studies have demonstrated that exercise-induced menstrual dysfunction with loss of menses occurs due to the loss of the LH surge. This is caused by a disruption in the pulsatile secretion of GnRH by the hypothalamus. The specific factors that cause this disruption are still unknown. However, it is shown to be linked to an energy deficit, which disrupts the normal brain function; therefore, C is the correct answer. Answers A and D are incorrect because exercise-induced menstrual dysfunction is not related to testosterone or prolactin. Answer B is incorrect because there is a relative decrease in LH, not an increased LH.

1. Beals KA, Meyer NL. Female athlete triad update. Clin Sports Med 2007 Jan;26(1):69-89.
2. Joy L, Macintyre JG. Women in sports. In: Mellion MB, Walsh MW, Madden C, Putukian M, Shelton GL (eds). Team Physician's Handbook. 3rd ed. Philadephia: Hanley and Belfus, 2002:79-81.

166. A 22-year-old male wrestler presents to your clinic after falling awkwardly in a match approximately four hours earlier in the day, injuring his left wrist. The patient appears uncomfortable and states the pain has been getting worse since the time of the injury despite ice and immobilization. On exam, he has swelling and is tender over the distal radius. His neurovascular exam is intact, but he is unwilling to allow extension of his wrist or fingers because of pain. An x-ray is done and shows a minimally displaced extra-articular fracture of the distal radius. Which of the following complications of this injury is most likely at this time?

   A. Stretch injury of the median nerve
   B. Compartment syndrome
   C. Malunion
   D. Complex regional pain syndrome

Correct Answer: B

Compartment syndrome of the antebrachium may present with pain out of proportion to the injury, tenseness of the forearm, swelling, and pain with passive movement of the fingers and wrist. Early on, the patient usually has an intact radial pulse and good refill as these changes tend to occur late after significant tissue damage has already occurred. Median nerve injury may occur as pressures within the compartment continue to rise. The median nerve and extensor pollicis longus tendon may be damaged with this injury because of their close proximity to the distal radius. In this case, the patient has normal neurologic function; therefore, Answer A is incorrect.

While malunion is a concern with any fracture, it is unlikely with minimal displacement noted on x-ray. This complication should be monitored with routine follow-up (Answer C is incorrect). Answer D is incorrect because complex regional pain syndrome (CRPS) can occur with a distal radius fractures. This complication is associated with lack of physical activity after a period of immobilization. CRPS should be monitored for during follow-up visits and can usually be prevented with the appropriate ROM exercises during the complete treatment period.

1. Compartment syndromes of hand and forearm. Wheeless' Textbook of Orthopaedics. Accessed December 12, 2011 at www.wheelessonline.com/ortho/compartment_syndromes_of_hand_and_forearm.
2. Eiff MP, Hatch RL, Calmbach WL. Fracture Management for Primary Care. 2nd ed. Philadelphia: Saunders, 2003:123-124.

167. You are evaluating a 27-year-old recreational tennis player. She felt some searing chest wall pain on her dominant side while extending for a forehand shot three days ago. On her exam today, you notice substantial bruising along the anterior chest wall, suggesting some soft tissue injury. You begin by palpating the pectoralis major muscle. Of the following points, which one is helpful when trying to palpate the pectoralis minor?

    A. Sternum
    B. Clavicle
    C. Ribs 2 through 6
    D. Humerus
    E. Coracoid process

Correct Answer: E

Answer E refers to the insertion of the pectoralis minor, which has its origin on the third to fifth ribs, and also inserts on the scapula. Answers A and C (sternum and ribs 2 through 6) are the origins of the sternal head of the pectoralis major. For Answer B, the medial clavicle is the origin of the clavicular head. The humerus, Answer D, is the insertion of the muscle on the intertubercular groove (outer lip).

1. Standring S, Williams PL, Warwick R (eds). Gray's Anatomy. 37th ed.: Longman Group UK Limited, 1989:610-611.
2. Minnesota State University, Mankato, Department of Human Performance, Athletic Training. Manual muscle testing: pectoralis minor. Accessed December 13, 2011 at http://ahn.mnsu.edu/athletictraining/spata/shouldermodule/muscletesting.html.

Test 1 Answers, Critiques, and References

168. Which of the following regarding injury prevention is correct?

   A. Single-hinge knee braces can prevent knee injuries in American football
   B. Lace-up braces for ankles can reduce recurring ankle injuries in athletes with previous ankle injuries
   C. Headgear (scrum caps) can decrease the incidence of concussions in rugby
   D. Eyewear with corrective lenses can prevent injury to the orbit

Correct Answer: B

Injury prevention is an important area of research, but unfortunately, good-quality controlled and blinded studies are lacking. In addition, there are conflicting results within this area of research. Hinged knee braces, overall, have not been consistently shown to reduce knee injuries. Single-hinge knee braces have actually been shown to increase injury to the ipsilateral ankle and foot. The effectiveness of custom functional knee braces has not been shown to consistently reduce injury, as they offer little protection to rotational stress.

Protective headgear for soccer and scrum caps for rugby do not consistently prevent concussions. They may provide some reduction in facial trauma. In order for eyewear to be protective for low-risk sports, certain specifications must be met. If using street-wear frames, they must meet American National Standards Institute (ANSI) standards with a securing strap and polycarbonite or CR-39 lenses. For high-risk sports, the use of fitted goggles with polycarbonite lenses are recommended because they are stronger than CR-39. Lace-up braces have been shown to help reduce future ankle injuries, especially with athletes with previous ankle injuries. Proprioceptive training has also shown to be effective at reducing ankle injuries.

1. Paluska SA, McKeag DB. Knee braces: current evidence and clinical recommendations for their use. Am Fam Physician 2000 Jan 15;61(2):411-418, 423-424.
2. Pedowitz DI, Reddy S, Parekh SG, Huffman GR, Sennett BJ. Prophylactic bracing decreases ankle injuries in collegiate female volleyball players. Am J Sports Med 2008 Feb;36(2):324-327.
3. McIntosh AS, McCrory P. Effectiveness of headgear in a pilot study of under 15 rugby union football. Br J Sports Med 2001 Jun;35(3):167-169.
4. Withnall C, Shewchenko N, Wonnacott M, Dvorak J. Effectiveness of headgear in football. Br J Sports Med 2005 Aug;39(Suppl 1):i40-48.
5. Protective eyewear for young athletes. American Academy of Pediatrics Committee on Sports Medicine and Fitness and American Academy of Ophthalmology Committee on Eye Safety and Sports Ophthalmology. Pediatrics 1996 Aug;98(2 Pt 1):311-313, 314.
6. Hootman JM. Is it possible to prevent sports and recreation injuries: a systematic review of randomized controlled trials with recommendations for future work. In: MacAuley D, Best T (eds). Evidence-Based Sports Medicine. 2nd ed. Hoboken, NJ: Wiley & Sons, 2007.

169. According to the ATLS guidelines, which of the following is the estimated minimum systolic blood pressure with a palpable radial pulse?

A. 40 mm Hg
B. 100 mm Hg
C. 80 mm Hg
D. 120 mm Hg

Correct Answer: C

ATLS courses teaches the blood pressures can be predicted based on which pulses are palpable. Femoral pulses indicate a SBP of 60 to 70, carotid pulses indicate a SBP of 70 to 80, and radial pulses indicate a SBP of greater than 80 mm Hg. One study evaluated these estimations but used non-invasive blood pressure measurements, which have a tendency to underestimate systemic arterial blood pressure during hypotension. Further study shows these may be overestimations.

1. Collicott PE. Advanced Trauma Life Support Course for Physicians. Chicago: American College of Surgeons, 1985.
2. Deakin CD, Low JL. Accuracy of the advanced trauma life support guidelines for predicting systolic blood pressure using carotid, femoral, and radial pulses: observational study. BMJ 2000 Sep 16;321(7262):673-674.

170. A 19-year-old female basketball player tries to deflect a pass and sustains a hyperextension injury to the PIP joint of her middle finger. Her finger dislocates dorsally. You reduce the dislocation on the sideline. Radiographs taken after the game are negative for bony injury and show good alignment. Which of the following is the most appropriate next step?

A. No further treatment is necessary
B. The finger should be splinted in full extension
C. The finger should be splinted in 20 to 30 degrees of flexion
D. The finger and hand should be placed in a short arm cast

Correct Answer: C

Due to the high likelihood of a volar plate rupture during the hyperextension injury the finger should be splinted in 20 to 30 degrees of flexion to allow the volar plate to heal. Splinting in extension would be correct for a volar dislocation at the PIP, but not for dorsal dislocation. Short arm casting is not indicated for a PIP dislocation.

1. Hodge DK. Sideline management of common dislocations. Curr Sports Med Rep 2002 Jun;1(3):149-155.
2. Leggit JC, Meko CJ. Acute finger injuries: part II. fractures, dislocations, and thumb injuries. Am Fam Physician 2006 Mar 1;73(5):827-834.

171. What has been shown to give patients—with moderate to severe symptomatic knee osteoarthritis—better pain relief according to the glucosamine/chondroitin arthritis intervention trial (GAIT)?

    A. Glucosamine with chondroitin
    B. Glucosamine
    C. Chondroitin
    D. Placebo
    E. Glucosamine with chondroitin and MSM

Correct Answer: A

Glucosamine and chondroitin sulfate are dietary supplements that have attracted much interest; however, until recently, there have not been many scientific studies assessing its efficacy. A large multicenter, randomized, double blind, placebo-controlled study of 24 weeks duration published in the New England Journal of Medicine found that for patients with symptomatic knee osteoarthritis, oral glucosamine and chondroitin sulfate, alone or in combination, taken for 24 weeks, did not reduce pain or improve other outcomes better than placebo. However, in patients with moderate to severe osteoarthritis, combination therapy was better than placebo.

1. Clegg DO, Reda DJ, Harris CL, Klein MA, O'Dell JR, Hooper MM, et al. Glucosamine, chondroitin sulfate, and the two in combination for painful knee osteoarthritis. N Engl J Med 2006 Feb;354(8):795-808.
2. Hart L. Are glucosamine and/or chondroitin sulfate effective for knee osteoarthritis? Clin J Sport Med 2006 Nov;16(6):528-529.
3. Q&A: NIH glucosamine/chondroitin arthritis intervention trial primary study. Accessed December 12, 2011 at http://nccam.nih.gov/research/results/gait/qa.htm.

172. Which of the following statements about open and closed kinetic chain exercises is correct?

    A. Open kinetic chain exercises occur when the distal aspect of the extremity is fixed and cannot move
    B. Closed kinetic chain exercises typically involve functional weight-bearing activities
    C. Knee extensions and straight leg raises are examples of closed kinetic chain exercises
    D. During open kinetic chain exercises, motion occurs simultaneously at all joints comprising the kinetic chain
    E. Closed kinetic chain exercises produce shearing forces, while open kinetic chain exercises produce compressive forces

Correct Answer: B

Knee extensions and straight-leg raises are examples of open kinetic chain exercises. Open kinetic chain exercises involve free movement of the distal segment and are typically non-weight bearing. Examples include knee extensions and straight-leg raises. Conversely, closed kinetic chain exercises involve fixation of the distal aspect of the extremity, and they are important during functional weight bearing activities (Answer B). Answer A is incorrect because it describes closed kinetic chain exercises. Answer D is incorrect since simultaneous motion at all joints occurs during closed kinetic chain exercises. Answer E is incorrect because open chain exercises produce shearing forces, while closed chain exercises produce compressive forces.

1. McMahon PJ. Current Diagnosis and Treatment in Sports Medicine. New York: McGraw-Hill, 2007:272.
2. Augustsson J, Esko A, Thomeé R, Svantesson U. Weight training of the thigh muscles using closed vs. open kinetic chain exercises: a comparison of performance enhancement. J Orthop Sports Phys Ther 1998 Jan;27(1):3-8.

173. A 20-year-old basketball player falls on a pronated right hand. He was initially treated by the athletic trainer, noted to have prominence of the ulnar head and loss of supination. The trainer reduced it with supination of the forearm. You see him in the training room, he has full range of motion, neurovascular exam is intact, radiographs do not show fracture, dislocataion, or widening of the distal radioulnar joint (DRUJ). This injury should subsequently be treated in which manner?

   A. Thumb spica splint for two weeks
   B. Short arm cast for four weeks
   C. Long arm cast for six weeks
   D. Ulnar gutter splint

Correct Answer: C

The injury is an uncomplicated dorsal dislocation of the DRUJ. The athletic trainer was able to successfully reduce it with supination (moving ulnar head volarly). The normal exam, lack of fracture or evidence of chronic subluxation/dislocation allows conservative treatment. This is with a long arm cast (including elbow) for four to six weeks. All the other methods are insufficient for optimal protection of the DRUJ, and preventing pronation or supination. Orthopedic consultation can be arranged; percutaneous pin fixation may augment stability.

1. Radial ulnar joint instability. Wheeless' Textbook of Orthopedics. Accessed December 12, 2011 at www.wheelessonline.com/ortho/radial_ulnar_joint_instability.
2. Ozer K, Luis R. Scheker LR. Distal radioulnar joint problems and treatment options. Orthopedics 2006 Jan;29(1):38-49.

174. Where is the purest area for sensory testing of the radial nerve on the hand located?

    A. Dorsal web between the thumb and the index finger
    B. Radial side of the hand
    C. Dorsum of the wrist
    D. Thenar eminence

Correct Answer: A

The radial nerve provides sensation to the radial side of the hand. Thus, secondary to significant overlap the purest area for testing the radial nerve is the web space between the thumb and index finger. Answer B is incorrect due to overlap. Answer C is incorrect because the posterior interosseous nerve supplies this area. Answer D is incorrect because the palmer cutaneous branch of the median nerve supplies innervation to this area.

1. Cohe PH, Aish B. The acutely injured wrist. In: Puffer J (ed). 20 Common Problems Sports Medicine. New York: McGraw-Hill, 2002:76-78.
2. Doyle J, Botte M. Surgical anatomy of the hand and upper extremity. Lippincott Williams & Wilkins, 2002:214-218.

175. A climber in the Himalayas crests 2,500 m (approximately 8,200 feet) and experiences headache, nausea, fatigue, significant confusion, and ataxia. The most appropriate treatment option for this condition is which of the following?

    A. Rapid descent
    B. Corticosteroid (prednisone)
    C. Calcium channel blockers
    D. Non-steroidal anti-inflammatories

Correct Answer: A

In this clinical scenario, the climber is suffering from high altitude cerebral edema (HACE), which is distinguishable from acute mountain sickness (AMS) due to the mental status changes and ataxia. Many therapies have been suggested for AMS and HACE. Rapid descent and supplemental oxygen are the mainstays of treatment for both conditions and are critically important for climbers suffering presumed HACE.

1. Hackett PH, Roach RC. High-altitude illness. N Engl J Med 2001 Jul 12;345(2):107-114.
2. High altitude cerebral edema. Climbing High: The Climbing Guide. Accessed December 12, 2011 at www.climbing-high.com/high-altitude-cerebral-edema.html.
3. Acute mountain sickness. A.D.A.M. Medical Encyclopedia. Accessed December 12, 2011 at www.ncbi.nlm.nih.gov/pubmedhealth/PMH0001190.

176. Which of the following is an absolute contraindication to collision sports participation?

   A. Torg-Pavlov ratio < 0.8
   B. Recurrent cervical cord neuropraxia
   C. Healed-displaced-stable fracture of C3-C7 at posterior ring
   D. Clay shoveler's fracture
   E. Healed herniated nucleosis pulposis

Correct Answer: B

Cervical cord neuropraxia is defined as bilateral neurologic symptoms of the upper or lower extremities that lasts under 15 minutes and is typically caused by hyperflexion or hyperextension of the cervical spine. A Torg-Pavlov ratio of < 0.8 correlates with the diagnosis of cervical spine stenosis; however, this finding is not an absolute contraindication to participation in collision sports. An isolated incidence of cervical cord neuropraxia remains a relative contraindication to return to collision sports. Both Cantu and Torg recommend that athletes with recurrent cervical cord neuropraxia not participate in collision sports. A healed-displaced-stable C3-C7 fracture at the posterior ring, healed-herniated nucleosis pulposis, and clay shoveler's fracture are all viewed as stable fractures and have no contraindication in participation in collision sports.

   1. Cantu RC. Cervical spine injuries in the athlete. Semin Neurol 2000;20(2):173-178.
   2. Torg JS, Guille JT, Jaffe S. Injuries to the cervical spine in American football players. J Bone Joint Surg 2002 Jan;84-A(1):112-122.

177. A 13-year-old female soccer player sustains a groin strain when performing a sliding tackle in a game. Her evaluation in the emergency room is remarkable for an avulsion of the lesser trochanter with 1 cm displacement. Appropriate management would include which of the following?

    A. Refer immediately for surgical management
    B. Start physical therapy
    C. Place on crutches and make her non-weight bearing
    D. Rest for one week and clear for sports when her pain has resolved

Correct Answer: C

Apophyseal avulsions are common pediatric injuries around major joints. Key apophyses include the iliac crest, ischium, greater and lesser trochanter, medial elbow, tibial tubercle, and calcaneous. Because these avulsions involve the disruption of major tendons the long-term consequences of improper healing can be devastating to future performance. Avulsions of the lesser trochanter and insertion of the iliopsoas muscle can generally be managed with non-weight bearing with crutches with progression to weight bearing as tolerated. As pain improves, therapy to work on range of motion, stretching and strengthening should begin. Return to sports may take two to four months. Avulsions with displacement > 1 cm should be referred for open fixation and reduction.

1. Morelli V, Smith V. Groin injuries in athletes. Am Fam Physician 2001 Oct 15;64 (8):1405-1414.
2. Davenport M. Hip fracture in emergency medicine. Medscape. Accessed December 12, 2011 at http://emedicine.medscape.com/article/825363.
3. Theologis TN, Epps H, Latz K, Cole WG. Isolated fractures of the lesser trochanter in children. Injury 1997 Jun-Jul;28(5-6):363-364.

178. Which of the following is true regarding commotio cordis?

A. Little League baseball now requires the batter to wear chest protectors for prevention in children under 12
B. The apparent mechanism for death is ventricular fibrillation induced by an abrupt blunt precordial blow during a specific time in the cardiac cycle
C. Baseballs thrown at 20 mph, a blow in the left area of the heart, and blunt impacts are associated with more deadly outcomes in commotio cordis
D. With rapid defibrillation, cardiac support, and AED maneuvers, greater than 25% of individuals may survive commotio cordis
E. Impact must occur within the QRS of the cardiac cycle in order for ventricular fibrillation to occur and cause commotio cordis

Correct Answer: B

Ventricular fibrillation is the mechanism of death for commotio cordis and is induced by the blunt precordial blow that occurs in the upslope of the T wave (Answer E) and causes sudden death in athletes. Little League baseball (Answer A) has discussed chest protectors and reviewed comfort, fit, and effectiveness, but no requirements are currently in place. Baseballs thrown at more than 40 mph (Answer C) and blows in the center of the chest and precordial area are associated with more deadly outcomes. Despite rapid defibrillation and AED maneuvers (Answer D), less than 10% of patients with commotio cordis survive.

1. Madias C, Maron BJ, Weinstock J, Estes NA III, Link MS. Commotio cordis: sudden cardiac death with chest wall impact. J Cardiovasc Electrophysiol. 2007 Jan;18(1):115-122.
2. Classie JA, Distel LM, Borchers JR. Safety baseballs and chest protectors: a systematic review on the prevention of commotio cordis. Phys Sportsmed. 2010 Apr;38(1):83-90.
3. Maron BJ, Estes NA III. Commotio cordis. N Engl J Med 2010 Mar 11;362(10):917-927.

179. Which of the following statements regarding exercise testing in individuals with coronary artery disease (CAD) or risk factors for CAD is true?

   A. Excessive ST depression of >2 mm horizontal or downsloping is an absolute indication to terminate an exercise test
   B. Recommendation to get a graded exercise test for a 25-year-old with type 1 diabetes (diagnosed with IDDM for at least 10 years)
   C. During an exercise test, a change of less than or equal to 12 beats per minute from peak exercise HR to HR two minutes into recovery is strongly predictive of mortality
   D. MET level or exercise duration is not an important predictor of adverse cardiac events after MI

Correct Answer: C

ST depression is not an absolute indication to stop an exercise test, but a relative indication. Among other relative indications to terminate an exercise test are a drop more than or equal to 10 mm Hg in SBP from baseline during increased workload without other evidence of ischemia, arrythmias other than sustained VT, such as multifocal PVCs, triplets of PVCs, supraventricular tachycardia, heart block, or bradyarrythmias, hypertensive response, increasing chest pain, symptoms of fatigue, shortness of breath, claudication, and development of bundle branch block or IVCD which resembles VT.

Absolute indications to terminate an exercise test are a drop in SBP more than or equal to 10 mm Hg from baseline during increase workload with other evidence of ischemia, moderate to severe angina, neurological symptoms such as dizziness, near-syncope, signs of poor perfusion, inability to monitor ECG or SBP, sustained VT, ST elevation > 1 mm without diagnostic Q waves, and the subjects desire to stop.

Exercise tolerance testing is recommended in any diabetic individual more than 35 years of age, or for those older than 25 years of age with a history of diabetes of 15 years or more.

The abnormal heart rate recovery pattern after exercise testing has prognostic importance. A change in HR of less than 12 bpm from peak to two minutes into recovery is strongly predictive of all-cause mortality in six years. MET level and exercise duration is an important predictor of adverse cardiac events after MI and inability to reach five METs during treadmill testing is associated with worse prognosis.

1. Gibbons RJ, Balady GJ, Bricker JT, Chaitman BR, Fletcher GF, Froelicher VF, et al. ACC/AHA 2002 guideline update for exercise testing: summary article: a report of the American College of Cardiology/American Heart Association Task Force on Practice Guidelines (Committee to Update the 1997 Exercise Testing Guidelines). Circulation 2002 Oct 1;106(14):1883-1892.
2. Dexter W, Rahman S. Endocrine considerations. In: O'Connor FG, Sallis RE, Wilder RP, St. Pierre P (eds). Sports Medicine: Just the Facts. New York: McGraw-Hill, 2005:97, 186-203.

180. A female runner with knee pain presents after running a 10K and has a mildly swollen knee. Which of the following is true?

   A. Voshell's bursitis is an inflamed bursa between the medial collateral ligament and the tibia and may be treated with rest, anti-inflammatory medicines, and cross training
   B. Bursitis in the knee should be drained and sent for culture for proper antibiotic coverage
   C. Pes anserine bursitis is less often associated with pes planus than prepatellar bursitis
   D. Voshell's bursa is one of two bursas in the body that can become infected, most commonly by staphylococcus aureus
   E. Prepatellar bursitis often presents as medial knee pain that is more common after long periods of sitting and long trips

Correct Answer: A

Voshell's bursa is less commonly discussed and lies between the MCL and the tibia. Usual methods of conservative care are often effective. Not all bursitis complaints need to have fluid obtained for culture (Answer B), but the prepatellar bursa is one of two bursas that can become infected and may need to be drained (Answer D). The other bursa is the olecranon bursa in the elbow. Pes anserine bursitis (Answer C) is often associated with pes planus and treatment includes orthotics or supportive shoe inserts. Prepatellar bursitis is caused more by trauma and overuse rather than anatomical risk factors. Patellofemoral pain syndrome often presents as medial knee pain that is more common after sitting and long trips. Prepatellar bursitis is more common after microtrauma and is located anterior rather than medial.

1. Dodds WN. Soft tissue injuries in sports medicine. BMJ 1996;313:827.1.
2. Sheon RP. Bursitis: an overview of clinical manifestations, diagnosis, and management. UpToDate. Accessed December 12, 2011 at www.uptodate.com/contents/bursitis-an-overview-of-clinical-manifestations-diagnosis-and-management.
3. Glencross PM. Pes anserine bursitis. Medscape. Accessed December 12, 2011 at http://emedicine.medscape.com/article/308694.

181. A 15-year-old rugby player presents with a left fourth finger injury. She is unable to flex the DIP, and there is fullness along the flexor tendon. Which of the following is the appropriate course of treatment?

    A. Ice and NSAIDs
    B. Early surgical intervention
    C. Custom splint during games
    D. Buddy taping to left third finger

Correct Answer: B

A jersey finger injury is caused by the avulsion of the flexor digitorum profundus tendon (FDP), and the athlete would be unable to flex the DIP, most commonly occurring in the ring finger. The mechanism of injury would include hyperextension of the DIP joint on attempted flexion of the finger. There may be fullness at the flexor tendon sheath from hematoma formation. Treatment is operative and requires reattachment of the FDP tendon to its insertion in the distal phalanx.

The flexion deformity of the DIP joint, which presents as an inability to extend the DIP joint, is called a mallet finger. This is usually caused by the sudden forceful flexion of the DIP joint. It can be treated non-operatively by splinting in complete extension for six to eight weeks. Operative management is usually only with large fractures of the distal phalanx. Ice, NSAIDs, and buddy taping would not be adequate treatment alone for this injury.

1. Peterson JJ, Bancroft LW. Injuries of the fingers and thumb in the athlete. Clin Sports Med 2006 Jul;25(3):527-542, vii-viii.
2. Leggit JC, Mekc CJ. Acute finger injuries: part 1. Tendons and ligaments. Am Fam Physician 2006 Mar 1;73(5):810-816.

182. Regarding pediatric injury and Salter-Harris fractures, which of the following creates the greatest risk to joint integrity?

    A. Salter-Harris Type I
    B. Salter-Harris Type II
    C. Salter-Harris Type III
    D. Salter-Harris Type IV
    E. Salter-Harris Type V

Correct Answer: B

Saltar-Harris Type III injuries create the greatest risk to joint integrity. Proper joint reduction and alignment must be maintained to insure the least amount of challenge is given to the cartilage and as an attempt to prevent future joint degeneration.

   1. Kelly AW, Adirim T. Special populations. In: O'Connor FG, Sallis RE, Wilder RP, St. Pierre P (eds). Sports Medicine: Just the Facts. New York McGraw-Hill, 2005:559.
   2. Maffulli N. The younger athlete. In: Brukner P, Khan K. Clinical Sports Medicine. 3rd ed. Sydney: McGraw Hill, 2007:654.

183. It is well known that the weather can play a significant role in the outcomes at endurance races. Which wet bulb globe temperature (WBGT) is the threshold that would warrant a black flag warning on race day?

    A. 78 degrees Fahrenheit (25.6 degrees Celsius)
    B. 88 degrees Fahrenheit (31 degrees Celsius)
    C. 82 degrees Fahrenheit (27.8 degrees Celsius)
    D. 85 degrees Fahrenheit (29.4 degrees Celsius)

Correct Answer: C

With a WBGT of 82 degrees Fahrenheit (27.8 degrees Celsius), it is advised that race directors alert participants to the black flag status. This is equivalent to extreme risk and the event should be cancelled, postponed, or modified according to ACSM guidelines.

   1. Jaworski CA. Medical concerns of marathons. Curr Sports Med Rep 2005 Jun;4(3):137-143.
   2. IAAF Competition Medical Handbook. Accessed December 12, 2011 at www.iaaf.org/medical/info/index.html.

184. A 25-year-old male presents with thumb pain after a fall while skiing. On exam, his MCP joint is grossly unstable and MRI reveals a Stener lesion. Optimal management of this injury requires which of the following?

    A. Thumb splinted in extension for four weeks
    B. Thumb spica splint for six weeks
    C. Short arm cast for six weeks
    D. Surgical repair

Correct Answer: D

A Stener lesion is an abnormality seen in as many as 29% of cases of gamekeeper's thumb. In addition to disruption of the ulnar collateral ligament at the first MCP joint, there is an abnormal folded position of the torn end of the ulnar collateral ligament superficial to the adductor aponeurosis. Spontaneous ligament healing is inhibited by the interposition of the thumb extensor mechanism between torn fragments of the ulnar collateral ligament. Only operative intervention allows apposition and healing of the traumatically displaced ligament.

1. Peterson JJ, Bancroft LW. Injuries of the fingers and thumb in the athlete. Clin Sports Med 2006 July; 25(3):527-542, vii-viii.
2. Rectenwald J. Stener lesion. Medscape. Accessed December 12, 2011 at http:// emedicine.medscape.com/article/1240710.

185. A 20-year-old male patient presents to your office with a history of anterior shoulder dislocation which occurred during a pick-up basketball game last week. This was the athlete's first such injury, and the report from the emergency department stated that the dislocation was reduced without difficulty. Which of the following findings would lead you to recommend surgical evaluation for the patient?

    A. Persistent anterior capsular pain one week after the injury
    B. Decreased range of motion on your initial examination
    C. Positive apprehension test on your initial examination
    D. Avulsion of the anterior capsulolabral complex on radiographic evaluation

Correct Answer: D

Traumatic shoulder dislocations normally occur in the anterior or inferior direction. After dislocation, the patient may experience pain for several weeks due to the accompanying stretching of the capsular and ligamentous structures that stabilize the shoulder. It is not uncommon during the initial healing phase to have decreased range of motion or a subjective sense of instability as manifested by a positive apprehension test. Management of first anterior dislocations is somewhat controversial, with some studies showing benefit from surgical stabilization, and others showing no difference in outcomes between surgical and non-surgical management. However, radiographic evidence of anterior capsulolabral complex avulsion (Bankhart lesion) should lead the physician to at least recommend a surgical consultation for the patient.

1. Hudson VJ. Evaluation, diagnosis, and treatment of shoulder injuries. Clin Sports Med 2010;29(1):19-32.
2. Welsh S. Shoulder dislocation surgery. Medscape. Accessed December 12, 2011 at http://emedicine.medscape.com/article/1261802.

186. At a college tennis tournament, you are caring for a 22-year-old male tennis player from Italy who passed out in the middle of his match. He denies chest pain. You order an ECG, which shows some T-wave inversions in leads V_1 to V_3 and an incomplete right bundle branch block. When asked about family history, he recalls his grandfather died at a young age of some heart problem. You are most worried about sudden cardiac death in this patient from which of the following?

A. Coronary artery disease
B. Hypertrophic cardiomyopathy
C. Prolonged QT syndrome
D. Arrhythmogenic right ventricular dysplasia

Correct Answer: D

The overall incidence of sudden cardiac death in athletes is fairly low. The most common cause for those over 35 years old is coronary artery disease (CAD). For younger patients in the U.S., the most common cause is hypertrophic cardiomyopathy (HCM). However, European studies have shown very different statistics. One Italian study showed arrhythmogenic right ventricular dysplasia (ARVC) as the most common cause (22%), premature CAD was second (18%), while HCM was very rare (2%). With ARVC, athletes can perform at high levels of exertion with ventricular fibrillation most likely secondary to ventricle irritation. The right ventricle is replaced with adipose tissue becoming very thin. The history is of syncope and positive family history of premature cardiac sudden death. The EKG can show inverted T waves in the precordial leads, PVCs with left bundle-branch block, and right bundle-branch block. Echocardiogram may show abnormal, hypokinetic right ventricular dilatation.

1. Pigozzi F, Rizzo M. Sudden death in competitive athletes. Clin Sports Med 2008 Jan;27(1):153-181, ix.
2. Madden C, Putkian M. Preparticipation physical evaluation. In: Mellion MB, Walsh MW, Madden C, Putukian M, Shelton GL (eds). Team Physician's Handbook. 3rd ed. Philadephia: Hanley and Belfus, 2002:20-35.
3. Maron BJ, Shirani J, Polia LC, Mathenge R, Roberts WC, Mueller FO. Sudden death in young competitive athletes. Clinical, demographic and pathological profiles. JAMA 1996 Jul 17;276(3):199-204.
4. Corrado D, Basso C, Schiavon M, Thiene G. Screening for hypertrophic cardiomyopathy in young athletes. N Engl J Med 1998 Aug 6;339(6):364-369.

187. A volleyball player complains of shoulder pain with overhead activity. She denies any new trauma to the shoulder. Physical examination shows pain with impingement testing, but no anatomical deformities are visualized. Normal strength of the rotator cuff is noted, and radiographs are negative for fracture and dislocation. Which of the following is the most likely diagnosis?

    A. Subacromial bursitis
    B. Hill-Sachs lesion
    C. Complete rotator cuff tear
    D. Acromioclavicular (AC) separation

Correct Answer: A

Subacromial bursitis often presents as pain on overhead activity and can be worse at night. Pain often is focused along the anterolateral aspect of the shoulder and does not radiate past the elbow. Repeated stresses from overhead motions like throwing or setting can lead to fatigue of the muscles that stabilize the humeral head and prevent anterior subluxation. MRI may show an inflammation of the bursa, but diagnosis is mostly clinical.

A Hill-Sachs lesion can be missed on x-ray and is more commonly found on MRI with a history of shoulder dislocations. The Hill-Sachs lesion is a bony defect in the posterolateral portion of the humeral head, and it occurs in more than 50% of patients with a primary dislocation. The exam will demonstrate tenderness over the posterior aspect of the shoulder, and the anterior apprehension test usually causes more pain than apprehension. She does not have a history of recent shoulder trauma or complaints of past dislocations.

Rotator cuff tears occur with trauma in this age group. Tears would present with weakness of the cuff and pain during exam. Older patients with chronic impingement may also suffer from rotator cuff tears. MRI complements physical exam findings in order to diagnose a complete rotator cuff tear. Impingement testing may also be painful with a complete rotator cuff tear, but weakness in provocative shoulder testing is key to the diagnosis.

AC separation is most common after a direct blow to the superior aspect of the shoulder or a lateral blow to the deltoid area. It also may occur after falling onto an outstretched hand. The exam and history rules out an AC separation, but anteroposterior x-rays of the shoulder will confirm a separation greater than a grade I.

1. Woodward TW, Best TM. The painful shoulder: part I. Clinical evaluation. Am Fam Physician 2000 May 15;61(10):3079-3088.
2. Woodward TW, Best TM. The painful shoulder: part II. Acute and chronic disorders. Am Fam Physician 2000 Jun 1;61(11):3291-3300.

188. Which of the following is a current American Heart Association (AHA) recommendation regarding cardiac evaluation during the preparticipation exam?

    A. Auscultate for heart murmur during provocative maneuvers
    B. Palpate bilateral brachial pulses
    C. Obtain bilateral brachial blood pressure with the athlete standing
    D. Perform electrocardiogram on all athletes

Correct Answer: A

In addition to medical and family history screening in the preparticipation exam, the AHA recommends that the cardiovascular screening physical exam include recognition of physical stigmata related to Marfan syndrome, seated brachial blood pressure, palpation of radial and femoral pulses, and ausculatory cardiac exam, including provocative maneuvers for murmurs. ECG remains optional and is usually reserved for those found to have abnormal findings on screening history or exam.

1. Maron BJ, Thompson PD, Ackerman MJ, Balady G, Berger S, Cohen D, et al. Recommendation and considerations related to preparticipation screening for cardiovasular abnormalities in competitive athletes: 2007 update: a scientific statement from the American Heart Association Council on Nutrition, Physical Activity, and Metabolism: endorsed by the American College of Cardiology Foundation. Circulation 2007 Mar 27;115(12):1643-1655.
2. Pigozzi F, Spataro A, Fagnani F, Maffulli N. Preparticipation screening for the detection of cardiovascular abnormalities that may cause sudden death in competitive athletes. Br J Sports Med 2003 Feb;37:4-5.
3. Bernhardt D, Roberts B (eds). Preparticipation Physical Exam. 4th ed. American Academy of Pediatrics, 2010:51-70.

189. A female cross country runner complains of right-sided heel pain. She states the pain has been present for two weeks. Initially, the pain only occurred with long runs, but now hurts most of the time. On exam, pain is elicited by squeezing the heel. X-rays confirm the diagnosis. Which of the following statements about this condition is true?

    A. Surgical intervention is required
    B. Posterior night splints should be used
    C. She should be sent for injection therapy
    D. Patient can expect to return to activity in four to six weeks
    E. Extracorporal shock wave therapy should be used

Correct Answer: D

Calcaneal stress fractures are not considered a high-risk injury. They typically heal four to six weeks after injury with activity modification, including crutches with weight bearing as tolerated. In more severe cases, a cam walker boot and crutches are used. Radiographs, often delayed in recognizing the injury often show a line perpendicular to the trabeculated pattern, running from posterior-superior to anterior inferior, best seen on lateral. Bilateral pain to calcaneous (squeeze test) is positive. Surgery is usually not required and most improve prior to season's end. Low body weight, as often seen in cross country runners can increase the risk of stress fractures. Extracorporal shock wave therapy, posterior night splints, and injection therapy are all used at various stages in treating plantar fasciitis.

1. Aldridge T. Diagnosing heel pain in adults. Am Fam Physician 2004 Jul 15;70(2):332-338.
2. Thomas JL, Christensen JC, Kravitz SR, Mendicino RW, Schuberth JM, Vanore JV, et al. The diagnosis and treatment of heel pain: a clinical practice guideline-revision 2010. J Foot Ankle Surg 2010 May-Jun;49(3 Suppl):S1-19.
3. Calcaneal stress fractures. Wheeless' Textbook of Orthopaedics. Accessed February 12, 2012 at www.wheelessonline.com/ortho/calcaneus_fatigue_fractures.
4. Calcaneal stress fracture. Accessed February 11, 2012 at www.learningradiology.com/archives2011/COW%204/0-Stress%20Fx-Calcaneous/stressfxcorrect.htm.

190. A 23-year-old thin marathon runner is diagnosed with a stress fracture of the second metatarsal bone. She recently recovered from a similar stress fracture of the contralateral extremity. Which of the following is most important in the management for this patient?

    A. Arch supports to correct pes planus and evaluation of running shoes
    B. Increased training as tolerated after appropriate respite period
    C. Proper screening for female athlete triad
    D. A bone scan to differentiate stress fracture from stress reaction
    E. Intramedullary screw fixation for an elite athlete

Correct Answer: C

The female athlete triad includes eating disorders, amenorrhea, and osteoporosis. After obtaining a thorough history and physical, lab, and screening tests, a multidisciplinary approach may be required to manage this patient. Metatarsal stress fractures are found more commonly in patients with high arches, not pes planus. MRI is now the gold standard for diagnosis because of the low specificity of bone scan. Screw fixation of the elite athlete is described for the fifth metatarsal fracture, not the medial four metatarsals.

1. Beals KA, Meyer NL. Female athlete triad update. Clin Sports Med 2007 Jan;26(1):69-89.
2. Nattiv A, Loucks AB, Manore MM, Sanborn CF, Sundgot-Borgen J, Warren MP, et al. American College of Sports Medicine position stand. The female athlete triad. Med Sci Sports Exerc 2007 Oct;39(10):1867-1882.
3. Gottschlich LM. Female athlete triad. Medscape. Accessed December 11, 2011 at http://emedicine.medscape.com/article/89260.

191. Which of the following statements is true regarding pronator syndrome?

    A. The most common cause is mechanical compression by the pronator teres
    B. Athletes with pes planus are at increased risk for pronator syndrome
    C. Athletes with pronator syndrome are at increased risk for ankle sprains
    D. An MRI is often helpful in making the diagnosis
    E. Pronator syndrome is caused by compression of the radial nerve

Correct Answer: A

Pronator syndrome (median nerve compression syndrome) is an entrapment neuropathy of the median nerve (Answer E is incorrect). Sites of compression include:
  • Supracondylar process/ligament of Struthers
  • Lacertus fibrosus
  • Pronator teres
  • Flexor digitorum superficialis arcade

Repetitive elbow motions such as sculling often trigger pronator syndrome. Patients present with anterior proximal forearm pain and numbness in the volar forearm and radial three-and-a-half digits. Electromyogram (EMG) and nerve conduction studies of the median nerve around the elbow can be technically difficult, and they are often normal. They can be made more sensitive by testing after a session of the inciting activity. MRI is usually not helpful in making the diagnosis except in the rare case of a mass compressing the nerve (Answer D is incorrect). Answers B and C are incorrect because they refer to the lower extremity.

1. Mehlhoff TL, Bennett JB. Elbow injuries. In: Mellion MB, Walsh MW, Madden C, Putukian M, Shelton GL (eds). Team Physician's Handbook. 3rd ed. Philadelphia: Hanley and Belfus, 2002:421.
2. Keefe DT, Linter DM. Nerve injuries in the throwing elbow. Clin Sports Med 2004 Oct;23(4):732-736.
3. Wilhelmi BJ. Nerve compression syndromes of the hand. Medscape. Accessed December 12, 2011 at http://emedicine.medscape.com/article/1285531.
4. Morris HH, Peters BH. Pronator syndrome: clinical and electrophysiological features in seven cases. J Neurol Neurosurg Psychiatry 1976 May;39(5):461-464.

192. Which of the following statements is true concerning the respiratory system during pregnancy?

    A. Tidal volume decreases
    B. Vital capacity is unchanged
    C. Minute ventilation is unchanged
    D. Reserve volumes increase

Correct Answer: B

During pregnancy, both tidal volume and minute ventilation increase while reserve volumes decrease. As a result, the vital capacity remains unchanged.

1. Christian JS, Christian SS, Stamm CA, Mc Gregor JA. Pregnancy physiology and exercise. In: Ireland ML, Nattiv A (eds). The Female Athlete. Philadelphia: Saunders, 2002:186.
2. Trupin SR. Common pregnancy complaints and questions. Medscape. Accessed December 12, 2011 at http://emedicine.medscape.com/article/259724.

193. A 36-year-old female recreational soccer player presents with insidious onset of left posterior heel pain and a limp. She is wearing flip-flops because shoes make the pain worse. Examination reveals swelling and erythema of the posterior heel. There is no palpable defect in the Achilles tendon, and a Thompson test is negative. The most likely diagnosis is which of the following?

    A. Stress fracture of the calcaneus
    B. Plantar fasciitis
    C. Achilles tendon avulsion
    D. Sural neuritis
    E. Retrocalcaneal bursitis

Correct Answer: E

Retrocalcaneal bursitis (Haglund's syndrome) is associated with overuse and presents with pain behind the calcaneus. Examination reveals swelling and erythema of the posterior heel. A prominence, called a "pump bump," may be noticeable. Retrocalcaneal bursitis is associated with pain and tenderness anterior to the Achilles tendon, along the medial and lateral aspects of the posterior calcaneus. Plantar flexion of the foot and/or squeezing the bursa from side to side reproduces the patient's complaint. A stress fracture of the calcaneus produces mid-calcaneal bony tenderness and occurs with acute overuse. The symptoms of plantar fasciitis include tenderness and pain underneath (plantar surface), rather than behind the heel. A pop is generally heard and felt along with a palpable defect in the tendon and a positive Thompson test with an Achilles tendon avulsion injury. Sural neuritis is rare and the result of direct trauma. A positive percussion sign over the nerve lateral to the Achilles tendon is diagnostic of sural neuritis.

1. Snider RK. Posterior heel pain. In: Greene WB (ed). Essentials of Musculoskeletal Care. 2nd ed. Rosemont, IL: American Academy of Orthopaedic Surgeons, 2001:493-494.
2. Retrocalcaneal bursitis insertional heel pain. A.D.A.M. Medical Encyclopedia. Accessed December 12, 2011 at www.ncbi.nlm.nih.gov/pubmedhealth/PMH0002068.

194. Which item would a sports medicine physician want in a game bag to help emergently reduce a symptomatic posterior sternoclavicular dislocation in the field?

    A. Trainer's Angel
    B. Towel roll
    C. Towel clamp
    D. Sling and swathe

Correct Answer: C

Closed reduction can be attempted using traction in abduction and extension. Reduction of an acute injury usually occurs with an audible pop or snap, and the relocation can be noted visibly. However, if not successful, an assistant can grasp or push down on the clavicle in an effort to dislodge it from behind the sternum. Occasionally, in a stubborn case—especially in a thick-chested person or a patient with extensive swelling—it is impossible for the assistant's fingers to obtain a secure grasp on the clavicle. The skin should then be surgically prepared, and a sterile towel clip should be used to gain purchase on the medial clavicle percutaneously. The towel clip is used to grasp completely around the shaft of the clavicle. The dense cortical bone prevents the purchase of the towel clip into the clavicle. Then, the combined traction through the arm plus the anterior lifting force on the towel clip will reduce the dislocation. After the reduction, the sternoclavicular joint is stable, even with the patient's arms at the sides. However, the shoulders should be held back in a well-padded figure-of-eight clavicle strap for three to four weeks to allow for soft tissue and ligamentous healing. A Trainer's Angel is used to cut off a face mask.

1. Roipal CE, Wirth MA, Da Silva Leitao IC, Rockwood CA. Section B Injuries to the sternoclavicular joint in the adult and child. DeLee JC, Drez D, Miller MD (eds). DeLee & Drez's Orthopaedic Sports Medicine. 3rd ed. Philadelphia: Saunders, 2003:791-825.

195. A 54-year-old male presents to your office today, complaining of bilateral knee pain. He was diagnosed with osteoarthritis in both his knees after he was referred by his primary care provider to see an orthopedic surgeon. He was given a prescription for an anti-inflammatory medication and told that he may need knee replacement surgery some day. He does not like taking medications and has come to see you regarding non-pharmacologic treatment options. Which of the following statements regarding exercise and osteoarthritis is true?

   A. Aerobic exercise should be discouraged because it will increase the patient's pain
   B. This patient's x-ray findings are moderate to severe; therefore, exercise is unlikely to be helpful
   C. Strengthening exercises may be helpful in preventing osteoarthritis and may also alter disease progression
   D. Aquatic exercise has not been shown to be beneficial for patients with osteoarthritis

Correct Answer: C

Answer C is correct. Improvements in muscle strength and proprioception gained from exercise programs may prevent and reduce the progression of osteoarthritis. Answer A is incorrect. For people with osteoarthritis, both high intensity and low intensity aerobic exercise have been shown to be effective in improving a patient's functional status, gait, pain, and aerobic capacity. Different exercise types have different effects; thus, an individualized approach to exercise prescription is recommended, based on presenting symptoms, problems, and the needs of the patient. For people with osteoarthritis of the knee, land-based therapeutic exercise has been shown to reduce pain and improve physical function. Optimal exercise type or dosage has not clearly been defined. Supervised exercise classes appeared to be as beneficial as treatments provided on a one-to-one basis. Answer B is incorrect. The effectiveness of exercise is independent of the severity of x-ray findings. Answer D is incorrect because there is evidence to support aquatic exercise for the treatment of knee osteoarthritis and/or hip, at least in the short term. Although no long-term effects have been documented (very few studies performed at this point), the short-term benefits make it a viable option for your patients.

1. Bartels EM, Lund H, Hagen KB, Dagfinrud H, Christensen R, Danneskiold-Samsøe B. Aquatic exercise for the treatment of knee and hip osteoarthritis. Cochrane Database Syst Rev 2007 Oct 17;(4):CD005523.
2. Roddy E, Zhang W, Doherty M, Arden NK, Barlow J, Birrell F, et al. Evidence-based recommendations for the role of exercise in the management of osteoarthritis of the hip or knee—the MOVE consensus. Rheumatology (Oxford) 2005 Jan;44(1):67-73.
3. Brosseau L, MacLeay L, Robinson V, Wells G, Tugwell P. Intensity of exercise for the treatment of osteoarthritis. Cochrane Database Syst Rev 2003;(2):CD004259.

196. Which of the following statements is true regarding nail disorders in athletes?

A. The risk of ingrown toenails can be minimized by having the athlete wear shoes that are snug and minimize the sliding of the foot inside the shoe

B. Trimming the toenails in a curved arc just distal to the free edge will minimize the risk of ingrown toenails

C. Any collections of dark fluid beneath the nail bed should be immediately drained with a red-hot paper clip

D. The persistence of a linear black band or streak running the length of the nail warrants further evaluation

E. The treatment of choice for onychomycosis is a topical antifungal

Correct Answer: D

The persistence of a linear black band or streak running the length of the nail may represent a melanocytic nevus or malignant melanoma of the proximal melanoma and warrants further evaluation. The risk of reoccurring ingrown toenails and subungual hematoma can be minimized by having the athlete wear shoes that are at least 2 cm longer than the longest toe. Cutting the toenail straight across and with enough length to clear the nail bed minimizes the risk of ingrown toenails. While subungual hematomas may be drained by pressing a red-hot paper clip end (as well as drilling with an 18 gauge needle or the use of an electrocautery), there is no need to do so unless the patient is having symptoms. Asymptomatic onychomycosis does not need to be treated; however, if treatment is chosen, oral antifungals are the treatment of choice.

1. Batts KB. Dermatology in sports medicine. In: O'Connor FG, Sallis RE, Wilder RP, St. Pierre P (eds). Sports Medicine: Just the Facts. New York: McGraw-Hill. 2005;149-157.

2. Tanzi EL, Scher RK. Managing common nail disorders in active patients and athletes. Phys Sportsmed 1999 Sep;27(9):35-47.

197. Which of the following statements is true regarding scapular fractures?

   A. Reduction of an isolated displaced glenoid neck fracture is usually not necessary to achieve a good clinical outcome
   B. Non-surgical treatment is an option for glenoid fractures that involve 50% or less of the articular surface
   C. Non-operative treatment of glenoid fractures consists of immobilization with a sling and swathe for at least two weeks
   D. Non-operative treatment of glenoid fractures consists of immobilization with a sling for at least two weeks
   E. Sports-related injury is responsible for almost half of the cases of scapular fractures

Correct Answer: A

Because of the large range of motion of the glenohumeral joint, reduction of an isolated displaced glenoid neck fracture is usually not necessary to achieve a good clinical outcome. Association of a glenoid neck fracture with a displaced clavicle fracture or coracoclavicular ligament tears usually results in an unstable injury and therefore will require operative management. Surgical treatment should be strongly considered for involvement of more than 25% of the articular surface. Non-operative treatment of glenoid fractures involves use of a sling for comfort and early mobilization. Motor vehicle accidents are the most common cause of scapular fractures; they are relatively rare in sports since they require a high level of force to occur.

1. Eiff MP, Hatch RL, Calmbach WL. Clavicle and scapula fractures. Fracture Management for Primary Care. 2nd ed. Philadelphia: Saunders, 2003:198-210.
2. Schmidt JC. Scapular fracture. Medscape. Accessed December 12, 2011 at http://emedicine.medscape.com/article/826084.

198. A college athlete presents with fever, myalgias, and rhinorrhea for three days. Which of the following treatments are banned by NCAA standards?

    A. Phenylephrine
    B. Pseudoephedrine
    C. Antipyretic agents
    D. Ephedrine
    E. Antihistamines

Correct Answer: D

Answer D is specifically on the NCAA banned list and should not be used. The remainder may be used for symptom relief. For Answers A and B, although considered stimulants, they are not on the banned list.

1. 2011-2012 NCAA Banned Drug List. Accessed December 11 at www.ncaa.org/wps/wcm/connect/public/NCAA/Student-Athlete+Experience/NCAA+banned+drugs+list.

199. A 55-year-old female presents to your clinic after a fall during a hike earlier in the day. You obtain an x-ray and see a fracture through the surgical neck of the proximal humerus. Which motor function corresponds to the nerve that may have been damaged as a result of this injury?

   A. Abduction of the arm
   B. Wrist extension
   C. Finger abduction
   D. Wrist flexion and abduction

Correct Answer: A

The axillary nerve innervates teres minor and deltoid. It comes in contact with the humerus at the surgical neck. Injury to the axillary nerve results in loss of abduction of the shoulder and external rotation. The radial nerve innervates triceps brachii, anconeus, brachioradialis, extensor carpi radialis longus, extensor carpi radialis brevis, extensor digitorum, extensor digiti minimi, extensor carpi ulnaris, abductor pollicis longus, extensor pollicis brevis, extensor pollicis longus, extensor indicis. It comes in contact with the humerus at the radial groove. The ulnar nerve innervates flexor carpi ulnaris, flexor digitorum profundus (medial half), hypothenar muscles opponens digiti minimi, abductor digiti minimi, flexor digiti minimi brevis, adductor pollicis, the third and fourth lumbrical muscles, dorsal interossei, palmar interossei and the palmaris brevis. It comes in contact with the distal end of the humerus. The median nerve innervates most of the flexors in the forearm except flexor carpi ulnaris and the medial two digits of flexor digitorum profundus, which are supplied by the ulnar nerve. Muscles include the pronator teres, flexor carpi radialis, palmaris longus, and flexor digitorum superficialis muscle. The anterior interosseus branch supplies the following muscles lateral (radial) half of flexor digitorum profundus, flexor pollicis longus, pronator quadratus. Innervation is provided to the first and second lumbricals and the muscles of the thenar eminence of the hand by a recurrent thenar branch. It comes in contact with the humerus at the medial epicondyle.

1. Axillary nerve. Wheeless' Textbook of Orthopedics. Accessed December 12, 2011 at www.wheelessonline.com/ortho/axillary_nerve.
2. Steinmann SP, Moran EA. Axillary nerve injury: diagnosis and treatment. J Am Acad Orthop Surg 2001 Sep-Oct;9(5):328-335.
3. Moore K, Dalley A. Clinically Oriented Anatomy. 5th ed. New York: Lippincott Williams & Wilkins, 2006.

200. A 20-year-old endurance athlete presents to your clinic complaining of a generalized, itchy, papular rash that occurs only during exercise. You would recommend that he do which of the following?

A. Use unscented laundry detergent
B. Take a hot shower the night before a long run or try an antihistamine tablet one hour prior to exercise
C. Use topical steroids on the rash during exercise
D. Use sunscreen with PABA (para-aminobenzoic acid) at least half an hour prior to exercise

Correct Answer: B

This athlete has cholinergic urticaria, which is characterized by papular wheals with surrounding erythema occurring during and after heat exposure or exercise. A hot shower prior to a long run may deplete histamine and provide a refractory period for the athlete. H1 antihistamines are effective when taken one hour prior to activity. Sunscreen with PABA or PUVA has no effect on cholingeric urticaria. If it would be a contact dermatitis from the laundry detergent, it would be expected to appear all the time and not just during exercise.

1. Batts KB. Dermatology. In: O'Connor F, Sallis RE, Wilder RP, St. Pierre P (eds). Sports Medicine: Just the Facts. New York: McGraw-Hill, 2005:152.
2. Hosey RG, Carek PJ, Goo A. Exercise-induced anaphylaxis and urticaria. Am Fam Physician 2001 Oct 15;64(8):1367-1372.
3. Grattan CE, Humphreys F. Guidelines for evaluation and management of urticaria in adults and children. Br J Dermatol 2007 Dec;157(6):1116-1123
4. Magerl M, Borzova E, Giménez-Arnau A, Grattan CE, Lawlor F, Mathelier-Fusade P, et al. The definition and diagnostic testing of physical and cholinergic urticarias—EAACI/GA2LEN/EDF/UNEV consensus panel recommendations, Allergy 2009 Dec;64(12):1715-1721.

4

Test 2
Answers, Critiques,
and References

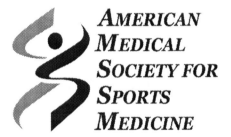

AMERICAN
MEDICAL
SOCIETY FOR
SPORTS
MEDICINE

Leading Sports Medicine into the Future

1. A 25-year-old male tennis player has noted loss of strength and power in his backhand stroke. He denies injury, and only mild pain with range of motion, specifically cross-arm adduction of his dominant arm. Exam reveals infraspinatus atrophy and weakness with external rotation. You diagnose infraspinatus syndrome, involving which of the following nerves?

    A. Long thoracic nerve
    B. Dorsal scapular nerve
    C. Radial nerve
    D. Suprascapular nerve
    E. Axillary nerve

Correct Answer: D

Infraspinatus syndrome is defined as a condition of painless atrophy of the infraspinatus muscle secondary to suprascapular neuropathy. The course of the nerve through the suprascapular notch and the spinoglenoid notch makes it vulnerable to injury from repetitive stretch, compression (e.g., ganglion cyst), or adjacent clavicle fracture. Overhead athletes are more at risk, and may present with dull aching posterior shoulder pain or loss of power in external rotation movements.

1. Reeser JC, Milne L, Talavera F, Whitehurst JB. Suprascapular neuropathy. Medscape. Accessed November 15, 2011 at http://emedicine.medscape.com/article/92672.
2. Bencardino JT, Rosenberg ZS. Entrapment neuropathies of the shoulder and elbow in the athlete. Clin Sports Med 2006 Jul;25(3):465-487, vi-vii.

2. An 18-year-old male novice crew athlete presents to the athletic training room with a one-week history of low back pain. He just started crew about three weeks ago and is trying to keep up with the strength and conditioning as well. He points to the lumbosacral junction as the point of maximal pain. His pain is more right-sided and occurs when he pulls back the oar. He denies groin pain. He denies numbness or tingling, radicular signs and symptoms, bowel or bladder incontinence. Ibuprofen does help him somewhat; however, the symptoms return the next day in the boat. On physical exam, he has full range of motion and 5/5 strength on forward flexion and extension. His DTRs are +2/4 bilaterally. His leg lengths are equal. His straight leg raise is negative. FABER is positive on the right and negative on the left. FADIR is negative bilaterally. His lumbosacral and thoracolumbar junctions are equivocal. He has no gluteal tenderness to the point. What is your working diagnosis, and what is the best treatment option for the patient?

   A. Sacroiliac dysfunction: perform a corticosteroid injection, continue to evaluate
   B. Lumbar radiculopathy: obtain a plain film and subsequently an MRI
   C. Sacroiliac dysfunction: improve lumbar core strength and stability with ATCs, osteopathic manipulation (if available)
   D. Femoral neck stress fracture: stop crew, and remain non-weight-bearing
   E. Piriformis syndrome: exercise program with ATCs

Correct Answer: C

SI joint dysfunction is a very common presentation to the athletic training room for the primary care sports medicine physician. It can occur in almost any type of athlete. In this case, the novice crew athlete is not used to the stressors of the boat and the core strengthening program. Sacroiliac joint dysfunction is typically diagnosed by history and physical exam only with no images necessary. The FABER test (Patrick test) is the classic test, but not very specific to diagnose sacroiliac joint dysfunction. Also useful is the standing flexion test and Gillet test (one-leg stork test). Looking for pelvic symmetry is also useful. A femoral stress reaction or fracture typically presents as groin pain, and an athlete would experience pain on FADIR (flexion adduction internal rotation). It is also more common in female athletes. The patient is not experiencing piriformis symptoms and does not have any gluteal pain. Management can include increasing core strength, osteopathic manipulation, and occasional NSAIDs. Injection therapy may be considered in chronic cases; however, it should not be an initial step to treatment. The patient is not experiencing discogenic symptoms on history or physical exam.

1. Sherman AL, Gotlin R. Sacroiliac joint injury. Medscape. Accessed November 15, 2011 at http://emedicine.medscape.com/article/96054.
2. Kuhlman GS, Domb BG. Hip impingement: identifying and treating a common cause of hip pain. Am Fam Physician 2009 Dec 15;80(12):1429-1434.
3. Rouzier, P. Sacroiliac dysfunction. Sports Medicine Patient Advisor. Amherst, MA: Sportsmed Press, 2010.

3. A 35-year-old third base coach is hit below the right breast by a line drive and collapses to the ground. He is in obvious pain and has difficulty speaking more than three words between breaths. He is transported by EMS for evaluation. His heartrate is 120, and breath sounds are decreased on the right side. Which other factor indicates need for urgent needle or tube thoracostomy?

A. A 10-pack-per-year history of smoking
B. Chest x-ray showing 1 cm of pleural space at the right apex
C. CT scan indicating a 20% pneumothorax
D. Tracheal deviation to the left

Correct Answer: D

Tracheal deviation with diminished unilateral breathsounds in a breathless patient indicates tension pneumothorax, a lifethreatening clinical diagnosis. Tension pneumothorax is a cause of cardiac arrest and PEA (pulseless electrical activity). Smoking history increases the risk of spontaneous pneumothorax by 20-fold but is irrelevant to determination of tension pneumothorax, and emergent CT findings of a < 20% pneumothorax indicate a good chance of resolution with observation. Emergent thoracostomy placement is not needed without hemodynamic compromise. Plain chest x-ray is useful to establish the diagnosis, but CT is required to precisely define extent of pneumothorax in simple—not tension—pneumothorax.

1. Bascom R. Pneumothorax. Medscape. Accessed November 15 2011 at http://emedicine.medscape.com/article/424547.
2. Chest trauma: pneumothorax tension. Trauma.org. Accessed November 15, 2011 at trauma.org/archive/thoracic/CHESTtension.html.
3. Legome E, Marx JA, Grayzel J. General approach to blunt thoracic trauma in adults. UpToDate. Accessed November 15, 2011 at www.uptodate.com/contents/general-approach-to-blunt-thoracic-trauma-in-adults.

4. Which of the following is a physiologic change associated with aging?

    A. Skin, tendon, and ligamentous elasticity increases
    B. Basal metabolic rate and caloric needs increase
    C. VO_2max remains unchanged
    D. Muscle mass decreases due to loss of type II muscle fibers

Correct Answer: D

Sarcopenia is a physiologic change in aging that is caused by a loss of type II muscle fibers and, therefore, a loss in muscle mass. Other changes with aging include a decrease in VO_2max, decreased basal metabolic rate and energy expenditure causing decreased caloric need, and loss of elasticity of the skin, tendons, and ligaments. Aerobic and resistance training in combination have been shown to be beneficial as a primary prevention to counter the affects of aging as well as show benefits in those who are frail or sedentary.

1. Foster C, Wright G, Battista RA, Porcari JP. Training in the aging athlete. Cur Sports Med Rep 2007 Jun;6(3):200-206.
2. American College of Sports Medicine position stand. Exercise and physical activity for older adults. Med Sci Sports Exerc 1998;30(6):992-1008.

5. A recreational diver develops stupor, confusion, focal weakness, visual loss, and seizures 10 minutes after ascent. What is the most likely diagnosis?

    A. Middle ear barotrauma
    B. Diving migraine
    C. Oxygen toxicity
    D. Arterial gas embolism
    E. Spinal cord decompression syndrome

Correct Answer: D

Pulmonary barotrauma is the most severe form of barotrauma and occurs during ascent. Arterial gas embolism (AGE) is the most dangerous form of pulmonary barotrauma and accounts for nearly one fourth of fatalities per year among recreational divers. Neurologic symptoms predominate over pulmonary symptoms and include stupor, confusion, coma, seizures, focal weakness, and visual loss.

Middle ear barotrauma is the most common type of diving injury and may involve hemorrhage and rupture of the tympanic membrane. Symptoms include acute onset of pain, vertigo, and conductive hearing loss.

Diving migraine headache is a common symptom in divers. Migraines are not often precipitated by diving but can be severe when they occur. Symptoms include pounding, throbbing pain, nausea, emesis, and photophobia.

The most likely cause of oxygen toxicity is diving with oxygen-enriched air (Nitrox). Symptoms develop at depth without warning and consist of focal seizures (facial or lip twitching), vertigo, nausea, emesis, paresthesias, and respiratory changes.

Spinal cord decompression syndrome is a neurologic decompression sickness that can present with a wide spectrum of symptoms. The most severe presentation is partial myelopathy to the thoracic spinal cord (spinal cord decompression syndrome). Patients complain of paresthesias and sensory loss in the trunk and extremities, tingling or constriction around the thorax, ascending leg weakness, pain in the lower back or pelvis, and loss of bowel/bladder control.

1. Newton, HB. Neurologic complication of scuba diving. Am Fam Physician 2001 Jun 1;63(11):2211-2218.
2. Melamed Y, Shupak A, Bitterman H. Medical problems associated with underwater diving. N Engl J Med 1992 Jan 2;326(1):30-35.
3. Moon RE. Treatment of diving emergencies. Crit Care Clin 1999 Apr;15(2):429-456.

6. A 20-year-old male basketball player collapses and dies suddenly during a recreational basketball game. He was evaluated by a physician prior to participation in division I college athletics, and family reports the doctor noted no cardiac problems and "cleared him" for all sports. His height was 6'7". The family reports his grandfather was also tall and died of "heart problems" in his 60s. Which of the following is the most likely cause of death?

   A. Hypertrophic cardiomyopathy
   B. Coronary anomalies
   C. Myocarditis
   D. Aortic dissection
   E. Arrhythmia

Correct Answer: A

The most likely cardiovascular cause of exercise-related sudden death in young athletes is hypertrophic cardiomyopathy (HCM). The other choices are possibilities but much less common. HCM is autosomal dominant, affects males slightly more than females, and is bimodal in peak occurrence. The most common presentation is in the third decade of life, but it may present in persons of any age, from newborns to elderly individuals. In children, inherited cases are found in an age range from newborn (i.e., stillborn babies) to adult. The peak incidence in these cases is in the second decade of life. In adults, the peak incidence is in the third decade of life with the vast majority of cases occurring in the age range between the third and sixth decades of life.

1. Thompson PD, Franklin BA, Balady GJ, Blair SN, Corrado D, Estes M, et al. Exercise and acute cardiovascular events: placing the risks into perspective. Med Sci Sports Exerc 2007 May;39(5):886-897.
2. Sander GE. Hypertrophic cardiomyopathy. Medscape. Accessed November 15, 2011 at http://emedicine.medscape.com/article/152913.

7. A tennis player you previously diagnosed with ulnar neuropathy and referred for surgical decompression returns six months post-surgery with complaints of recurrent paresthesias of the hand in an ulnar distribution. Exam reveals no tenderness with a normal Tinel's at Guyon's canal. Imaging demonstrates normal bony structures of the wrist and hand. Review of the patient's surgical records and physical exam reveal that the patient underwent a submuscular transposition of the ulnar nerve. Which of the following would most likely explain the patient's persistent symptoms?

    A. Hypermobility of the ulnar nerve at the cubital tunnel
    B. Accessory anconeous epitrochlearis muscle compressing the ulnar nerve
    C. Compression by the medial head of the triceps
    D. Compression in the distal upper arm by the Arcade of Struthers

Correct Answer: D

The Arcade of Struthers is the most common area of recurrent ulnar nerve symptoms after ulnar nerve transposition. The Arcade of Struthers is a thick, fibrous raphe present in 70% of the population. Hypermobility of the ulnar nerve at the cubital tunnel is a common cause of ulnar neuropathy that is resolved by transposition of the ulnar nerve out of the cubital tunnel. An accessory anconeous epitrochlearis and compression of the ulnar nerve by the medial head of the triceps are both rare causes of ulnar neuropathy.

1. Keefe DT, Lintner DM. Nerve injuries in the throwing elbow. Clin Sports Med 2004 Oct;23(4):723-742, xi.
2. Bencardino JT, Rosenberg ZS. Entrapment neuropathies of the shoulder and elbow in the athlete. Clin Sports Med 2006 Jul;25(3):465-487, vi-vii.

8. A 46-year-old workers' compensation case manager presents to your clinic, complaining of pain over her lateral elbow. After appropriate workup, the diagnosis of lateral epicondylitis is made. Which of the following comments is correct in regards to evidence-based medicine?

   A. Topical anti-inflammatory medications (NSAIDs) are as effective as placebo
   B. Oral NSAIDs are as effective as placebo
   C. A corticosteroid injection is as effective as a wait-and-see approach at 52 weeks
   D. For six weeks, a corticosteroid injection is more effective than physiotherapy

Correct Answer: D

Topical or oral nonsteroidal anti-inflammatory medications (NSAIDs), corticosteroid injection, and acupuncture are more helpful than placebo in treating lateral epicondylitis, or tennis elbow (strength of recommendation) (SORT B). A corticosteroid injection is more effective for short-term therapy—as long as six weeks—but produces no long-term improvement. Physiotherapy or a wait-and-see approach are superior to corticosteroid injection at 52 weeks (SORT B). There is insufficient evidence to support specific physiotherapy methods or orthoses (braces), shock wave therapy, ultrasound, or deep friction massage (SORT B). Surgery may succeed in refractory cases that have failed extensive conservative (SORT C) measures.

1. Beard JM. Safranek S. Clinical inquiries. What treatment works best for tennis elbow? J Fam Pract 2009 Mar;58(3):159-161.
2. Green S, Buchbinder R, Barnsley L, Hall S, White M, Smidt N, et al. Non-steroidal anti-inflammatory drugs (NSAIDs) for treating lateral elbow pain in adults. Cochrane Database Syst Rev 2002;(2):CD003686.
3. Smidt N, Assendelft WJ, Van der Windt DA, Hay EM, Buchbinder R, Bouter LM. Corticosteroid injections for lateral epicondylitis: a systematic review. Pain. 2002 Mar;96(1-2):23-40.

9. A 16-year-old male is found to have an elevated blood pressure at a mass preparticipation physical exam (PPE) to participate in high school football. Which of the following is the next-best step in management for this athlete?

    A. Restrict him from playing this season if the blood pressure was above 140/90
    B. Restrict him from playing this season if the blood pressure was above the 95% for his age, sex, and height
    C. Restrict him from playing this season if the blood pressure falls within the stage 2 (moderate) category of hypertension
    D. Arrange for the patient to receive follow-up care with his personal physician to obtain three different readings on three different days
    E. Start the patient on an antihypertensive medication in order to control his blood pressure, and allow him to play

Correct Answer: D

The correct answer is D because the diagnosis of hypertension is made after three different measures on three different days using properly fitting cuffs. The measures are then averaged, and either the systolic or diastolic pressure falling into the higher category is used to classify the athlete's blood pressure status. This ensures that hypertension is not overdiagnosed after only one reading. Answer A is incorrect because only one reading has been done, and children and adolescents are classified into stages of hypertension using age, sex, and height. Answer B is incorrect because only one reading has been done and stage 2 hypertension athletes can be allowed to play if blood pressure is well controlled and there is no target organ damage or heart disease. Drug therapy may be needed to accomplish control. Blood pressure should be rechecked every two to four months. Answer C is incorrect because only one reading has been done and Stage 2 hypertension athletes can be allowed to play if blood pressure is well controlled and there is no target organ damage or heart disease. Drug therapy may be needed to accomplish control. Blood pressure should be rechecked every two to four months. Answer E is incorrect because there has been only one reading and follow-up with the patient would be difficult after a mass PPE event. If medication is needed this should be done by his personal physician with proper follow-up.

1. American Academy of Family Physicians, American Academy of Pediatrics, American College of Sports Medicine, American Medical Society for Sports Medicine, American Orthopedic Society for Sports Medicine, American Osteopathic Academy of Sports Medicine. Preparticipation Physical Examination. 3rd ed. Minneapolis, MN: McGraw-Hill, 2004:1-82.
2. Saglimbeni AJ, Young C. Sports physicals. Medscape. Accessed November 15, 2011 at http://emedicine.medscape.com/article/88972.
3. Hergenroeder AC, Chorley J, Triedman JK, Torchia MM. The preparticipation sports examination in children and adolescents. UpToDate. Accessed November 15, 2011 at www.uptodate.com/contents/the-preparticipation-sports-examination-in-children-and-adolescents.

10. Which of the following patient conditions is not an absolute contraindication to starting an exercise program?

    A. Unstable angina
    B. Severe symptomatic aortic stenosis
    C. Left main coronary artery stenosis
    D. Uncontrolled symptomatic heart failure

Correct Answer: C

Left main coronary artery stenosis is a relative contraindication to starting an exercise program, and a program should be considered if the benefits outweigh the risks, and exercise is begun at a low level. All other answers are absolute contraindications, which also include: a recent significant change in resting ECG suggesting significant ischemia, recent myocardial infarction within two days or other acute cardiac event, uncontrolled cardiac arrhythmias causing symptoms or hemodynamic compromise, acute pulmonary embolus or pulmonary infarction, acute myocarditis or pericarditis, suspected or known dissecting aneurysm, and acute infections.

1. Gibbons RA, Balady GJ, Beasley JW, Bricker JT, Duvernoy WFC, Froelicher VF, et al. ACC/AHA guidelines for exercise testing: executive summary. A report of the American College of Cardiology/American Heart Association Task Force on Practice Guidelines (Committee on Exercise Testing). Circulation 1997 Jul 1;96(1):345-354.
2. Braun LT, Wenger NK, Rosenson RS. Components of cardiac rehabilitation and exercise prescription. UpToDate. Accessed November 15, 2011 at www.uptodate.com/contents/components-of-cardiac-rehabilitation-and-exercise-prescription.

11. Which of the following statements is true?

    A. Panner's disease occurs in children ages four to eight and is a self-limiting condition managed by conservative treatment
    B. Panner's disease is a defect of the wrist in gymnasts and most commonly needs casting
    C. Panner's disease occurs as a result of a traumatic injury that usually requires surgical repair
    D. Panner's disease is a congenital problem involving the hips and usually presents with a limp
    E. Panner's disease involves the medial elbow

Correct Answer: A

Panner's disease is osteochondrosis of the capitellum that occurs in children age four to eight and is usually a self-limiting condition. It does not usually occur as a result of trauma and does not usually require surgery. Panner's disease is only found in the elbow. Slipped capital femoral epiphysis (SCFE) may present with a limp and is a congenital problem involving the hips.

1. Kobayashi K, Burton KJ, Rodner C, Smith B, Caputo AE. Lateral compression injuries in the pediatric elbow: Panner's disease and osteochondritis dissecans of the capitellum. J Am Acad Orthop Surg 2004 Jul-Aug;12:246-254.
2. Chorley J. Elbow injuries in the young athlete. UpToDate. Accessed November 15, 2011 at www.uptodate.com.

12. A right-hand-dominant 16-year-old female tennis player complains of chronic aching pain distal to the lateral epicondyle of the elbow. Her symptoms are worse after tennis practice. She denies any numbness or tingling. On exam, she has weakness with supination and wrist extension. Pulses and neurological exam are within normal limits. The remainder of the hand exam is unremarkable. She has entrapment of which nerve?

   A. Posterior interosseous nerve
   B. Anterior interosseous nerve
   C. Superficial radial nerve (Wartenberg's disease)
   D. Ulnar nerve

Correct Answer: A

A is the correct answer. Posterior interosseous nerve entrapment causes pain in the lateral extensor mass of the forearm distal to the elbow and a pure motor deficit with weakness of extension of the wrist and fingers. It can be misdiagnosed as lateral epicondylitis. Answer B is incorrect because AIN entrapment causes weakness of the flexor pollicis longus, flexor digitorum profundus to the index and long fingers, and pronator quadratus. Answer C is incorrect because Wartenberg disease, which is caused by entrpament of the superficial radial nerve, causes sensory symptoms of burning, numbness, and tingling over the dorsal radial aspect of the wrist and hand. Answer D is incorrect because ulnar nerve entrapment also causes sensory symptoms and parasthesias. Additionally, there may be weakness and atrophy of the intrinsic muscles of the hand.

1. Stern M. Radial nerve entrapment. Medscape. Accessed November 26, 2011 at http://emedicine.medscape.com/article/1244110.

2. Bencardino JT, Rosenberg ZS. Entrapment neuropathies of the shoulder and elbow in the athlete. Clin Sports Med 2006 Jul;25(3):465-487, vi-vii.

3. Kennedy J. Neurologic injuries in cycling and bike riding. Neurol Clin 2008 Feb;26(1):271-279, xi-xii.

13. When covering an athletic event, it is recommended that the team physician do all of the following except?

   A. Assess the playing conditions of the venue
   B. Introduce yourself to the opposing team medical staff, and review emergency protocols
   C. Choose a location in the stands that allows good visibility of the game action
   D. Meet with ambulance personnel and assess their capability and available equipment
   E. Document the care provided

Correct Answer: C

According to the consensus statement on sideline preparedness for the team physician: "Sideline preparedness is the identification and planning for medical services to promote the safety of the athlete, to limit injury and to provide medical care at the site of practice or competition." During the athletic event, the team physician should be in a location that allows quick and ready access to the field of play. That location is generally on the sidelines at a location that allows good visibility. Locating in the stands is seldom appropriate. The other answers are all part of the game day preparation checklist for the team physician.

1. Herring SA, Bergfeld JA, Bernhardt DT, Boyajian-Oneill L, Gregory A, Indelicato PA, et al. Selected issues for the adolescent athlete and the team physician: a consensus statement. Med Sci Sports Exerc 2008 Nov;40(11):1997-2012.

14. A 19-year-old lacrosse player first presented to the training room with a two-day history of persistent left axillary pain and swelling. He noted the pain was exacerbated by weight lifting activities. He denied fevers, chills, rash, left arm numbness, or constitutional or respiratory symptoms. There was no recent history of direct trauma. His symptoms persisted for two days despite ibuprofen and a significant reduction in upper extremity resistance training (he remained active in lacrosse practice). He has no known sick contacts and denied recent unprotected intercourse. No change in hygiene or deodorant. He denies leg swelling or shortness of breath. Physical exam reveals localized area of swelling and tenderness in the left axilla with some firmness on palpation. No increased warmth. Distal pulses were strong. When supine, prominent superficial venous structures were noted in both extremities and were slightly more dilated in the left upper extremity. Which of the following is the presumed diagnosis?

   A. Superficial phlebitis
   B. Pectoralis major tear
   C. Labral tear
   D. Effort-induced thrombosis
   E. Lymphangitis

Correct Answer: D

Thoracic outlet syndromes are caused by compression of the neurovascular structures passing through the thoracic outlet. Venous thrombosis may be categorized into primary and secondary thrombosis based on the etiology. Primary venous thoracic outlet syndrome, or primary venous thrombosis, is also called Paget-Schroetter syndrome. Other terms for this condition include effort thrombosis, spontaneous thrombosis, and traumatic thrombosis.

Patients may describe a history of trauma or, more frequently, strenuous use of the arm (> 50% of cases). Common precipitating activities involve repeated hyperabduction and external rotation of the arm or backward and downward rotation of the shoulder. Causative activities may include participating in cricket, tennis, wrestling, lifting weights, water polo, gymnastics, baseball, or chopping wood. Because the symptoms of subclavian stenosis are fairly dramatic, most patients present promptly to the emergency department, usually within 24 hours. They may report dull ache in the shoulder or axilla, and the pain often is worsened by activity.

External compression of the axillary-subclavian vein has been suggested to contribute to the stasis of blood that engenders thrombosis. The factors that cause external compression include:
- Anomalous subclavius or anterior scalene muscle, long transverse process of cervical spine, cervical rib, abnormal insertion of the first rib, congenital fibromuscular bands, or narrowing of the costoclavicular space from depression of the shoulder

- Stress from exercise temporarily, causing hypercoagulability
- Repetitive shoulder-arm motion, causing microscopic intimal tears in the vessel wall

These factors, taken together, satisfy the classic Virchow triad for thrombosis. The initial treatment of subclavian vein thrombosis is conservative management, which includes rest, elevation of the limb, and application of heat or warm compresses. Currently, most investigators favor using thrombolytic therapy to rapidly restore patency of the vein. Thrombolytic therapy should be initiated within five to seven days of venous thrombosis. Fortunately, this syndrome occurs in fairly young individuals who do not have multiple medical illnesses that may contraindicate thrombolytic therapy. Thrombolytic therapy is preferred over thrombectomy because it does not carry the risks of an operation and the possibility of an intimal tear related to the embolectomy catheter.

In some cases, therapy may involve diagnostic venography, followed by thrombolysis, followed by several weeks of anticoagulation. If symptoms recur, a repeat venography may be indicated, possibly followed by balloon dilatation with or without stenting of the subclavian vein, and more anticoagulation. The desired international normalized ratio is 2:3. Labral tear and pectoralis injury would not involve the venous system. Superficial phlebitis would be associated with fevers, ertheyma, and warmth.

1. Haire WD. Arm vein thrombosis. Clin Chest Med 1995 Jun;16(2):341-351.
2. Atasoy E. Thoracic outlet compression syndrome. Orthop Clin North Am 1996 Apr;27(2):265-303.
3. Hendrickson CD, Godek A, Schmidt P. Paget-Schroetter syndrome in a collegiate football player. Clinic J Sports Med 2006 Jan;16(1):79-80.
4. Bhimji S. Subclavian vein thrombosis. Medscape. Accessed November 15, 2011 at http://emedicine.medscape.com/article/424777.

15. Which of the following statements is true about what happens during muscle contraction?

    A. Actin filaments on the thick filament bind to the myosin thin filament
    B. Sarcomere length increases during a concentric muscle contraction
    C. During muscle action and contraction calcium binds to myosin
    D. During muscle action and contraction ATP binds to myosin, allowing the thin and thick filaments to slide past each other
    E. When muscle stimulation increases intercellular calcium levels decrease and there is less calcium available for the actin and myosin filaments

Correct Answer: D

Muscle excitation-contraction is based on the sliding filament theory. ATP binds to the myosin thick filaments, which provides the necessary energy to allow the thin and thick filaments to slide by each other. Thick filaments are made of myosin, and the thin filaments are made of actin, troponin, and tropomyosin. As the thick and thin filaments slide past each other in muscle contraction, the sarcomere length decreases. Calcium binds to troponin on the thin filament, while ATP binds to myosin on the thick filament. When muscle stimulation increases, intercellular calcium levels increase so there is more calcium to bind to the troponin calcium binding sites. Higher calcium levels means muscles can contract to produce more force.

1. McArdle WD, Katch FI, Katch VL. Exercise Physiology. 6th ed. Williams & Wilkins, 2006.
2. Baechle TR, Earle RW (eds). Essentials of Strength Training and Conditioning. 3rd ed. Champaign, IL: Human Kinetics, 2008.

16. A 67-year-old male runner presents to the office complaining of right knee pain for several months. He denies mechanical symptoms. An MRI demonstrates osteoarthritis and a degenerative meniscal tear. Which of the following treatments is least likely to result in significant long-term reduction of pain?

    A. NSAID medication
    B. Activity modification
    C. Physical therapy
    D. Arthroscopic debridement
    E. Acetaminophen

Correct Answer: D

According to one of the few studies in the orthopedic literature properly designed to evaluate a surgical procedure, there is no difference at two years with regard to pain following arthroscopic debridement. Patients (n = 180) with osteoarthritis of the knee, moderate pain, no recent arthroscopy, and no suspected ligament damage were included. Half received standard arthroscopic debridement, and half were subjected to sham arthroscopy. There was no long-term difference in pain between groups at two years. Answers A, B, C, and E are all standard treatments for osteoarthritis with proven benefits.

1. Moseley JB, O'Malley K, Petersen NJ, Menke TJ, Baruch BA, Kuykendall DH, et al. A controlled trial of arthroscopic surgery for osteoarthritis of the knee. N Engl J Med 2002 Jul 11;347(2):81-88.
2. Fransen M, McConnell S, Bell M. Exercise for osteoarthritis of the hip or knee. Cochrane Database Syst Rev 2003;(3):CD004286.

17. The most reliable magnetic resonance imaging (MRI) finding, signifying osteitis pubis that is chronic and has likely been present for greater than six months, is which of the following?

    A. Subchondral sclerosis
    B. Fluid in the symphysis pubis joint
    C. Subchondral bone marrow edema
    D. Periarticular edema of the symphysis pubis joint
    E. Symphyseal disc extrusion

Correct Answer: A

In a study by Kunduracioglu, et al, MRI findings have been shown to have a strong correlation with duration of symptoms in osteitis pubis. Subchondral sclerosis, subchondral resorption and bony margin irregularities along with osteophytes correlated cases of osteitis pubis of greater than six months. Fluid in the symphysis pubis joint, subchondral bone marrow edema, and periarticular edema correlated with acute cases of osteitis pubis. Symphyseal disc extrusion and symphysis instability do not consistently correlate with either acute or chronic cases. Of note, associated other pathologies—especially adductor tendon injuries—were noted in more than half of the chronic cases.

1. Kunduracioglu B, Yilmaz C, Yorubulut M, Kudas S. Magnetic resonance findings of osteitis pubis. J Magn Reson Imaging 2007 Mar;25(3):535-539.
2. Radic R, Annear P. Use of pubic symphysis curettage for treatment-resistant osteitis pubis in athletes. Am J Sports Med 2008 Jan;36(1):122-128.

18. Encouraging patients to lead an active lifestyle is important to reduce the risk of developing a variety of different medical conditions including obesity, diabetes, and hyperlipidemia. There is also strong medical evidence to show that physical activity reduces the risk of development of which of the following types of cancer?

    A. Breast cancer
    B. Melanoma
    C. Prostate cancer
    D. Ovarian cancer

Correct Answer: A

The available evidence suggests that physical activity offers the strongest protective effect for breast and colon cancer. The Nurses' Health Study additionally documented a dose-response relationship between physical activity and breast cancer risk. The biological mechanism for this protective effect is unclear. It has been theorized that it may be due to alteration of menstrual cycle patterns and, therefore, exposure to sex hormones, enhancement of immune function, better energy balance, or changes in insulin (or insulin-like) growth factors, although no mechanism has been proven. The other cancers listed have not been studied, or have not yet shown a clear protective effect from physical activity.

1. Katzmarzk PT. Physical activity status and chronic diseases. In: Kaminsky L (ed). ACSM's Resource Manual for Guidelines for Exercise Testing and Prescription. 5th ed. Lippincott Williams & Wilkins, 2006:122-135.
2. Rockhill B, Willett WC, Hunter DJ, Manson JE, Hankinson SE, Colditz GA. A prospective study of recreational physical activity and breast cancer risk. Arch Intern Med 1999 Oct 25;159(19):2290-2296.

19. A 35-year-old experienced male diver with a history of hypertension has just returned from a week of recreational scuba diving in the Carribean and comes to your office. He reports feeling ill the last couple of days with episodes of nausea, vomiting, and tingling in his hands and feet. He states that when he washes his hands in cold water, it feels oddly warm. He denies fevers, chills, or diarrhea. He states during his week-long stay that he stayed in a resort and participated in four recreational dives over two consecutive days. He reported dive times and depths well within the safety parameters set by PADI. His last dive was over 36 hours before his departure. His symptoms started on the last day of his trip. He denies using any alcohol or drugs around the times of his dives. He takes lisinopril 10 mg a day for HTN and has been on it for seven years. He has no allergies. He denies eating any sushi or raw fish, but did eat some locally caught fish (i.e., eel). His vitals are stable with BP 132/86. Rest of exam is remarkably normal, including full neuro exam. This patient is most likely suffering from which of the following?

A. Arterial gas embolism
B. Pulmonary barotrauma of ascent
C. Scombroid poisoning
D. Decompression illness
E. Ciguartera poisoning

Correct Answer: E

The correct answer is ciguartera poisoning due to the duration of symptoms 1 to 14 days after eating tropical fish, reef fish, barracuda, moral eel. Hot/cold reversal is pathognomonic symptom of this condition. The answer is not arterial gas embolism or pulmonary barotrauma of ascent because 90% of those symptoms occur within five minutes of surfacing. It is not decompression illness because those symptoms start with 10 to 60 minutes of surfacing. It is not scombroid poisoning due to the symptoms listed, and the patient did not eat mackerel or tuna. Scombroid poisoning occurs one hour after ingestion and includes nausea vomiting diarrhea, headache, and abdominal cramps.

1. Bove AA. Diving Medicine. 3rd ed. Philadelphia: W.B.Saunders, 1997.
2. Schilling CW. The Physician's Guide to Diving Medicine, New York: Plenum, 1984.
3. Plantz SH. Scombroid poisoning. Medscape. Accessed November 15, 2011 at www.emedicinehealth.com/wilderness_scombroid_poisoning/article_em.htm.
4. Trojian TA. Environment. In: McKeag D, Moeller J. ACSM's Primary Care Sports Medicine. 2nd ed. Philadelphia: Lippincott Williams & Wilkins, 2007:286-287.
5. Marcus EN. Marine toxins. UpToDate. Accessed November 14, 2011 at www.uptodate.com.
6. Bove AA. Diving Medicine. 3rd ed. Philadelphia: W.B. Saunders, 1997.
7. Schilling CW. The Physician's Guide to Diving Medicine. New York: Plenum, 1984.

20. A 21-year-old male ice hockey player is struck in the mouth by a hockey puck during a game. After initially being evaluated by the team athletic trainer, the player is escorted off the ice for you to evaluate his injury. The patient is alert and oriented. Your examination reveals a single dental fracture. The exposed surface of the fractured tooth appears to be yellow with a discrete, central pink-red focus, exhibiting a slow seepage of blood. The athletic trainer has retrieved the fracture fragment for you. Assuming no cervical injuries, concussion, or other fractures, the best next step in treatment is which of the following?

A. Apply a wax dressing to the exposed surface of the fractured tooth, have the athlete wear a mouthpiece, and allow him to return-to-play

B. Restrict the athlete from continued participation, referring him to see his dentist the next day

C. Restrict the athlete from continued participation, referring him to see a dentist immediately for urgent evaluation, root canal, and/or crown (cap) placement

D. Place the fractured tooth fragment in cold milk, allow him to return to play, and refer the athlete to see a dentist immediately following the conclusion of the game for splinting

E. Restrict the athlete from continued participation, and attempt to reapproximate the fractured tooth fragment as soon as possible, taking care to achieve anatomic reduction

Correct Answer: C

Maxillofacial and dental trauma make up as much as 12% of ice hockey injuries. Uncomplicated crown fractures are the most common dental fractures, making up to 43.5% of all hockey maxillofacial injuries. Dental fractures may involve only the enamel; the enamel and dentin; or the enamel, dentin, and pulp. Enamel-only fractures are not considered dental emergencies and are often asymptomatic. They may be addressed on the sidelines with wax or gauze dressing to avoid tongue abrasions against the rough fracture surface; no restrictions to participation are necessary. Smoothing and contouring of the enamel-only fracture surface can be accomplished by a dentist at a later time. Enamel-dentin fractures are painful with sensitivity of the fractured tooth to air, cold, or contact.

Upon examination, both the white enamel and yellow dentin may be observed at the fracture site. In addressing enamel-dentin fractures on the sidelines, the fracture fragment should be located; rinsed and placed in milk, Hank's balanced salt solution, or carried in the patient's mucobuccal fold; and brought with the patient to see a dentist as soon as possible. The fragment may be amenable to reattachment, or a prosthetic crown (cap) may be placed by the treating dentist. Enamel-dentin-pulp fractures—such as the one seen in this patient—may or may not be painful and sensitive as in enamel-dentin fractures. Upon examination, the white enamel, yellow dentin, and pink-red exposed pulp are visible at the fracture site—and in the case of a vital pulp, blood may be seen oozing from the pulp canal. Enamel-dentin-pulp fractures are dental emergencies, and should prompt immediate evaluation and treatment by a qualified dentist, due to both the threat to tooth viability, as well as the risk of secondary pulpitis. Fragment reattachment and fixation are appropriate only if the pulp is vital and should be performed in the dental office, clinic, or emergency department, and only by a qualified dental professional. In many cases, the pulp is not vital, prompting root canal and/or crown (cap) placement.

1. Ranalli DN. Dental injuries in sports. Curr Sports Med Rep 2005 Feb;4(1):12-17.
2. Lahti H, Sane J, Ylipaavalniemi P. Dental injuries in ice hockey games and training. Med Sci Sports Exerc 2002 Mar;34(3):400-402.
3. Sane J, Ylipaavalniemi P, Leppänen H. Maxillofacial and dental ice hockey injuries. Med Sci Sports Exerc 1988 Apr;20(2):202-207.

21. A 12-year-old competitive female gymnast presents to your office after sustaining an inversion injury to her right foot 10 days earlier. At that time, she saw her athletic trainer in the training room and was advised to ice, elevate, and rest the ankle. Her father reports that she has been very diligent in following these instructions. However, her ankle remains swollen and painful, and she reports difficulty bearing weight. On physical exam, you find exquisite tenderness over the lateral malleolus, the anterior talofibular ligament, the talar dome, and the midfoot section. The remainder of the exam is unremarkable.

X-rays of the ankle reveal no acute bony abnormality. The decision is made to make her nonweightbearing in a pneumatic boot for two weeks.The patient returns to you after two weeks of nonweightbearing, complaining that the pain in her ankle is still present. Physical exam reveals marked tenderness over the distal tip of the fibula with no remaining tenderness over the ATFL, the talar dome, or the midfoot section. At this time you order an MRI, which supports your suspicion of which of the following?

A. Complete rupture of the deltoid ligament
B. Salter-Harris I fracture of the lateral malleolus
C. Munchhausen syndrome
D. Sever's disease

Correct Answer: B

This is a typical presentation of an initially missed growth plate injury. On initial presentation, the diffuse pain from the ankle sprain may overshadow the fracture of the distal fibula tip. Radiographs may not show this type of injury unless the fracture ends are displaced. In pediatric patients, ligaments are often more stabile than the physeal growth plates. Among children, fractures occur much more frequently than ligament sprains. Among rapidly growing adolescents, the growth plate often fails before the attached ligament tears. Adolescents may sustain fractures of the distal fibular growth plate from the inversion mechanism that causes sprains in young adults. Unrecognized and untreated, simple distal fibular physeal fractures may cause chronic pain.

The deltoid ligament is attached to the medial malleolus and would be damaged by an eversion rather than an inversion injury. The diagnosis of a Munchhausen syndrome cannot be made based on the information provided. Sever's disease, or calcaneal apophysitis, is common in this age group but involves the hindfoot with insertiona of the Achilles tendon.

1. Hecht SS, Gymnastics. In: Mellion MB, Walsh WM, Madden C, Putukian M, Shelton GL (eds). Team Physician's Handbook. 3rd ed. Philadelphia: Hanley and Belfus, 2002:668-677.
2. Micheli, LJ. Sports injuries in children and adolescents. Clin Sports Med 1995 Jul;14(3)727-745.
3. Krueger-Franke M, Siebert CH, Pfoerringer W. Sports-related epiphyseal injuries of the lower extremity. J Sports Med Phys Fitness 1992 Mar;32(1):106-111.

22. Which of the following is true regarding children and sports activity?

    A. Preteen athletes most commonly injure lower limbs, whereas teenagers injure upper limbs
    B. Salter-Harris II fractures generally require surgical intervention
    C. Joint dislocations and ligamentous injuries are more common than buckle and other types of fractures
    D. Physes close on average at 14.5 years in girls and 16.5 years in boys
    E. Non-unions fractures are common in the immature skeleton

Correct Answer: D

After physeal closing, injury patterns are similar to those in adults, but physes close at about 15 years of age in girls and 17 years of age in boys. Preteens have injuries in the upper limbs (Answer A), including contusions, strains, and simple fractures, whereas teenagers more commonly injure the lower limbs—knee injury being the most common. Salter-Harris II fractures (Answer B) are the most common type of physeal fracture at the transphyseal location with extension into the epiphysis and exiting from the joint. These do not often require surgical intervention. Open epiphyses are three to five times weaker than the surrounding capsular and ligamentous tissues so fractures are more common than dislocations and ligamentous injuries (Answer C). Non-union is rare because the immature skeleton forms callous early and heals quickly. Non-unions are more common in adults than children.

1. Miner C, Berg K. Youth sports issues. In: Mellion MB, Walsh WM, Madden C, Putukian M, Shelton GL (eds) . Team Physician's Handbook. 3rd ed. Philadelphia: Hanley and Belfus, 2002:61-67.
2. Pray WS, Pray JJ. Sports injuries in children. Medscape Family Medicine. Accessed November 15, 2011 at www.medscape.com/viewarticle/492435.

23. An otherwise healthy 12-year-old boy presents to the office for evaluation of left foot pain. He states that it occurred while training for soccer. He states the pain is worse with activity and totally resolves by the next day. No night pain. On exam, he has mild point tenderness over the proximal fifth metatarsal. You confirm your diagnosis with foot radiographs that show a fragment of bone running parallel to the fifth metatarsal diaphysis bilaterally. Initial treatment would include which of the following?

A. Supportive shoes with a narrow toe box
B. Short leg cast in 30 degrees of plantar flexion
C. Holding the child out of activities that cause pain
D. Referral to a surgeon to correct the deformity

Correct Answer: C

The condition that is described in this case is Iselin's disease, or fifth metatarsal aphophysitis. It affects girls age 9 to 11 and boys age 11 to 14. Included in the differential diagnosis is a fracture to the base of the fifth metatarsal. While a fracture runs oblique or perpendicular to the shaft of the fifth metatarsal, the apophyseal fragment runs parallel to the fifth metatarsal diaphysis. The initial treatment is relative rest, including limitation of activities; therefore, the correct answer is C. Answer A is incorrect, as you would want to avoid narrow shoe wear. While immobilization may be necessary if the patient is non-compliant with activitiy limitation, it would not be initial treatment. Also, you would cast him in neutral and not 30 degrees of plantar flexion. This condition usually responds to treatment and rarely requires surgery. Ice and anti-inflammatory medications, as well as physical therapy, may be used.

1. McBryde AM, Locke MD, Batson JP. Foot and ankle injuries. In: Micheli LJ, Purcell L (eds): The Adolescent Athlete: A Practical Approach. New York: Springer, 2007:377.
2. Strayer SM, Reece SG, Petrizzi MJ. Fractures of the proximal fifth metatarsal. Am Fam Physician 1999 May 1;59(9):2516-2522.

24. A right-hand-dominant 20-year-old college baseball pitcher feels a pop in his elbow while throwing followed by medial elbow pain. He experiences persistent pain and decreased throwing velocity. On exam, he has pain and mild opening on valgus stress of the elbow. Which of the following is the test of choice?

    A. MRI
    B. CT scan
    C. Ultrasound
    D. MRI arthrogram

Correct Answer: D

The diagnosis until proven otherwise in this patient is an ulnar collateral ligament tear. Answer D is the best answer, as MRI arthrogram is 97% sensitive in detecting UCL injuries. MRI alone is only 57% sensitive. CT alone is not a good choice for soft tissue injury. Ultrasound has promise but needs more studies to show its effectiveness for UCL injury detection. Presently, MRI arthrogram is the gold standard. Level of evidence is expert opinion.

1. Safran MR. Ulnar collateral ligament injury in the overhead athlete: diagnosis and treatment. Clin Sports Med 2004 Oct:23(4):643-663, x.
2. Tuite MJ, Kijowski R. Sports-related injuries of the elbow: an approach to MRI interpretation. Clin Sports Med 2006 Jul;25(3):387-408, v.

25. Regarding training at altitude, which of the following statements is true?

    A. Maximal aerobic power is reduced by 5% for every 100 m above 1500 m elevation in normal individuals
    B. Acclimatized individuals demonstrate lower peak lactate levels at altitude than at sea level for a given workload
    C. Reduction in maximal aerobic power is less severe in endurance trained athletes
    D. Living at lower elevations but training at higher elevations introduces the greatest physiological adaptation to altitude

Correct Answer: B

Maximal aerobic power is reduced by 1% for every 100 m above 1500 m elevation in normal individuals. The lactate paradox describes a phenomenon whereby acclimatized individuals demonstrate lower peak lactate levels at altitude than at sea level for a given workload, despite the physiologic challenges inherent to training at altitude. The reduction in maximal aerobic power is actually more severe in endurance trained athletes, most likely due to greater pulmonary blood flow (cardiac output). This further limits the ability to exchange oxygen in the diffusion limited condition of altitude. The greatest adaptation is obtained by living at elevation and training near sea level.

1. Levine BD, Stray-Gunderson J. High altitude training and competition. In: Mellion MB, Walsh WM, Madden C, Putukian M, Shelton GL (eds) . Team Physician's Handbook. 3rd ed. Philadelphia: Hanley and Belfus, 2002:159-165.
2. Mazzeo RS, Fulco CS. Physiological systems and their responses to conditions of hypoxia. In: ACSM's Advanced Exercise Physiology. Philadelphia: Lippincott Williams & Wilkins, 2006:564-580.

26. A 20-year-old female soccer athlete complains of pain and pressure over the anterior aspect of her shin with exercise. Physical exam that is performed just after exercise reveals a tense anterior compartment, weakness in great toe extension and ankle dorsiflexion, as well as decreased sensation in the first toe web space. Which nerve is involved?

    A. Superficial peroneal nerve
    B. Sural nerve
    C. Deep peroneal nerve
    D. Tibial nerve
    E. Obturator nerve

Correct Answer: C

The case described defines chronic exertional compartment syndrome of the anterior compartment. The anterior compartment contains the extensor digitorum longus, extensor hallucis longus, and the tibialis anterior muscle, which explains the weakness noted on exam. The nerve that is contained in the anterior compartment and effected in this case is the deep peroneal nerve.

1. Netter FH. Carpal bones. In: Brueckner JK, Carmichael SW, Gest TR, Granger NA, Hansen JT, Walji AH (eds). Atlas of Human Anatomy. Philadelphia: Saunders, 2006: 510-512.
2. Rowdon GA. Chronic exertional compartment syndrome. Medscape. Accessed November 17, 2010 at http://emedicine.medscape.com/article/88014.

27. Of the following, identify the false statement regarding acute patella dislocations?

    A. Often associated with hemarthrosis or effusion
    B. Requires disruption of the medial patella restraints
    C. Frequently associated with chondral injury or loose bodies
    D. Rarely responds to non-operative treatment

Correct Answer: D

Acute dislocation of the patella in the adult requires disruption of the medial patellar restraints. Swelling associated with the acute injury is often rapid, and a significant hemarthrosis frequently develops, especially if there is an associated osteochondral fracture. This swelling may mask a persistent lateral subluxation of the patella within the trochlea, which may be noted on physical examination. Loose chondral or bony fragments may be palpable in the joint, and attached osteochondral fragments may be palpable in the medial parapatellar retinaculum. A thorough palpation of the knee should be performed to detect focal areas of maximum tenderness that suggest soft tissue injury. The examiner may find a palpable defect at the medial patellar margin, tenderness along the course of the MPFL and the other medial retinacular ligaments, or tenderness near the medial femoral epicondyle at the MPFL insertion site.

The treatment for an initial patellar dislocation varies between simple immobilization and operative repair or reconstruction. Current evidence from the literature suggests that about half of all adults suffering an acute primary dislocation do reasonably well with nonoperative treatment. The only problem is that this leaves another 50% who do not do as well. Recent studies have shown that many patients with APD are young and active, and there is some evidence that young, active patients suffer a greater degree of prolonged impairment. Some authors have stated that regardless of treatment type, between 30% and 50% of patients will continue to have symptoms of instability or anterior knee pain. Given the multitude of studies of patellar dislocation in the literature, no definitive work yet has recommended for or against conservative or operative treatment.

1. Atkin DM, Fithian DC, Marangi KS, Stone ML, Dobson BE, Mendelsohn C. Characteristics of patients with primary acute lateral patellar dislocation and their recovery within the first 6 months of injury. Am J Sports Med 2000 Jul-Aug;28(4):472-479.
2. Hawkins RJ, Bell RH, Anisette G. Acute patellar dislocations: The natural history. Am J Sports Med 1986 Mar-Apr;14(2):117:120.

28. A sophomore female college soccer player tests positive for amphetamines on an NCAA drug test. She requests a medical exemption for the positive result because her physician prescribes Ritalin for her ADHD. The medical exemption will be approved only if which of the following is the case?

A. The athletics medical administrator has medical records proving that Ritalin is prescribed by her primary care physician or team physician
B. The athletics medical administrator has medical records proving that she has undergone standardized testing for ADHD and is prescribed Ritalin by her team physician or primary care physician
C. She makes an appointment to undergo standardized testing for ADHD, tests positive for ADHD, and the team physician or her primary care physician prescribes Ritalin and she sends the records to the NCAA
D. Her primary care physician and/or team physician has medical records proving that she has a documented improvement in ADHD symptoms with Ritalin and that they prescribe the Ritalin

Correct Answer: B

As of August 2009, stricter guidelines go into effect for the use of stimulants, finasteride (Propecia®), and testosterone. In order for the student-athlete to receive a medical exemption for ADHD medications, the student-athlete must declare the use of the substance to his athletics administrator responsible for keeping medical records, present documentation of the diagnosis of the condition with standardized testing, and provide documentation from the prescribing physician explaining the course of treatment and the current prescription. Answer A does not include standardized testing for ADHD. Just documentation of a prescription is not enough for a medical exemption. In Answer C, the testing needs to occur prior to testing positive for the banned drug. The records are not sent to the NCAA unless they are asked for. The athletics medical administrator keeps copies of the records in case of a positive drug test. In Answer D, improvement in symptoms and documentation of prescription is no longer enough for a medical exemption. Standardized testing must be performed.

1. The National Collegiate Athletic Association. NCAA Drug Testing Education Programs, March 11, 2008.
2. Green GA, Puffer JC. Drugs and doping in athletes. In: Mellion MB, Walsh WM, Madden C, Putukian M, Shelton GL (eds). Team Physician's Handbook. 3rd ed. Philadelphia: Hanley and Belfus, 2002:180-196.
3. NCAA banned drugs and medical exceptions policy guidelines regarding medical reporting for student-athletes with attention deficit hyperactivity disorder (ADHD) taking prescribed stimulants. Accessed November 26, 2011 at www.ncaa.org/wps/wcm/conn ect/67e423804e0b8a1d9978f91ad6fc8b25/NCAA+Guidelines+to+Document+ADH D+Treatment+with+Banned+Stimulant+Medications+01302009.pdf?MOD=AJPERES& CACHEID=67e423804e0b8a1d9978f91ad6fc8b25.

29. Which of the following training interventions, if used alone, has been proven to be most effective in reducing injuries, including ACL tears in athletes?

   A. Eccentric hamstring strength training
   B. Plyometrics
   C. Warm-up stretching
   D. Flexibility training

Correct Answer: A

While warm-up and stretching have been major players in the traditional injury prevention programs, only eccentric hamstring strength exercises have consistently been able to show a decrease in injuries of the lower extremity. Flexibility training alone shows no difference in the incidence of hamstring strains between teams that use the flexibility training and those who do not.

   1. Arnason A, Andersen TE, Holme I, Engebretsen L, Bahr R. Prevention of hamstring strains in elite soccer: an intervention study. Scand J Med Sci Sports 2008 Feb;18(1):40-48.
   2. Gabbe BJ, Branson R, Bennell KL. A pilot randomised controlled trial of eccentric exercise to prevent hamstring injuries in community-level Australian football. J Sci Med Sport 2006 May;9(1-2):103-109.
   3. Holcomb WR, Rubley MD, Lee HJ, Guadagnoli MA. Effect of hamstring-emphasized resistance training on hamstring:quadriceps strength ratios. J Strength Cond Res 2007 Feb;21(1):41-47.

30. A severe varus injury to the knee can result in an injury to which of the following nerves?

   A. Femoral
   B. Common peroneal
   C. Tibial
   D. Sural
   E. Deep peroneal

Correct Answer: B

The common peroneal nerves is the most commonly injured nerve in the lower limb. The common peroneal nerve may be severely stretched subsequent to the rupture of the fibular (lateral) collateral ligament.

   1. Peroneal nerve. Wheeless' Textbook of Orthopaedics. Accessed February 16, 2012 at www.wheelessonline.com/ortho/peroneal_nerve.
   2. Pritchett JW. Foot drop. Medscape. Accessed November 17, 2011 at http://emedicine.medscape.com/article/1234607.

31. You are covering a marathon on a slightly warm day. You are presented with a male runner who collapsed shortly after crossing the finish line about one minute ago. You are able to determine that he is conscious and has no mental status changes. His racing bib did not indicate any underlying medical conditions. His temperature was 101 degrees Fahrenheit (38 degrees Celsius). He was able to orally rehydrate. His pulse was 142. His blood pressure was not elevated, and demonstrated a 26 mm Hg systolic drop between supine and standing. There are no recent illnesses reported. The runner completed the race and sprinted to the finish for a personal best, and decided during the race to skip a few water stops to keep his record time. He reported no nausea or vomiting. Which of the following is the best statement regarding this scenario?

A. The runner is withholding information
B. The runner is hyponatremic
C. The runner has experience exertional heat illness
D. The runner suffered an episode of exercise-associated collapse

Correct Answer: D

Answer A may or may not be true. Answer B is unclear. This runner did not experience any mental status changes, which should be present in cases of hyponatremia. Additionally, he skipped water stops. This would make it unlikely for this runner to have had excessive fluid intake, which is common in hyponatremic episodes. It is unlikely he suffered exertional heat illness with his temperature under 104 degrees Fahrenheit (40 degrees Celsius), and so Answer C is incorrect. The best answer is D. This runner had all the hallmarks of EAC: Collapse after the finish, orthostatic, no mental status changes, improved in a short period, and an environment fit for this (warm, decreased fluid, and high effort with a sudden stop).

1. Jaworski CA. Medical concerns of marathons. Curr Sports Med Rep 2005 Jun;4(3):137-143.
2. Sallis RE. Fluid balance and dysnatremias in athletes. Curr Sports Med Rep 2008 Jul-Aug;7(4):S14-S19. doi: 10.1249/JSR.0b013e31817f381b.
3. Noakes TD. Hyponatremia in distance athletes: pulling the IV on the 'dehydration myth.' Phys Sportsmed 2000 Sep;28(9):71-76.

32. Which of the following is thought to play the most significant role in the increased risk of anterior cruciate ligament (ACL) injury for female athletes?

    A. Cyclical hormonal changes
    B. Decreased femoral notch width
    C. Imbalances in neuromuscular control
    D. Shoe-playing surface interactions
    E. Greater participation in high-risk sports

Correct Answer: C

ACL injury occurs with a four- to six-fold greater incidence in female athletes compared to male athletes. Several mechanisms have been explored to explain this gender disparity, including extrinsic (physical perturbations, bracing, shoe-surface interactions) and intrinsic (hormonal, anatomical, neuromuscular, and biomechanical) variables. Although the increased risk of injury for female athletes is likely multifactorial, the most convincing evidence points toward gender differences in neuromuscular control and proprioception (Answer C). With regard to hormonal (Answer A), anatomical (Answer B), and environmental (Answer D) risk factors, there is no conclusive evidence that any single variable correlates directly with injury risk. Answer E is also incorrect since there is no evidence that women have greater participation in high-risk sports.

1. Hewett TE, Myer GD, Ford KR. Anterior cruciate ligament injuries in female athletes: Part 1, mechanisms and risk factors. Am J Sports Med 2006 Feb;34(2):299-311.
2. Hewitt TE. Why women have an increased risk of ACL injury: decreased neuromuscular control of the trunk leads to valgus torques. AAOS Now 2010 Nov. Accessed November 26, 2011 at www.aaos.org/news/aaosnow/nov10/research3.asp.

33. A 25-year-old female presents to your office with the chief complaint of right thigh pain. She is training for her first marathon and shows you her detailed training log. It documents a gradual increase in her running intensity and length of training runs. She ran on a park trail and was comfortably running eight miles. Three weeks prior to her appointment, friends from her local running club encouraged her to run a half marathon road race with them. Upon finishing the race, she became aware of a nagging pain in her thigh. She presumed it was "just a strain" and continued on her usual training schedule. The thigh pain significantly limited the length of her runs, and by the time she presents to your office, she is having pain with walking.

On exam, she is limping, favoring her right leg. Range-of-motion testing of the hip and knee is full and pain-free both actively and passively. Palpation of the right thigh reveals a poorly localized area of pain in the midshaft of the femur. There is no difference in circumferential measurement of the right and left thighs. Strength testing of the right quadricep with resisted straight leg raise does not exacerbate her pain. Radiographs performed in the office of the right hip and femur are negative. What is the most likely diagnosis?

A. Quadriceps tear
B. Anterior superior iliac spine (ASIS) avulsion fracture
C. Femur stress fracture
D. Myositis ossificans

Correct Answer: C

This patient most likely has a femoral shaft stress fracture. Her history presents some important clues. She had an abrupt increase in her distance of running, from eight to 13 miles, and her intensity of running in a race was likely an abrupt increase as well. The surface change from a trail to asphalt road is also notable. She reported no acute onset of pain during the race, which would have been more likely with an ASIS avulsion fracture. Additionally, this patient at 25 years of age no longer has an open apophysis at the ASIS. A quadriceps tear would present with a discrete painful and swollen area in the thigh. Resisted strength testing would have revealed both pain and weakness. Range of motion would also have been limited with knee extension, and passive stretch would have reproduced pain. Likewise, myositis ossificans, representing heterotopic bone formation in muscle tissue, would have caused limited range of motion, especially with passive knee flexion with the patient in the prone position. A well-defined area of pain would have been palpated, and at three weeks, a firm mass in the area may have been felt as well.

1. DeFranco MJ, Recht M, Schils J, Parker RD. Stress fractures of the femur in athletes. Clin Sports Med 2006 Jan;25(1):89-103, ix.
2. O'Kane JW, Matsen LJ. Mid-third femoral stress fracture with hip pain. J Am Board Fam Pract 2001 Jan-Feb;14(1):64-67.
3. Sanderlin BW, Raspa RF. Common stress fractures. Am Fam Physician 2003 Oct 15;68(8):1527-1532.

34. An 18-year-old Division I wrestler presents for skin checks at the NCAA National Championships. He reports having been diagnosed three days prior with primary orolabial herpes. He was started on acyclovir 200 mg by mouth five times daily. He denies any current constitutional symptoms or new lesions since his diagnosis. On physical examination, there is a cluster of well-dried lesions on the left lower lip and chin area. In accordance with NCAA regulations, which of the following is the most appropriate return-to-play decision?

A. Allow the wrestler to participate because he is currently asymptomatic
B. Allow the wrestler to participate since he has not developed new lesions for the past 72 hours
C. Allow the wrestler to participate if he covers the lesions
D. Disqualify the wrestler because of an inadequate treatment course
E. Disqualify the wrestler because of an inappropriate dosage of systemic antiviral

Correct Answer: D

Per the NCAA guidelines, herpes infection requires a minimum of 120 hours (five full days) of antiviral therapy prior to competition, no new active blisters may be present for 72 hours pre-competition, and dry, crusted lesions are permissible if after five full days of antiviral therapy.

1. NCAA Sports Medicine Handbook 2011, p. 63. Accessed November 17, 2011 at fs.ncaa. org/Docs/health_safety/2011_12_Sports_Medicine_Handbook.pdf.

35. A 12-year-old male soccer player presents to your clinic with right anterior hip pain after feeling a pop in this area after taking a strong shot to score a goal. His radiographs reveal an avulsion of the anterior inferior iliac spine apophysis. The muscle that attaches here is which of the following?

   A. Sartorius
   B. Rectus femoris
   C. Gracilis
   D. Tensor fascia lata

Correct Answer: B

In the adolescent competitive athlete, the pelvis is a common location of apophyseal avulsion injury. In a study of 203 avulsion fractures seen on radiographs, the most commonly affected apophyses were:
   • The ischial tuberosity: the origin of the hamstrings
   • The anterior inferior iliac spine (AIIS): the origin of the straight head of the rectus femoris
   • The anterior superior iliac spine (ASIS): the origin of the sartorius and some fibers of the tensor fascia lata
   • A portion of the pubic symphysis: the origin of the adductor brevis and longus as well as the gracilis

   1. Hip avulsion fracture. Family Practice Notebook. Accessed November 17, 2011 at www. fpnotebook.com/Ortho/Hip/HpAvlsnFrctr.html.
   2. Rossi F, Dragoni S. Acute avulsion fractures of the pelvis in adolescent competitive athletes: prevalence, location and sports distribution of 203 cases collected. Skeletal Radiol 2001 Mar;30(3):127-131.

36. A collegiate level rower presents to your office after exercise-associated syncope. Your workup includes detailed personal and family histories and further cardiovascular testing, including ECG and 2D-echocardiogram with color Doppler. Which of the following most favors the diagnosis of athlete's heart rather than hypertrophic cardiomyopathy?

    A. Left ventricular cavity dilation
    B. Altered echocardiographic parameters in first degree relatives
    C. EGG patterns including extremely elevated voltages, Q waves, and negative T waves
    D. Maintenance of wall thickness after deconditioning
    E. Marked left atrial enlargement

Correct Answer: A

Of the given choices, only Answer A increased left ventricular (LV) cavity dilation is consistent with athlete's heart syndrome rather than hypertrophic cardiomyopathy (HCM). Eccentric remodeling of myocardium increases ventricular volumes, whereas concentric remodeling as seen in HCM does not. However, diagnosis should not be made solely on this feature.

HCM is usually an autosomal dominant disorder and first-degree relatives may show similar cardiac morphology as affected patients. Unusual and bizarre ECG patterns with strikingly increased voltages, prominent Q waves, or deep, negative T waves are most characteristic of HCM and represent evidence favoring this diagnosis. A deconditioning period of several months may induce remodeling with a reduction in LV wall thickness; such changes are inconsistent with a pathologic state such as HCM. Marked atrial enlargement is not seen in the athlete's heart syndrome.

1. Maron BJ. Distinguishing hypertrophic cardiomyopathy from athlete's heart: a clinical problem of increasing magnitude and significance. Heart 2005 Nov;91(11):1380-1382.
2. Maron BJ. Distinguishing hypertrophic cardiomyopathy from thlete's hear physiological remodelling: clinical significance, diagnostic strategies and implications for preparticipation screening. Br J Sports Med 2009 Sep;43(9):649-656.

37. A senior high school athlete with college aspirations comes to your clinic for a pre-participation physical exam. He states that he was syncopal while running on a hot day, preparing for the upcoming football season. He was seen at the emergency room, but he was only given intravenous fluids since he was felt to be dehydrated. He recovered well and has not had another syncopal episode. Since he had syncope with exertion, you decide to get an ECG, which is shown below. Which of the following is the best diagnosis?

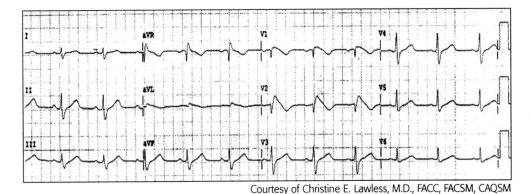

Courtesy of Christine E. Lawless, M.D., FACC, FACSM, CAQSM

A. Hypertrophic cardiomyopathy (HCM)
B. Arrythmogenic right ventricular dysplasia (ARVD)
C. Brugada syndrome
D. Long QT syndrome
E. Wolff-Parkinson-White syndrome (WPW)

Correct Answer: C

The correct answer is C. Brugada syndrome classically has "coved" ST segments with RBBB in leads V_1 and V_2. Long QT has a QT interval > 440 ms in males and > 460 ms in females. WPW has the classic delta wave (shortened up-sloping PR segment). HCM can have many ECG changes, but the most common are Q waves, T-wave inversions, left ventricular hypertrophy, and left axis deviation. ARVD has the classic epsilon wave (findings of electric potentials in the ST segment) with T wave inversions in the V leads.

1. Lawless CE, Best TM. Electrocardiograms in athletes: interpretation and diagnostic accuracy. Med Sci Sports Exerc 2008 May;40(5):787-798.

38. A 13-year-old male year-round soccer player presents for evaluation with a two-month history of knee pain. He denies any trauma or initial injury and reports that the pain initially was only after games and practices. Gradually, it began to bother him more toward the end of practice sessions, and now it starts to hurt within a few minutes of exercise. He localizes the pain to the inferior pole of the patella. This is most consistent with which of the following diagnoses?

    A. Quadriceps tendinitis
    B. Osgood-Schlatter's disease
    C. Anterior fat pad syndrome
    D. Sindig-Larsen-Johannson disease

Correct Answer: D

Sindig-Larsen-Johannson disease is an inflammatory process involving the inferior pole of the patella, caused by increased tension along the patellar tendon, and can occur in active young teens ages 10 to 14. Osgood-Schlatter's disease occurs by similar mechanism, in the same age group, and is treated the same way, but is an apophysitis of the tibial tuberosity. Quadriceps tendinitis involves the superior pole of the patella at the insertion of the quadriceps tendon. Fat pad syndrome is usually secondary to contusion and irritation to the anterior knee.

1. Minkoff J, Simonson BG. The patella: its afflictions in relation to athletics. In: Harries M, Williams C, Stanish WD, Micheli LJ (eds). Oxford Textbook of Sports Medicine. New York: Oxford University Press, 1994:402-404.
2. Stricker PR, Wasilewski C. Apophysitis. In: Puffer JC (ed). 20 Common Problems in Sports Medicine. New York: McGraw-Hill, 2002:357-358.

39. A 19-year-old offensive lineman sustained an injury to his right foot during a tackle. He developed forefoot swelling, ecchymosis, and has pain with weight-bearing. On physical examination, there is tenderness at the first MTP joint with limited range of motion. Routine standing AP and lateral foot radiographs are unremarkable. He was diagnosed with "turf toe." Which of the following is the most common mechanism of injury?

A. Hyperflexion of first MTP joint
B. Hyperextension of first MTP joint
C. Plantarflexion of forefoot
D. Valgus force to first MTP joint
E. Inversion of ankle

Correct Answer: B

Turf toe is most commonly seen in offensive lineman and running backs and associated with playing on artificial turf, wearing shoes with a flexible forefoot, and sports that require squatting and pushing off. The most common mechanism of injury is hyperextension of the first MTP joint while an axial load is applied to the hindfoot. Other mechanisms include hyperflexion and varus/valgus forces.

1. Mullen JE, O'Malley JM. Sprains-residual instability of subtalar, LisFranc joints and turf toe. Clin Sports Med 2004 Jan;23(1):97-121.
2. Glazebrook M, Annunziato A. Athletic foot disorders. In: Kibler WB (ed). Orthopaedic Knowledge Update: Sports Medicine 4. Rosemont, IL: AAOS, 2009:185-197.

40. Toward the middle of the season, a college soccer player suffers a lateral and syndesmosis ankle sprain, which prevents her from returning to play. Which of the following psychological issues needs to be addressed as it pertains to rehabilitation of her injury?

   A. Encourage a fear of reinjury so as to motivate the athlete in her rehabilitation program
   B. Share the basics about the injury, and encourage the athlete to look it up on the Internet to get a better understanding
   C. Foster an obsession with the question of return to play
   D. Prepare the coach for the injury recovery process, and encourage that the athlete not be isolated from the team

Correct Answer: D

The injury recovery and rehabilitation process is variable for each athlete. The coach should be educated about this particular athlete's injury based on the characteristic of the injury, the specific treatment required, the presence of complications and psychological issues. In addition, coaches should be encouraged to help the injured athlete stay involved with the team by being at practices and performing sport specific rehabilitation, attending team meetings, and being on the sidelines of games.

Unreasonable fears of reinjury or an obsession with the question of return to play are warning signs of poor adjustment to the injury. Goal setting, positive self-statements, cognitive restructuring, and visualization are strategies that can motivate the athlete and that are associated with faster recovery. Educating the athlete about the injury in terms that the injured athlete can understand and assessing the athlete's understanding of the information provided is essential and will help build trust and rapport.

1. Psychological issues related to injury in athletes and the team physician: a consensus statement. Med Sci Sports Exerc 2006 Nov;38(11):2030-2034.

41. A volleyball player presents with right shoulder pain after attempting to spike the ball in practice. The player is holding her arm in slight abduction and external rotation. The humeral head is palpated anteriorly. Before proceeding, it is important to first evaluate which of the following?

    A. Supraclavicular nerve by testing sensation over the clavicular area
    B. Axillary nerve by testing sensation over lateral aspect of the shoulder
    C. Radial nerve by testing sensation over inferolateral arm
    D. Medial cutaneous nerve by testing sensation over medial aspect of arm

Correct Answer: B

Axillary nerve injury is a known complication of anterior dislocations of the shoulder. Before proceeding with x-ray and/or reduction, it is important to document neurovascular status by specifically checking sensation over the superior lateral aspect of arm (i.e., over the deltoid).

1. Thompson JC. Netter's Concise Atlas of Orthopaedic Anatomy. Teterboro, NJ: Icon Learning Systems, 2002:47.
2. Seade LE. Shoulder dislocation clinical presentation. Medscape. Accessed November 17, 2011 at http://emedicine.medscape.com/article/93323.

42. Which of the following is not true of hepatitis B infection?

    A. Concurrent HDV infection increases risk of fulminent infection
    B. Enteric precautions will be necessary to avoid transmission
    C. Sexual contact increases the risk of transmission
    D. E-antigen-positive status is of concern for possible transmission
    E. Symptoms begin two to four months post exposure

Correct Answer: B

While there is conflicting evidence regarding saliva as a mode of transmission, there is no question regarding blood, sharing needles, and sexual contact as known modes of transmission. Because hepatitis B has never been isolated from stool, enteric precautions are not necessary. Concurrent hepatitis D infection does increase risk of fulminent infection. While the symptoms—including fever, malaise, jaundice, abdominal pain, nausea, vomiting, anorexia and puritis among others—may not start until two to four months, the chronic carrier who is E-antigen positive poses the greatest concern for transmission.

1. Mrtin TJ. Infections in athletes. In: Mellion MB, Walsh M, Madden C, Putukian M, Shelton G (eds.) Team Physicians Handbook. 3rd ed. Philadelphia: Hanley and Belfus, 2002:231-232.

2. Scuderi GR, McCann PD, Bruno PJ. Sports Medicine Prinicples of Primary Care. St Louis, MO: Mosby, 1997.

3. Broderick A, Jonas MM. Overview of hepatitis B virus infection in children. UpToDate. Accessed November 17, 2011 at www.uptodate.com/contents/search?search=hepatitis+sports&sp.

43. Which of the following statements is true regarding exertional headache?

    A. Factors associated with increased risk of exertional headaches include hot weather and high altitude
    B. Exertional headaches are always benign
    C. Exertional headaches most commonly occur in young women
    D. The typical duration of exertional headaches is seconds to minutes
    E. The athlete typically describes the pain from exertional headache as "the worst headache of my life"

Correct Answer: A

Factors that increase the risk of exertional headache include hot weather, dehydration, and high altitude. Exertional headache can be related to intracranial bleeding, brain tumors, and myocardial infarction. Benign exertional headache occurs most frequently in men over 40 years old. Typically, exertional headaches last from five minutes to 24 hours. Headaches that are described as "the worst headache of my life" are suspicious for subarachnoid hemorrhage.

1. Putukian M. Headaches in the athlete. In: Mellion MB, Walsh WM, Madden C, Putukian M, Shelton GL (eds). Team Physician's Handbook. 3rd ed. Philadelphia: Hanley and Belfus, 2002:299-311.
2. Cutrer FM. Primary exertional headache. UpToDate. Accessed November 17, 2011 at www.uptodate.com/contents/primary-exertional-headache.

44. Which of the following is a normal ECG response to exercise?

    A. Increase of T-wave amplitude
    B. Depression of the J point
    C. Increase of the QRS duration
    D. ST-segment depression

Correct Answer: B

A gradual decrease in T-wave amplitude is usually observed in all leads during early exercise. At maximal exercise, the T-wave amplitude begins to increase. The J point is the point at which the QRS complex meets the ST segment. Depression of the J point is a normal ECG response to exercise. QRS duration tends to decrease slightly with exercise (and increasing heart rate) in normal subjects. However, QRS duration may increase in patients with either angina or LV dysfunction. ST-segment depression is the most common manifestation of exercise-induced myocardial ischemia.

1. American College of Sports Medicine. Guidelines for Exercise Testing and Prescription. 7th ed. Baltimore, MD: Williams & Wilkins, 2005.
2. Yanowitz FG. Electrocardiographic changes during exercise ECG testing. UpToDate. Accessed November 17, 2011 at www.uptodate.com/contents/electrocardiographic-changes-during-exercise-ecg-testing.

45. In 2009, the NCAA recommended that all athletes with a diagnosis of attention deficit disorder be started on a non-stimulant medication unless contraindicated. Which of the following medications would be an appropriate initial therapy within those guidelines?

    A. Methylphenidate (Ritalin)
    B. Dextroamphetamine (Adderall)
    C. Atomoxetine (Strattera)
    D. Lisdexamfetamine (Vyvanse)

Correct Answer: C

In 2009, the NCAA Committee on Competitive Safety mandated tighter control over the use of stimulant medications to treat attention deficit disorder. The NCAA guideline suggests a trial of non-stimulant medication to manage this disorder. Of the medications listed, only atomoxetine is a non-stimulant medication.

1. NCAA Sports Medicine Handbook 2009. Accessed November 17, 2011 at www.ncaa.org/wps/wcm/connect/00e85e004e0b8a619ae5fa1ad6fc8b25/ADHD_QA2009.pdf?MOD=AJPERES&CACHEID=00e85e004e0b8a619ae5fa1ad6fc8b25.

46. You are performing a preparticipation physical exam on a 17-year-old male football player. In the process of questioning him about his history of concussion and neurological injuries, he reports an event last season when he had a few hours of weakness and numbness in his arms and legs after being tackled. He reports that he had negative C-spine x-rays at that time. He also had an MRI, but does not recall the findings. As part of your discussion with this athlete and his parents about this episode of transient quadriparesis (also referred to as transient neurapraxia and cervical cord neurapraxia), which of the following options would most represent an absolute contraindication to returning to contact sports?

    A. This was his second episode of transient quadriparesis
    B. His Pavlov-Torg ratio was less than 0.8
    C. He was found to have associated intervertebral disk disease with some degenerative changes
    D. He was found to have an associated type II Klippel-Feil deformity involving the interspace at C3

Correct Answer: A

Transient quadriparesis is associated with sensory or motor functional changes or a combined sensorimotor deficit. The episodes, by definition, are not permanent, and complete sensory and motor recovery occurs in 10 minutes to 36 hours. Answer A is correct because most agree that a multiple episodes are a contraindication to return to contact sports. Other absolute contraindications are ligamentous instability, MRI evidence of cord defect or edema, or symptoms lasting greater than 36 hours. Answers B through D are all relative contraindications. The Pavlov-Torg ratio is the ratio of the spinal canal to the sagittal midbody diameter of the vertebral body at the same level. The Pavlov-Torg ratio does indicate significant spinal stensois with high sensitivity, but is a poor predictor or who will suffer transient quadriparesis. A loss of CSF around the spinal cord on MRI is a more accurate method of determining spinal stenosis and an increased risk for transient quadriparesis. A type II Klippel-Feil deformity is a fusion of one or two vertebral bodies. This congenital abnormality in the absence of other findings—such as limited cervical spine motion, instability, disk disease, or spondylosis—is not considered a contraindication to contact sports.

1. Allen C, Kang J. Transient quadriparesis in the athlete. Clin Sports Med 2002; 21(1):15-27.
2. Boden BP. Cervical spine injuries. In: Beutler A, Seidenberg P (eds). The Sports Medicine Resource Manual. Philadelphia: Saunders Elsevier, 2008:272-284.

47. A 16-year-old with Down syndrome presents to the clinic with his parents. They are concerned with the patient's increasing weight. When considering an exercise program for this individual, you need to consider which of the following?

    A. A normal $\dot{V}O_2$max is commonly found in individuals with Down syndrome
    B. There is no evidence supporting exercise as an intervention to improve fitness in Down syndrome individuals
    C. Low exercise tolerance exists in the majority of Down syndrome individuals
    D. There is a normal muscle tone in individuals with Down syndrome

Correct Answer: C

Down syndrome patients are known to be at increased risk for obesity, low muscle tone, decreased $\dot{V}O_2$max, and low exercise tolerance. Despite this, there is some evidence of structured exercise programs and interventions improving certain parameters of fitness in studies of short duration.

1. Understanding intellectual disability and health. St. George's University of London. Accessed November 17, 2011 at www.intellectualdisability.info.
2. Rimmer JH, Heller T, Wang E, Valerio I. Improvements in physical fitness in adults with Down syndrome. Am J Ment Retard 2004 Mar;109(2):165-174.

48. You diagnose a patient with rotator cuff dysfunction. Which of the following would be least beneficial in the rehabilitative treatment of rotator cuff syndrome and dysfunction?

    A. Eccentric strengthening of the biceps
    B. Stretching of the posterior glenohumeral joint capsule and increasing internal rotation range-of-motion
    C. Scapular retraction postural training, with periscapular strengthening and stretching
    D. Strengthening of the teres minor, subscapularis, and infraspinatus, followed by strengthening of the supraspinatus
    E. Scapular protraction postural training, with stretching of the scalenes

Correct Answer: E

Rotator cuff syndrome and dysfunction encompasses a number of more traditional diagnoses—such as rotator cuff tendinitis (tendinosis), subacromial bursitis, partial rotator cuff tears and strains, and rotator cuff impingement—into a more appropriate clinical diagnosis, since distinguishing between the other, more traditional terms based on history, physical examination, and plain film radiographs is not particularly accurate. It also reflects the multi-factorial, complex nature of rotator cuff pathology and the need for a comprehensive evaluation and rehabilitation of rotator cuff problems. While the rehabilitation of any injury should be individualized to the specific patient, there are several common biomechanical factors that contribute to most cases of rotator cuff syndrome and should be addressed. Since the rotator cuff structures work primarily to help stabilize the glenohumeral joint throughout its active range of motion, it works with other stabilizing structures to provide a delicate balance between stability and motion. As such, the long head of the biceps is often overworked or strained in patients with subacute or chronic rotator cuff dysfunction. Glenohumeral internal rotational deficit—often due to posterior capsular and rotator cuff restrictions—has been shown to contribute to both rotator cuff injury and labral pathology. Altered scapular kinetics and scapular malpositioning contributes to two-thirds of patients with rotator cuff syndrome. All three of these issues should be addressed and treated as part of this patient's therapeutic exercise program. Rehabilitation of the rotator cuff is often more efficient with strengthening of all four muscle components as a single unit. However, when patients do not progress as desired, strengthening the uninjured or less-injured muscles before rehabilitation of the injured component—usually the supraspinatus—may be more beneficial.

Scapular retraction training helps correct many forms of scapular dyskinesis, but scapular protraction may place the rotator cuff at a mechanical disadvantage and potentially adversely affect shoulder rotation strength. This would, therefore, be unlikely to benefit this patient's condition. Stretching of the scalene muscles and scapular elevation training are two goals in the treatment of thoracic outlet syndrome.

1. Kennedy DJ, Visco CJ, Press J. Current concepts for shoulder training in the overhead athlete. Curr Sports Med Rep 2009 May-Jun;8(3):154-160.
2. Kibler, WB. Shoulder rehabilitation: principles and practice. Med Sci Sports Exerc 1998 Apr;30(4 Suppl):S40-50.

49. You are asked to set up a drug testing protocol for your school. You design a program that involves random testing, education, and rehabilitation. During the urine drug testing procedure, you ensure a chain of custody, which is defined as which of the following?

A. The record of a prescribing physician, who has given an athlete a banned substance for medical reasons
B. The witnessed observation of an athlete giving a urine sample
C. The order of procedures done during the testing
D. The physical barrier needed to ensure the athletes are kept in line
E. The chronological documentation showing the disposition of a sample from collection to testing

Correct Answer: E

A chain of custody (COC) is required to assure reliability of reported results. Maintaining a dependable COC can be laborious. It is the chronological documentation showing the possession of the sample from collection to testing. The COC documentation and testimony is presented to establish that the substance in evidence was in fact in the urine sample. The presence of a prohibited substance in an athlete's urine or the use of a prohibited method constitutes a doping offense, even if the substance is a pharmaceutical and is properly prescribed by a physician. The order of the procedure is the way the testing is done but is not the chain of custody. The chain is not a real chain that separates people. Witness observation is one aspect of a COC, but not all the steps.

1. Jaffee WB, Trucco E, Teter C, Levy S, Weiss RD. Focus on alcohol & drug abuse: ensuring validity in urine drug testing. Psychiatr Serv 2008 Feb;59(2):140-142.
2. Hilderbrand RL. The world anti-doping program and the primary care physician. Pediatr Clin North Am 2007 Aug;54(4):701-711, x-xi.
3. Tomlinson JJ, Elliott-Smith W, Radosta T. Laboratory information management system chain of custody: reliability and security. J Autom Methods Manag Chem 2006;2006:74907.

50. Your patient sustains an injury to his proximal forearm, and after exam you suspect pronator syndrome. Which of the following exam findings would support this suspicion?

    A. Decreased sensation over the lateral forearm
    B. Pain at night
    C. Positive Tinel's over the radial forearm
    D. Weakness of flexor pollicis longus

Correct Answer: C

The lateral forearm is served by the lateral cutaneous nerve, the terminal part of the musculocutaneous nerve. Tinel's that is positive over the radial side of the forearm may indicate pronator syndrome. Pain at night is typical with carpal tunnel syndrome, but not with pronator syndrome. The weakness of the flexor pollicis longus is secondary to the compression of the anterior interosseous motor nerve.

1. Younger DS. Entrapment neuropathies. Prim Care 2004 Mar;31(1):53-65.
2. Mehlhoff TL, Bennett JB. Elbow injuries. In: Mellion MB (ed). Team Physician's Handbook. 3rd ed. Philadelphia: Hanley and Belfus, 2002:159-165.

51. The placement of a methoxy group at position 8 of the quinolone antibiotics' chemical structure, as in gatifloxacin and moxifloxacin, has eliminated which of the following potential side effects of this class of antibiotic?

A. Tendinopathy
B. Seizures
C. QTc prolongation
D. Phototoxicity
E. Alterations in blood glucose levels

Correct Answer: D

The reason for the notable absence of phototoxicity has been determined to be the presence of the 8-methoxy group, which is possessed by both gatifloxacin and moxifloxacin and is a significant advancement in safety for this class of agents. The mechanism surrounding fluorquinolone associated tendinopathy is complex and poorly understood. Recent research indicates structural differences at position 7 may play a role. Position 7 accounts for differences in central nervous system adverse effects among agents in this class. Although it has been hypothesized that structural differences at position 5 of the quinolone nucleus affect cardiotoxicity, researchers have not yet identified an obvious structural moiety that increases an agent's risk for QTc prolongation. Researchers have not yet identified an obvious structural moiety that increases a drug's risk of causing dysglycemia.

1. Mehlhorn AJ, Brown DA. Safety concerns with fluoroquinolones. Ann Pharmacother 2007 Nov;41(11):1859-1866.
2. Owens RC Jr, Ambrose PG. Antimicrobial safety: focus on fluoroquinolones. Clin Infect Dis 2005 Jul 15;41(Suppl 2):S144-157.

52. Which of the following statements regarding carbohydrates and exercise is true?

    A. The optimal carbohydrate concentration in rehydration solutions is 6% to 8%
    B. Carbohydrate loading before a marathon is only recommended for novice runners
    C. Carbohydrate ingestion only has value in events lasting less than one hour
    D. Glycogen synthesis can be enhanced by ingesting a combination of carbohydrates and fats shortly after exercise

Correct Answer: A

Rehydration solutions with carbohydrate concentrations of 6% to 8% are optimal to maintain blood glucose levels and performance. This concentration provides around 30 to 80 g/hour if consumed at a rate of 1 L/hour. Answer B is incorrect. Carbohydrate loading is recommended for all levels of runners for the marathon distance of 42 km and any distance 30 km or greater. Answer C is incorrect. In fact, ingestion during an event lasting more than one hour has been shown to help maintain intensity and therefore has value. Benefits from ingestion in events less than one hour are not as clearly demonstrated. Answer D is incorrect. The combination of carbohydrates and protein at a ratio around 3:1 or 4:1 has been shown to be optimal for glycogen synthesis.

1. Burke LM, Millet G, Tarnopolsky MA. Nutrition for distance events. J Sports Sci 2007;25(Suppl 1):S29-38.
2. Sawka MN, Burke LM. American College of Sports Medicine position stand. Exercise and fluid replacement. Med Sci Sports Exerc 2007 Feb;39(2):377-390.
3. Millard-Stafford M, Childers WL, Conger SA, Kampfer AJ, Rahnert JA. Recovery nutrition: timing and composition after endurance exercise. Curr Sports Med Rep 2008 Jul-Aug:7(4):193-201.

53. During a session of free preparticipation physical exams offered at your local high school, you see a freshman who had a tibial osteotomy early in childhood. She is new to organized sports. After surgery, there had been no mention of the ACL, bracing, or care during sports participation. She has had no symptoms involving her knee. There is no knee effusion. Your full examination includes an abnormal Lachman test and a positive pivot-shift test, indicating absence of the anterior cruciate ligament. There is also a scar from her previous corrective tibial osteotomy. Concerning clearance for sports, you should do which of the following?

   A. Clear her to play sports without restrictions since she has had no symptoms over the years since her osteotomy
   B. Disqualify her from any fitness or athletic activities
   C. Prescribe physical therapy
   D. Refer her to an orthopedic surgeon experienced in handling teens with no anterior cruciate ligament
   E. Provide a brace and clear her to play sports

Correct Answer: D

Without her ACL, she is at risk of further damage to her knee, including meniscal injuries and articular cartilage damage that can contribute to chronic painful degenerative arthritis at an early age. It has been years since her surgery. She has not participated in organized sports, but she does not have to stop moving completely because of her newly assigned diagnosis. Straight running, weight training, and other activities can be safe for a patient with a chronically ACL-deficient knee. Twisting and cutting may be a problem for her. Sharing the specifics of her case with family, parents, gym teachers, and coaches can allow her to remain involved in safe fitness activities while her ACL is being evaluated further and options are discussed. Simply checking off the "not cleared" portion of her PPE form is not sufficient.

Whereas physical therapy may be an important component of her preparation for and recovery from ACL reconstruction, physical therapy alone cannot solve her ACL deficiency and her risk of further injury. A teen who plans to participate in sports and who is missing an ACL requires consultation with an orthopedist experienced in ACL reconstruction in teens. Braces have not been shown to provide adequate stability with twisting and cutting sports to be able to predict a good result in the majority of ACL-deficient patients.

1. Salter RB. Textbook of Disorders and Injuries of the Musculoskeletal System. 3rd ed. Baltimore: Williams & Wilkins, 1999:364.
2. Reider B. The Orthopedic Physical Examination. Philadelphia: Saunders, 1999:231-233.
3. Fowler PJ. Anterior cruciate ligament injuries in the child. In: DeLee JC, Drez D, Miller MD (eds). DeLee & Drez's Orthopaedic Sports Medicine. 2nd ed. Philadelphia: Saunders, 2003:2067-2074.

54. A 65-year-old male with past medical history of diabetes, who was recently seen in your office to discuss an exercise presciption prior to intiating a new exercise program, now presents to your office with a one-week history of left hip pain and numbness and tingling of the lateral thigh. The symptoms are aggravated by walking and relieved by sitting. Physical examination is normal with the exception of a sensory deficit on the lateral thigh area. Which of the following nerves is involved?

   A. Obturator nerve (L2-L4)
   B. Femoral nerve (L2-L4)
   C. Superior gluteal nerve (L5)
   D. Lateral femoral cutaneous nerve (L2-L3)
   E. Genitofemoral nerve (L1-L2)

Correct Answer: D

The patient is presenting with meralgia paresthetica, which is a painful mononeuopathy of the lateral femoral cutaneous nerve (LCFN). It is commonly due to entrapment of the nerve as it passes through the inguinal ligament. The LCFN is responsible for the sensation of the anteriorlateral thigh and is purely sensory with no motor component.

1. Sekul EA. Meralgia paresthetica. Medscape. Accessed November 17, 2011 at http://emedicine.medscape.com/article/1141848.
2. Luzzio C. Physical medicine and rehabiitation for meralgia paresthetica. Medscape. Accessed November 26, 2011 at http://emedicine.medscape.com/article/308199.
3. Netter FH. Atlas of Human Anatomy. 5th ed. Philadelphia: Saunders Elsevier, 2011.

55. A 22-year-old male presents complaining of pain following being hit in the nose about one hour ago. On exam, you find a soft and fluctuant mass that is seen at the nasal septum bilaterally. Which of the following statements is true of this patient's injury and treatment?

    A. Once drained, there is no risk of reaccumulation or need for nasal packing
    B. Hematoma does not occur without associated nasal fracture
    C. If treatment is delayed, there is increased risk for infection or abscess formation
    D. Hematoma formation is most commonly unilateral
    E. Treatment can be delayed up to 72 hours without increased risk for complication

Correct Answer: C

Septal hematoma follows nasal or facial trauma, with or without nasal fracture. Hematoma formation can be unilateral, but is more commonly bilateral. A soft, fluctuant hematoma forms between the nasal mucosa and the cartilaginous septum. This condition is urgent and should be treated within the first few hours of injury. Management options include needle aspiration or I&D followed by nasal packing to avoid reaccumulation. If treatment is delayed, abscess formation, infection, septal perforation, and saddle nose deformity can develop.

1. Kucik CJ, Clenney T, Phelan J. Management of acute nasal fractures. Am Fam Physician 2004 Oct 1;70(7):1315-1320.
2. Junnila J. Swollen masses in the nose. Am Fam Physician 2006 May 1;73(9):1617-1618.

56. In an adult heart transplant recipient, the donor heart is completely denervated. Which of the the following is correct concerning the heart rate during exercise following a heart transplant?

   A. The heart rate during exercise following a heart transplant is determined by circulating plasma catecholamines alone
   B. Complete denervation of the heart prior to transplant is followed by complete functional reinnervation after transplant
   C. The heart rate control mechanisms are exactly the same as prior to transplant
   D. Partial functional reinnervation allows some heart rate control by sympathetic and parasympathetic stimuli
   E. Increased sensitivity of myocardial adrenergic receptors completely replaces the role of sympathetic and parasympathetic innervation in determining heart rate during exercise

Correct Answer: D

Many other factors play a role, including pulmonary, muscular, hormonal, and partial reinnervation, allowing some neural control. Complete reinnervation is not achieved. Partial functional reinnervation has been shown in transplant patients. It was once believed that no reinnervation occurs. Denervation occurs when removing and transplanting the heart. The increased sensitivity of adrenergic receptors also occurs after transplant. Data show that there is some heart rate control from nerves even after transplant. This recovery has been shown to be partial and not complete. There is increased sensitivity of adrenergic receptors after transplant, but partial reinnervation allows some neural control of heart rate as well.

1. Ferretti G, Marconi C, Achilli G, Caspani E, Fiocchi R, Mamprin F, et al. The heart rate response to exercise and circulating catecholamines in heart transplant recipients. Pflugers Arch 2002 Jan;443(3):370-376.
2. Burke MN, McGinn AL, Homans DC, Christensen BV, Kubo SH, Wilson RF. Evidence for functional reinnervation of left ventricle and coronary arteries after orthotopic heart transplantation in humans. Circulation 1995 Jan 1;91(1):72-78.
3. Bengel FM, Ueberfuhr P, Hesse T, Shiepel N, Ziegler S, Scholz S, et al. Clinical determinants of ventricular sympathetic reinnervation after orthotopic heart transplantation. Circulation 2002 Aug 13;106(7):831-835.

57. A 12-year-old right-hand-dominant male baseball pitcher presents with right upper extremity pain after pitching his most recent game. He reports feeling severe pain after throwing a fastball, with immediate loss of strength in that arm. He admits to some vague discomfort for a week or so before the injury, and confesses that he "may have thrown more than 85 pitches" in the previous game, with only one day of rest between games. His father tells you that playoffs are in two weeks. After examination and radiographs (with comparison views), you determine he has "Little League shoulder" and recommend which of the following?

A. Complete rest from throwing for 6 to 12 weeks
B. One week rest, with return in time for playoffs
C. Moving to the catcher position for the next game, and return to pitching when pain-free
D. Ice, a rotator cuff rehabilitation program, and allow pitching with a pitch count of < 60 pitches per game through the playoffs
E. Referral for surgical evaluation of rotator cuff tear

Correct Answer: A

Proximal humeral epiphysiolysis (or "Little League shoulder") is an overuse injury of the adolescent athlete involved in overhead sports. It can be seen in swimmers or volleyball players, but is most often seen in baseball players, especially pitchers. Biomechanics may play a role, as certain throwing motions place more stress along the kinetic chain.

The diagnosis is made with a high clinical suspicion, and the patient may have limited ROM or strength, and tenderness to palpation or squeezing at the proximal humerus. Radiographs may show a widened proximal humeral physis compared with the unaffected side, but in cases where diagnosis is uncertain, an MRI can be helpful to visualize injury within the physis. The condition is considered a Salter-Harris type I injury, and absolute rest from throwing for a period of time is essential to healing, with full recovery expected. The length of time of rest before pain resolves with throwing can be up to three or four months.

Moving the player to another position that requires significant throwing (e.g., catcher) does not constitute arm rest, and therefore will prolong symptoms and recovery. Rotator cuff tear in this age group is extremely rare, and therefore is unlikely in this case. Pitch counts have been established by Little League and the American Sports Medicine Institute, and should be strictly adhered to at all levels.

1. Johnson JN, Houchin G. Adolescent athlete's shoulder: a case series of proximal humeral epiphysiolysis in nonthrowing athletes. Clin J Sport Med 2006 Jan;16(1):84-86.
2. Taylor DC, Krasinski KL. Adolescent shoulder injuries: consensus and controversies. J Bone Joint Surg Am 2009 Feb;91(2):462-473.
3. The little league pitch count questions and answers 2008. Little League. Accessed November 17, 2011 at www.littleleague.org/Assets/forms_pubs/PitchCount_faq_08.pdf.

58. A 17-year-old female volleyball player presents for her first college preparticipation exam. You note that she is 6'4' tall with long thin limbs, arachnodactyly, scoliosis, and a pectus excavatum. Which of the following would be considered a major eye criterion in assisting in making the clinical diagnosis of Marfan syndrome?

    A. Ectopia lentis
    B. Flat cornea
    C. Myopia
    D. Retinal detachment

Correct Answer: A

Marfan syndrome is currently diagnosed using criteria based on an evaluation of the family history, molecular data, and clinical evaluation. In 1995, a group of the world's leading clinicians and investigators in Marfan syndrome proposed revised diagnostic criteria. Known as the Ghent criteria, they identify major and minor diagnostic findings, which are largely based on clinical observation of various organ systems and on the family history. A major criterion is defined as one that carries high diagnostic precision because it is relatively infrequent in other conditions and in the general population. The Ghent criteria were intended to serve as an international standard for clinical and molecular studies and for investigations of genetic heterogeneity and genotype-phenotype correlations. In the evaluation of the ocular system, the major criterion is ectopia lentis. About 50% of patients have lens dislocation. The dislocation is usually superior and temporal. This may present at birth or develop during childhood or adolescence.

1. Chen H. Genetics of Marfan syndrome. Medscape. Accessed November 2011 at http://emedicine.medscape.com/article/946315.
2. Maron BJ, Ackerman MJ, Nishimura RA, Pyeritz RE, Towbin JA, Udelon JE. Task Force 4: HCM and other cardiomyopathies, mitral valve prolapse, myocarditis, and Marfan syndrome. J Am Coll Cardiol 2005 Apr 19;45(8):1340-1345.

59. The most common cause of sudden death in older athletes (> 35 years old) while running the marathon is which of the following?

    A. Hyponatremia
    B. Neurocardiogenic syncope
    C. Coronary artery disease
    D. Trauma
    E. Cerebral vascular accident

Correct Answer: C

Among older (> 35 years old) athletes, available estimates suggest that the frequency of sudden cardiac death is in the range of one in 15,000 joggers per year or one in 50,000 participants in marathon per year, with a marked predominance of deaths in men. Atherosclerotic coronary artery disease is the most common form of heart disease relevant to the masters population as a cause of nonfatal or fatal cardiovascular events.

1. Franklin BA, Fern A, Voytas J. Training principles for elite senior athletes. Curr Sports Med Rep 2004 Jun;3(3):173-179.
2. Noakes TD. Sudden death and exercise. In: Fahey TD (ed). Encyclopedia of Sports Medicine and Science. Nov 1998. Accessed November 26, 2011 at www.sportsci.org/encyc/suddendeath/suddendeath.html.

60. A 14-year-old male is hit in the left eye with a softball. He complains of blurry, double vision. On exam, he has numbness of his left cheek and is unable to look up with his left eye. The athlete still wants to play. Which of the following should you do next?

    A. Cover the left eye with a shield, and send the athlete to the emergency room
    B. Cover the left eye with a pad, and send the athlete to the emergency room
    C. Have the athlete wear sports goggles and return to play
    D. Cover the left eye with a pad, and return the athlete to play

Correct Answer: A

The numbness of the athlete's cheek and inability to look up suggest the athlete has an orbital floor fracture with entrapment of his ocular muscles and injury to the infraorbital nerve. Globe ruptures are associated with orbital fractures, and a shield is preferred over a pad because the shield applies no direct pressure onto the eye. Athletes with suspected orbital fractures are referred for immediate ophthalmologic evaluation.

1. Rodriguez JO, Lavina AM, Agarwal A. Prevention and treatment of common eye injuries in sports. Am Fam Physician 2003 Apr 1;67(7):1481-1488.
2. Cohen AJ. Orbital floor fractures (blowout). Medscape. Accessed November 26, 2011 at http://emedicine.medscape.com/article/1284026.

61. Which of the following responses during cardiopulmonary exercise testing would most likely indicate myocardial ischemic dysfunction?

    A. Decrease in systolic blood pressure
    B. Increase in systolic blood pressure
    C. Decrease in diastolic blood pressure
    D. Increase in diastolic blood pressure

Correct Answer: A

Blood pressure is dependent on cardiac output and peripheral resistance. As work increases, the systolic blood pressure normally had a corresponding increase that peaks at maximal exercise. A decrease in systolic blood pressure is suggestive of associated ischemic dysfunction, aortic outflow obstruction, severe LV dysfunction, and certain types of drug therapy (e.g., beta-blockers). Diastolic blood pressure normally remains the same or decreases with exercise. Increase in diastolic blood pressure > 10 mm Hg is consistent with a hypertensive response.

1. Fletcher GF, Balady GJ, Amsterdam EA, Chaitman B, Eckel R, Fleg J, et al. Exercise standards for testing and training: a statement for healthcare professionals from the American Heart Association. Circulation 2001 Oct 2;104(14):1694-1740.
2. Akinpelu D. Treadmill stress testing. Medscape. Accessed November 26, 2011 at http://emedicine.medscape.com/article/1827089.

62. A 21-year-old right-handed female collided with the shortstop during a softball game and injured her left elbow when she fell. She presents to you two days after the injury with lateral elbow pain. On exam, she is tender directly over the radial head and has some limitations in range of motion (ROM) with most pain during pronation/supination. An anterior and posterior fat pad are noted on her lateral x-ray from her initial four views of the left elbow, which showed overall normal alignment and no displaced fractures or fracture fragments. What single factor among the following choices would be an indication for orthopedic referral to discuss ORIF for this elbow?

A. Limited ROM in first two days following injury
B. Mechanical block to motion
C. < 2 mm displacement of radial head fracture
D. No dislocation or ligamentous injury
E. Posterior fat pad sign on lateral x-ray

Correct Answer: B

Within the first week of a minimally displaced radial head fracture with no associated dislocation or ligamentous instability, it is normal to have some degree of limited ROM, but the patient should be allowed to begin early ROM as tolerated and should only be immobilized for up to one week. On early plain films, the radial head fracture as well as other elbow fractures may be subtle, but a fat pad sign is a clue that a fracture is present. A posterior fat pad on x-ray is always abnormal. There are several classification systems for radial head fractures, including Mason's orginal classification system, which has since been modified by Hotchkiss (level V, expert opinion):

• Type I: minimally displaced, no mechanical block to rotation, intra-articular displacement < 2 mm
• Type II: fracture displaced > 2 mm or angulated, possible mechanical block to forearm rotation
• Type III: severely comminuted fracture, mechanical block to motion
• Type IV: radial fracture with associated elbow dislocation

In determining appropriate treatment, all associated injuries and their implications must be considered. Mason's type I fractures can be treated with early ROM, while Mason's type II fractures may require orthopedic referral if mechanical block of forearm rotation is present. Mason's types III and IV require ORIF or replacement arthroplasty. General guidelines for orthopedic referral include the following indications (level V, expert opinion):

• Fracture dislocation
• Mechanical block to motion
• Greater than 2 mm displacement
• More than one third articular surface involvement

- More than 3 mm depression
- More than 30 degrees angulated
- Severe comminution

1. Eiff MP, Hatch RL, Calmbach WL. Elbow fractures. Fracture Management for Primary Care. 2nd ed. Philadelphia: Saunders, 2003:148-156.

2. Pike JM, Athwal GS, Faber KJ, King GJ. Radial head fractures: an update. J Hand Surg Am 2009 Mar;34(3):557-565.

3. Rosenblatt Y, Athwal GS, Faber KJ. Current recommendations for the treatment of radial head fractures. Orthop Clin North Am 2008 Apr;39(2):173-185.

63. A 15-year-old male competitive soccer player falls to the ground during a tournament you are covering. He was running maximally without difficulty, but then loses muscle tone and falls to the ground in prone position. You do not remember witnessing any head trauma or collisions to the chest during the game. The trainer signals you to the field, and en route, you notice convulsions lasting two to five seconds. Rolled onto supine position with cervical spine protected, he is unresponsive to verbal and painful stimuli, not breathing spontaneously, and has no radial or carotid pulse.

You initiate rescue breathing and chest compressions while the trainer retrieves the AED and activates EMS. You perform CPR, and the AED delivers shocks twice. With pulse regained, the athlete is transported to the hospital, and he is admitted to you.

On admission, his urine drug screen, urine specific gravity, and serum sodium were normal. His cardiac enzymes, potassium, glucose, and liver enzymes are elevated. Further research reveals that he has had previous episodes of exertional syncope at ages six, seven, and 11, for which the ECG, echocardiogram, treadmill exercise test, and EEG were normal. Newborn screen for sickle cell was normal, and previous fasting glucose was normal. He has had no history of seizures nor syncopal episodes at rest. He had no history of abnormal heart sounds on exams. He does not taking any medication or supplements. There is no family history of sudden cardiac arrest or premature cardiovascular disease. Which of the following is the next appropriate step to arrive at a diagnosis?

A. Cardiac MRI
B. Three-hour 100 g glucose tolerance test
C. Video EEG
D. Psychiatric evaluation
E. Myocardial biopsy

Correct Answer: A

Anomalous coronary arteries are the second-most common cardiovascular cause of sudden death in young athletes (following hypertrophic cardiomyopathy). The most common of these malformations is anomalous origin of the left main coronary artery from the anterior (right) sinus of Valsalva, with acute angled bend coursing between the pulmonary trunk and anterior aspect of the aorta. Rare cases of right coronary artery originates from the left coronary sinus, congenitally hypoplastic coronary arteries, and anomalous origin of left main coronary artery from pulmonary trunk has been associated with sudden cardiac death. Diagnosis (during life) can be difficult because patients often do not exhibit warning signs, and resting/exercise ECG are usually normal. Coronary anomalies should be considered in athletes with exertional syncope or symptomatic ventricular arrhythmia. Transthoracic and transesophageal echocardiogram with Doppler mapping, cardiac MRI (Answer A is correct), and ultrafast CT can detect lesions originating from the wrong sinus, but can be missed. Coronary angiography would be appropriate if all other studies were normal, but certain lesions like acute angle take-off and ostial ridges can still be missed premortum. Sudden death in these cases are usually due to arrhythmias triggered by myocardial infarction during exercise. While there are case reports of exercise-induced syncope with neurological (seizure-like) symptoms in patients with conversion disorder, the firing of the AED in this case suggests a cardiac etiology with the presence of a shockable rhythm (Answer D is incorrect). This patient's seizure-like convulsions are more likely due to hypoxia/hypoxemia from cardiac arrest (and his abnormal lab values can be explained by his cardiac arrest). Uncontrolled seizure disorders can cause syncope during exercise, and seizures can threaten cardiopulmonary functions but such is more commonly observed during status epilepticus, which this athlete did not have. Video EEG, typically performed during rest, is likely to be abnormal post-cardiac arrest; but at this point in the case unlikely to contribute to the diagnosis of the primary cause (Answer C is incorrect). Hypoglycemia can cause syncope, and more information would be needed to rule out this possibility. That being said, the three-hour 100 g glucose tolerance test is used to detect hyperglycemia in the 24- to 28-week pregnant woman (Answer B is incorrect). Myocardial biopsy may be considered to establish the diagnosis of ARVD, cardiac amylodosis, or cardiac sarcoidosis (which can cause sudden cardiac death in athletes but occurs in lesser frequency than anomalous coronary arteries). However, at this point in the case, a less-invasive option is preferable to the biopsy which given the risks of sampling error and myocardial perforations (Answer E is less preferable).

1. Graham TP Jr, Driscoll DJ, Gersony WM, Newburger JW, Rocchini A, Towbin JA. Task Force 2: congenital heart disease. J Am Coll Cardiol 2005 Apr 19;45(8):1326-1333.

2. Kumpf M, Sieverding L, Gass M, Kaulitz R, Ziemer G, Hofbeck M. Anomalous origin of left coronary artery in young athletes with syncope. BMJ 2006 May 13; 332(7550):1139-1141.

3. Iskandar EG, Thompson PD. Exercise-related sudden death due to an unusual coronary artery anomaly. Med Sci Sports Exerc 2004 Feb;36(2):180-182.

64. Which of the following is the most common cause of airway obstruction in an unconscious athlete?

    A. Mouthguard
    B. The tongue
    C. Swelling from anaphylaxis
    D. Inhaled foreign body

Correct Answer: B

The tongue is the one answer that would be present in all athletes. A mouthguard would be present only in contact sports. Swelling from anaphylaxis is a valid answer, but it is not the most common cause. Inhaled foreign body is also a valid option, but the inhalation of foreign bodies is not that common.

1. Weiss EA. Wilderness 911: A Step-by-Step Guide for Medical Emergencies and Improvised Care in the Back Country. Seattle, WA: The Mountaineers Books, 1998.
2. American Heart Association. American Heart Association 2005 guidelines for cardiopulmonary resuscitation and emergency cardiac care.

65. A six-year-old soccer player twists his ankle and presents to you three hours later with a tender, swollen lateral ankle and limited weight bearing. Which of the following is true?

    A. Patients of this age more commonly have sprains than fractures
    B. The Ottawa Ankle Rules have been validated for patients of this age
    C. Salter I fractures are usually evident on plain radiographs at this time
    D. Sever's disease is the most likely diagnosis
    E. Childhood obesity is not associated with a greater risk of ankle injury

Correct Answer: B

Ottawa Ankle Rules have been validated for children greater than five years of age, presenting with ankle and midfoot injuries. The original rules were developed for adults in the early 1990s. Patients of this age more commonly sustain fractures than sprains due to the immaturity of bones and the relative strength of ligaments. Salter I fractures are often missed on plain radiographs. Sever's lesions would present with more heel pain and typically occur in adolescence. Childhood obesity is associated with increased ankle injuries.

1. Dowling S, Spooner CH, Liang Y, Dryden DM, Friesen C, Klassen TP, et al. Accuracy of Ottawa ankle rules to exclude fractures of the ankle and midfoot in children: a meta-analysis. Acad Emerg Med 2009 Apr;16(4):277-287.
2. Zonfrillo MR, Seiden JA, House EM, Shapiro ED, Dubrow R, Baker MD, et al. The association of overweight and ankle injuries in children. Ambul Pediatr 2008 Jan-Feb;8(1):66-69.

66. You are seeing a 13-year-old in follow-up one week after being kicked by a horse. He was transferred to an emergency department from the scene and was diagnosed with simple fractures of the sixth and seventh ribs and a right pulmonary contusion. He briefly received supplemental oxygen but did not require mechanical ventilation and was discharged from the hospital after two days. After seeing the patient, you are concerned that he is suffering from the most common complication of a pulmonary contusion. The clinical scenario most supportive of your suspicion would be which of the following?

    A. Severe respiratory distress and hemoptysis productive of copious amounts of bright red blood
    B. Orthopnea, pulsus paradoxus, muffled heart tones, and a friction rub auscultated over the precordium
    C. Hypoxia and diffuse, bilateral hazy ground-glass opacities on chest radiography
    D. Tympany on percussion of the affected side, tracheal shift to the contralateral side, and diminished breath sounds on the affected side
    E. Fever, tachypnea, cough productive of purulent sputum, and focal rhales

Correct Answer: E

The most common complication of a pulmonary contusion is pneumonia. Radiographically, the pneumonia can be indistinguishable from the contusion on x-ray. Therefore, it is important to monitor the patient for signs of worsening respiratory status and fever. Acute respiratory distress syndrome (ARDS) has been described as a complication also, but it is less common than pneumonia in this setting. Pulmonary hemorrhage, pericardial effusion, and tension pneumothorax are not common complications of pulmonary contusion.

1. Bliss D, Silen M. Pediatric thoracic trauma. Crit Care Med 2002 Nov;30(11 Suppl):S409-415.
2. Clark GC, Schecter WP, Trunkey DD. Variables affecting outcome in blunt chest trauma: flail chest vs. pulmonary contusion. J Trauma 1988 Mar;28(3):298-304.

67. A 16-year-old male high school wrestler presents to the ER after being accidentally kicked in the groin during a competition. Patient was unable to finish the competition because of nausea, vomiting, and difficulty walking due to pain. Examination revealed a tender and swollen right testicle and scrotal hematoma measuring 2 cm in diameter. A scrotal ultrasound with doppler revealed normal parenchymal echo pattern and intact testicular blood flow. His parents are very concerned about the patient's future fertility since he is their only child. The most appropriate next step would be which of the following?

A. Oral antibiotics
B. Exploration of hematocoele
C. Rest, pain control and ice packs on groin for 24 to 48 hours
D. Scrotal MRI
E. Microsurgery to diagnose/repair possible injury to vas deferens since this cannot be seen in the diagnostic studies

Correct Answer: C

With the scrotal ultrasound showing normal results and intact blood flow, it would be reasonable to treat this patient conservatively with rest, pain management, and ice packs to the groin. An MRI is usually reserved for equivocal findings on ultrasound, which is not the case in this situation. Antibiotics are usually not indicated in blunt testicular trauma. Exploration and microsurgery are also not necessary.

1. Terlecki RP. Testicular trauma. Medscape. Accessed November 22, 2011 at http://emedicine.medscape.com/article/441362.
2. Dogra VS. Testicular trauma imaging. Medscape. Accessed November 22, 2011 at http://emedicine.medscape.com/article/381131.

68. In order to diagnose the presence of a posterior tibialis injury, which of the following signs or symptoms would be present?

A. Poorly defined burning, tingling, or numbness sensation on the plantar surface, inferior to the medial malleolus and the plantar aspect radiating to the toes
B. Pain on toe-off or forefoot weight bearing
C. Pain with resisted dorsiflexion and eccentric inversion
D. Pain with passive pronation and active supination

Correct Answer: D

Burning, tingling, and numbness as noted above suggests tarsal tunnel sydrome. Pain in the toe-off or forefoot weight bearing suggests tendonopathy of the flexor hallicus longus tendon. Pain demonstrated by resisted dorsiflexion and eccentric inversion suggests extensor tendonopathy. Pain with passive pronation and active supination would suggest injury to the posterior tibialis.

1. Brown DE. Ankle and leg injuries. In: Mellion MB (ed). Team Physician's Handbook. 3rd ed. Philadelphia: Hanley and Belfus, 2002:509-520.
2. Holzer K. Ankle pain. In: Bruckner P, Khan D (eds). Clinical Sports Medicine. 3rd ed. Sydney: McGraw-Hill, 2007:632-645.
3. Persich G. Tarsal tunnel syndrome. Medscape. Accessed November 22, 2011 at http://emedicine.medscape.com/article/1236852.

69. When there is suspicion of a basilar skull fracture, one is told to look for Battle's Sign. Which of the following best describes Battle's Sign?

A. Ecchymosis around the eyes
B. Ecchymosis over the zygomatic arch
C. Ecchymosis at the base of the neck
D. Ecchymosis of the mastoid process

Correct Answer: D

Battle's Sign is ecchymosis of the mastoid process of the temporal bone seen with a basilar skull fracture. Raccoon eyes are the bruises seen around the eyes in a basilar skull fracture. Leakage of CSF from the ears or nose is also sometimes seen in a basilar skull fracture. Cranial nerve palsy of the facial (CN VII), oculomotor (CN III) or auditory-vestibular (CN VIII) nerve can also occur.

1. Qureshi NH. Skull fracture. Medscape. Accessed November 22, 2011 at http://emedicine.medscape.com/article/248108.
2. Duldner JE. Battle's Sign: behind the ear. MedlinePlus. Accessed November 22, 2011 at www.nlm.nih.gov/medlineplus/ency/imagepages/3067.htm.

70. Which of the following is correct regarding the tendon of the long head of the biceps muscle?

    A. The tendon traverses anteriorly across the glenohumeral joint and attaches to the coracoid process
    B. As the tendon traverses the intertubercular sulcus, it is held in place by the tendon of the pectoralis minor muscle
    C. Superiorly, the tendon is covered by the coracohumeral and superior glenohumeral ligaments
    D. The tendon remains extra-articular throughout its course

Correct Answer: C

The tendon of the long head of the arises from the biceps muscle and traverses through the intertubercular sulcus, where it then traverses superiorly to its attachment on the superior glenoid labrum. As it traverses the intertubercular sulcus, it is held in place by the tendon of the pectoralis major muscle and the transverse ligament, an extension of the subscapularis tendon. The tendon then becomes intra-articular until its attachment at the superior glenoid labrum. Superiorly, the tendon is covered by the coracohumeral and superior glenohumeral ligaments. The short head of biceps tendon traverses anteriorly and attaches at the coracoid process.

1. Erickson SJ, Fitzgerald SW, Quinn SF, Carrera GF, Black KP, Lawson TL. Long bicipital tendon of the shoulder: normal anatomy and pathologic findings on MR imaging. AJR Am J Roentgenol 1992 May;158(5):1091-1096.
2. Bicos J. Biomechanics and anatomy of the proximal biceps tendon. Sports Med Arthrosc 2008 Sep;16(3):111-117.
3. Gamradt SC, Warren RF. Glenohumeral linstability in adults. In: DeLee JC, Drez D, Miller MD (eds). DeLee & Drez's Orthopaedic Sports Medicine. 3rd. Philadelphia: Saunders Elsevier, 2010:909.

71. Which of the following statements is true regarding fungal infection in athletes?

    A. The most common cause of "jock itch" is candida
    B. Most cases of tinea pedis involve the toe web spaces
    C. An NCAA collegiate wrestler diagnosed with tinea corporis at a pre-meet skin-check, may be cleared for participation, as long as the lesions can be adequately covered
    D. Classical tinea corporis lesions present as weeping, red scaly patches surrounded by satellite lesions

Correct Answer: B

The best answer is B. Most cases of tinea pedis involve at least one web space. The most common cause of "jock itch" is a dermatophyte, not candida. Candidal infections may involve the scrotum; dermatophytic infections do not because of the fungistatic sebum produced by the scrotal skin. Classically, tinea corporis presents as a sharply demarcated, annular lesion with a reddened border and central clearing. Candidal infections often present with satellite lesions. The NCAA requires 72 hours of antifungal treatment in addition to adequate coverage of trunk lesions and two weeks of oral antifungal treatment for scalp lesions in order to clear a wrestler to participate.

1. Batts KB. Dermatology in sports medicine. In: O'Connor FG, Sallis RE, Wilder RP, St. Pierre P (eds). Sports Medicine: Just the Facts. New York: McGraw-Hill, 2005:149-157.
2. NCAA 2009-2010 Sports Medicine Handbook, p. 56. Accessed November 24, 2011 at www.ncaapublications.com/productdownloads/MD10.pdf.
3. Wiederkehr M. Tinea cruris. Medscape. Accessed November 23, 2011 at http://emedicine.medscape.com/article/1091806.

72. Which of the following has been shown to have the greatest risk reduction of cardiovascular disease?

    A. Resistance training
    B. Mild cardiovascular exercise
    C. Moderate cardiovascular exercise
    D. Vigorous cardiovascular exercise

Correct Answer: D

Vigorous intensity exercise has been shown to increase aerobic fitness more effectively than moderate intensity exercise, suggesting that the former may confer greater cardioprotective benefits. The epidemiologic studies consistently found a greater reduction in risk of cardiovascular disease with vigorous (typically $\geq$ 6 METs) than with moderate intensity physical activity and reported more favorable risk profiles for individuals engaged in vigorous, as opposed to moderate, intensity physical activity. Clinical trials generally reported greater improvements after vigorous (typically $\geq$ 60% aerobic capacity) compared with moderate intensity exercise for diastolic blood pressure, glucose control, and aerobic capacity, but reported no intensity effect on improvements in systolic blood pressure, lipid profile, or body fat loss. In conclusion, if the total energy expenditure of exercise is held constant, exercise performed at a vigorous intensity appears to convey greater cardioprotective benefits than exercise of a moderate intensity.

1. Swain DP, Franklin BA. VO(2) reserve and the minimal intensity for improving cardiorespiratory fitness. Med Sci Sports Exerc 2002 Jan;34(1):152-157.
2. Wenger HA, Bell GJ. The interactions of intensity, frequency and duration of exercise training in altering cardiorespiratory fitness. Sports Med 1986 Sep-Oct;3(5):346-356.
3. Swain DP, Franklin BA. Comparison of cardioprotective benefits of vigorous versus moderate intensity aerobic exercise. Am J Cardiol 2006 Jan 1;97(1):141-147.

73. An inability to supinate the forearm could be due to an injury to which of the following pairs of nerves?

   A. Suprascapular/axillary
   B. Musculocutaneous/median
   C. Axillary/radial
   D. Radial/musculocutaneous
   E. Median/ulnar

Correct Answer: D

Forceful supination of the forearm benefits from the combined contraction of the biceps brachii (musculo-cutaneus nerve) and the supinator muscle (deep branch of radial nerve). Pronation is performed primarily by the pronator quadratus (anterior interosseus nerve—branch of median nerve) and assisted by the pronator teres (median nerve).

1. Gordon KD. Electromyographic activity and strength during isometric pronation and supination efforts in healthy adults. J Orthop Res 2004 Jan;22(1):208-213.
2. Vicente DP, Calvet PF. Innervation of biceps brachii and brachialis: anatomical and surgical approach. Clin Anat 2005 Apr;18(3):186-194.
3. Kulshreshtha R, Singh R, Sinha J, Hall S. Anatomy of the distal biceps brachii tendon and its clinical relevance. Clin Orthop Relat Res 2007 Mar;456:117-120.

74. An 18-year-old college athlete sustains a traumatic injury to his lower leg during a football game. The physical exam reveals gross angular deformity of the lower leg and no sensation to the first dorsal web space. In addition to a fracture, which of the following is the most likely diagnosis?

   A. Acute compartment syndrome of the anterior compartment
   B. Acute compartment syndrome of the deep posterior compartment
   C. Acute and chronic compartment syndrome of the anterior compartment
   D. Acute compartment syndrome of the lateral compartment
   E. Acute compartment syndrome of the lateral and superficial posterior compartment

Correct Answer: A

The presentation of this athlete suggests a lower extremity fracture given the obvious deformity. Fractures of the tibia are associated with acute compartment syndromes and thus require early recognition. Any of the four compartments can be affected. The anterior compartment contains the deep peroneal nerve and thus decreased sensation between the first and second web space is an indicator of early anterior compartment syndrome. Pain on passive ankle or toe plantarflexion is also consistent with an acute anterior compartment syndrome. Pain with passive inversion of the foot and numbness of the lateral dorsum of the foot excluding the first web space indicates acute lateral compartment syndrome findings. Pain on dorsiflexion of the toes and numbness along the sole of the foot due to the tibial nerve are seen in deep posterior compartment. Patients with superficial posterior compartment have pain with passive ankle dorsiflexion and lateral numbness of the heel (sural nerve). The history does not suggest a chronic exertional compartment syndrome but rather an acute process due to trauma.

1. Rasul AT. Acute compartment syndrome. Medcsape. Accessed November 24, 2011 at http://emedicine.medscape.com/article/307668.
2. Pearse MF, Harry L, Nanchahal J. Acute compartment syndrome of the leg. BMJ 2002 Sep 14;325(7364):557-558.

75. A football player presents to your clinic with a long thoracic nerve injury on the right that has resulted in weakness of the muscle this nerve innervates. Which of the following do you expect to see on physical exam?

    A. Lateral winging of the right scapula
    B. Medial winging of the right scapula
    C. Weakness with internal rotation of the right humerus
    D. Weakness with right shoulder shrugs
    E. Weakness with abduction of the right shoulder

Correct Answer: B

The long thoracic nerve innervates the serratus anterior muscle. The action of the serratus anterior muscle is to draw the scapula forward, abducts and rotates the scapula to point the glenoid cavity superiorly, and stabilizes the vertebral boarder of the scapula to the thoracic cage. Paralysis or weakness of the serratus anterior muscle causes medial winging of the scapula. Weakness of the trapezius causes lateral winging of the scapula and difficulty with shoulder shrugs. The trapezius is innervated by branches of the ansa cervicalis and the spinal accessory nerves. Weakness of the subscapularis muscle causes weakness with internal rotation of the humerus. The subscapularis muscle is innervated by the subscapular nerve. Weakness of the deltoid muscle causes weakness with shoulder abduction. It is innervated by the axilary nerve.

1. Serratus anterior. Wheeless' Textbook of Orthopaedics. Accessed November 24, 2011 at www.wheelessonline.com/ortho/serratus_anterior.
2. Long thoracic nerve. Wheeless' Textbook of Orthopaedics. Accessed November 24, 2011 at www.wheelessonline.com/ortho/long_thoracic_nerve.
3. Wiater JM, Flatow EL. Long thoracic nerve injury. Clin Orthop Relat Res 1999 Nov;(368):17-27.

76. A 50-year-old female patient presents to your office with exertional pain in her right calf. She has noted the pain during exercise for the past several weeks. Which of the following historical and physical findings would you expect with a diagnosis of popliteal artery entrapment syndrome?

    A. Diminished foot pulses at rest

    B. Pain more closely associated with volume of exercise rather than intensity of exercise

    C. Slow resolution of symptoms at conclusion of exercise

    D. Normal pulses that disappear or decrease with plantar flexion or dorsiflexion of the foot

    E. Markedly elevated compartment pressure

Correct Answer: D

Popliteal artery entrapment syndrome causes calf pain during exercise due to compression of the popliteal artery by an abnormal relationship of the artery to the gastrocnemius and/or plantaris muscles. Unlike exertional compartment syndrome, symptoms are associated with intensity of exercise rather than volume. In addition, symptoms tend to resolve quickly after the conclusion of exercise until very late in the disease, when sclerosis of the artery creates a more chronic condition. Foot pulses tend to be normal at rest, but can be abnormal with dorsiflexion and plantarflexion of the foot. For this reason, diagnostic workup for the disorder includes Doppler ultrasonography or angiography in neutral position, dorsiflexion, and plantarflexion. Compartment pressures are usually normal or slightly elevated. This disorder is usually treated by cessation of causative activities followed by surgical release of the artery from the offending muscles. After surgical release, most patients can resume normal exercise.

1. Zetaruk M, Hyman J. Leg injuries. In: Bruckner P, Khan K (eds). Clinical Sports Medicine. 3rd ed. Sydney: McGraw Hill, 2007:451.
2. Wright LB, Matchett WJ, Cruz CP, James CA, Culp WC, Eidt JF, McCowan TC. Popliteal artery disease: diagnosis and treatment. Radiographics 2004 Mar-Apr; 24(2):467-479.

77. An 18-year-old female long distance runner has recently been diagnosed with her second tibial stress fracture and reports her last menstrual cycle occurred six months ago. You rule out other causes for amenorrhea and get a DEXA scan, which reports "low bone density below the expected range for age." Which of the following options is the first aim of treatment for this athlete?

   A. Begin an antidepressant to treat emotional issues and/or unhealthy thought processes that maintain her disorder
   B. Treat low bone density below the expected range for age with a bisphosphonate
   C. Restore regular menstrual cycles with hormone replacement therapy or oral contraceptive pill
   D. Optimize nutritional status by increasing energy intake and/or reduce energy expenditure

Correct Answer: D

Treatment of the female athlete triad should involve a multidisciplinary approach including a physician, dietician, and mental health professional (SORT C). The first aim of treatment should be to optimize nutritional status by increasing energy intake and/ or decreasing energy expenditure (SORT C). Cognitive, behavioral, individualized, group, or family therapy should be utilized for treatment of emotional issues and/or unhealthy thought processes that maintain her disorder (Evidence category B). Pharmacotherapy is not first line therapy, but antidepressants are often used to treat concomitant anxiety or depression and HRT/OCP can be considered in females age 16 whose BMD decreases despite adequate non-pharmacologic therapy (Evidence category C). Bisphosphonates are not recommended for young athletes due to unproven efficacy in this age group and risk of teratogenicity.

1. Nattiv A, Loucks AB, Manore MM, Sanborn CF, Sundgot-Borgen J, Warren MP, et al. American College of Sports Medicine position stand. The female athlete triad. Med Sci Sports Exerc 2007 Oct;39(10):1867-1882.
2. International Olympic Committee Medical Commission Working Group Women in Sport. Position stand on the female athlete triad, revised 8-06. Accessed November 25, 2011 at www.olympic.org/Documents/Reports/EN/en_report_917.pdf.
3. Manore MM, Kam LC, Loucks AB. The female athlete triad: components, nutrition issues, and health consequences. International Association of Athletics Federations. J Sports Sci 2007;25 Suppl 1:S61-71. Erratum in: J Sports Sci 2009 Apr;27(6):667.

78. An afebrile patient with acute low back pain notices pain going down the posterior-lateral aspect of their right thigh and leg. It is noted on your exam that she has the following: positive straight leg raise, a slight sensory deficit located on the lateral aspect of the right foot, a diminished ankle jerk, and weakness with plantar flexion of the great toe. It is also noted that it is hard for her to walk on her toes. Which nerve root is mostly likely the cause of her symptoms?

    A. L3
    B. L4
    C. L5
    D. S1
    E. L2

Correct Answer: D

This question focuses on knowing the dermatomes of the lumbo-sacral spine. The S1 nerve provides sensation to the lateral aspect of the foot, the achilles reflex and plantar flexion of the great toe.

   1. Humphreys SC, Eck JC. Clinical evaluation and treatment options for herniated lumbar disc. AFP 1999 Feb 1;59(3):575-582, 587-588.
   2. Kishner S. Dermatomes anatomy. Medscape. Accessed November 23, 2011 at http://emedicine.medscape.com/article/1878388.

79. Which of the following is true regarding eye protection in sports?

    A. Soft contacts or daily wear glasses can provide some eye protection
    B. Lensless eyeguards provide adequate protection
    C. Highly farsighted athletes may be more prone to retinal detachment injuries
    D. Radial keratotomy (RK) surgery can strengthen a cornea after healing
    E. Well-fitted, certified polycarbonate lenses provide adequate protection in sports

Correct Answer: E

Contact lenses and daily wear glasses provide no protection (and may actually increase injury severity). Lensless eyeguards offer no protection. Highly nearsighted (not farsighted) athletes are more prone to retinal detachment. History of incisional RK surgery weakens the cornea and excimer laser probably does not. Polycarbonate lenses and frames will not break and those that have passed the ASTM standard are the best available eye protectors for sports.

1. Rodriquez JO, Lavina AM, Agarwal A. Prevention and treatment of common eye injuries in sports. Am Fam Physician 2003 Apr 1;67(7):1481-1488.
2. Eime R, Finch C, Wolfe R, Owen N, McCary C. The effectiveness of a squash eyewear promotion strategy. Br J Sports Med 2005 Sep;39(9):681-685.
3. Jerffers JB. Sports-related eye injuries. In: Mellion MB, Putukian M, Madden C (eds). Sports Medicine Secrets. 3rd ed. Philadelphia: Hanley and Belfus, 2002:294.
4. Cass SP. Ocular injuries in sports. Curr Sports Med Rep 2012 Jan;11(1):11-15.
5. Heimmel MR, Murphy MA. Ocular injuries in basketball and baseball: what are the risks and how can we prevent them? Curr Sports Med Rep 2008 Sep-Oct;7(5):284-288.

80. A 12-year-old male pitcher collapses shortly after being struck in the chest by a baseball. Which of the following is true regarding commotio cordis (CC)?

    A. The use of chest protectors is proven to decrease the likelihood of CC
    B. Impact occurs during the QRS complex in the cardiac cycle
    C. Initial arrhythmia is atrial fibrillation
    D. Defibrillation is highly successful in reverting CC events
    E. Age appropriate safety balls have been proven to reduce CC events

Correct Answer: E

Commotio cordis (CC) involves blunt, non-penetrating trauma to the chest resulting in irregular heart rhythm and often leading to sudden death. Commercially available chest protectors are *not* effective in protecting against CC events; however, their use is recommended in high risk positions (i.e., catchers and goalies). Impact occurs during a vulnerable window in the cardiac cycle 10 to 30 milliseconds before the T-wave peak. The most common initial arrhythmia is ventricular fibrillation. Early defibrillation is critical for survival, but defibrillation even in optimal situations has a success rate of less than 50%. Survival rate with defibrillation within three minutes of occurrence is 25% (17 of 68 cases). Survival rate drops to 3% with prolongation of resuscitation beyond three minutes (1 of 38 cases). Use of age-appropriate safety baseballs is proven to reduce CC events, and they are used in leagues with participants under age 13.

1. Madias C, Maron BJ, Alsheikh-Ali AA, Estes NA III, Link MS. Commotio cordis. Indian Pacing Electrophysiol J 2007 Oct 22;7(4):235-245.
2. Palacio LE, Link MS. Commotio cordis. Sports Health 2009;1(2):174-179.

81. A 20-year-old male college basketball player presents for a preparticipation exam. He reveals that he is HIV+. He is asymptomatic, on appropriate medications, and has normal laboratory findings. If his health status remains stable, your recommendations should include which of the following?

   A. He discontinues playing basketball, and his previous teamates are tested for HIV

   B. He continues playing basketball, and his previous teamates are tested for HIV

   C. He discontinues playing basketball and his previous teamates should not be tested for HIV

   D. He continues playing basketball, and his previous teamates are not tested for HIV

Correct Answer: D

An otherwise healthy/asymtomatic patient infected with HIV without evidence of immune system dysfunction—either clinically or by laboratory analysis—does not need restriction on activities. HIV transmission by sports participation has not been documented in any validated report, and so testing for teamates is unwarranted.

1. McGrew CA. Acute infections In: McKeag DB, Moeller JL (eds). ACSM's Primary Care Sports Medicine. 2nd ed. Philadelphia: Lippincott William & Wilkins, 2007:251-260.
2. Brown LS Jr, Drotman DP, Chu A, Brown CL Jr, Knowlan D. Bleeding injuries in professional football: estimating the risk for HIV transmission. Ann Intern Med 1995 Feb 15;122(4):273-274.
3. NCAA guideline 2l: blood-borne pathogens and intercollegiate athletics. 2011-2012 NCAA Sports Medicine Handbook, p. 68. Accessed November 25, 2011 at fs.ncaa.org/Docs/health_safety/2011_12_Sports_Medicine_Handbook.pdf.

82. The four bones that make up the proximal carpal row of the wrist are which of the following?

    A. Capitate, hamate, trapezium, trapezoid
    B. Scaphoid, lunate, trapezoid, pisiform
    C. Lunate, triquetrum, scaphoid, pisiform
    D. Scaphoid, lunate, triquetrum, hamate

Correct Answer: C

The bones of the wrist consist of the proximal carpal row, which is made up of the scaphoid, lunate, triquetrum, and pisiform, which articulate with the distal radio-ulnar joint and the distal carpal row. The distal carpal row consists of the trapezium, trapezoid, capitate, and hamate.

1. Hoynak BC. Carpal bone injuries. Medscape. Accessed November 25, 2011 at http://emedicine.medscape.com/article/97565.
2. Richars L, Loudon J. Bone and joint structure. University of Kansas Medical Center, School of Allied Health. Accessed November 25, 2011 at http://classes.kumc.edu/sah/resources/handkines/bone/wrist.html.

83. Which of the following is a contraindication to hyaluronic acid viscosupplementation?

    A. Hip osteoarthritis
    B. Pregnancy
    C. Knee osteoarthritis
    D. Rheumatoid arthritis
    E. Glenohumeral osteoarthritis

Correct Answer: B

Hyaluronic acid therapy is approved by the FDA for treatment of knee osteoarthritis. Several trials have shown utility in treating osteoarthritis in alternate joints. Contraindications include avian allergy (except Euflexxa®), bacteremia, joint infection, local skin disease, nursing, pediatric patients, pregnancy, and protein allergy. Hyaluronic acid therapy may be used in rheumatoid arthritis patients with a diagnosis of knee osteoarthritis.

1. Strauss EJ, Hart JA, Miller MD, Altman RD, Rosen JE. Hyaluronic acid viscosupplementation and osteoarthritis: current uses and future directions. Am J Sports Med 2009 Aug;37(8):1636-1664.
2. Das A, Neher JO, Safranek S. Clinical inquiries. Do hyaluronic acid injections relieve OA knee pain? J Fam Pract 2009 May;58(5):281c-e.

84. Which of the following statements is true based on the image provided?

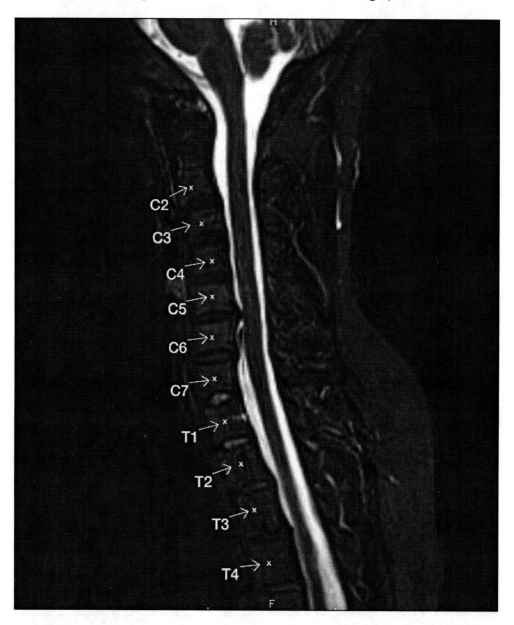

A. The patient is likely to present with complaints of numbness and tingling of the fourth and fifth digit

B. Testing the wrist flexors and finger extensors is likely to present with weakness

C. Reflex testing of the triceps will indicate an increased response

D. The patient may complain of pain and tingling to deltoid and shoulder

E. Atrophy of the thenar eminence may be a presenting symptom

Correct Answer: D

The image is an MRI of the cervical spine. It demonstrates a bulging disk at the C5-C6 level. It may present with decreased or heightened sensation of the deltoid, biceps, wrist extensors, and upper arm. The same muscles may demonstrate weakness on testing, depending on the neurological damage. Reflex testing of the biceps and brachoradialis may be decreased as a result of this injury or changes. Numbness and tingling of the fourth and fifth digit is most often due to a bulging disk or lesion at the C7-C8 neurological level or ulnar nerve. Wrist flexors and finger extensors are neurological testing of the C7 neurological level. This image does not indicate a pronounced effect at the C7 level. The triceps reflex tests C7 neurological level and is minimally affected in this MRI. Atrophy of the thenar eminence is most likely due to median nerve injury and carpal tunnel syndrome among other lesions affecting the median nerve and hand muscles.

1. Netter FH. Atlas of Human Anatomy. 5th ed. Philadelphia: Saunders Elsevier, 2011.
2. Greene WB, Snider RK (eds). Essentials of Musculoskeletal Care. 2nd ed. Rosemont IL: Am Academy Orthopedic Surgeons, 2001:518-550.
3. Kishner S. Dermatomes anatomy. Medscape. Accessed November 23, 2011 at http://emedicine.medscape.com/article/1878388.

85. A 12-year-old black male with sickle cell disease presents to your office for a preparticipation physical exam. He has had no recent hospitalizations, blood transfusions, or sickle cell crisis. He can be cleared for participation in which of the following sports?

   A. Football
   B. Baseball
   C. Soccer
   D. Basketball

Correct Answer: B

Athletes with sickle cell disease are at risk for sickle crisis. If the sickle cell disease is stable, the athlete is permitted to participate in all but high-exertion, collision, and contact sports. All of the given choices are collision/contact sports except for baseball, which is a limited contact sport. Overheating, dehydration, and chilling must be avoided, since these conditions can trigger a sickle crisis.

1. Saglimbeni AJ. Sports physicals. Medscape. Accessed November 25, 2011 at http://emedicine.medscape.com/article/88972.
2. NCAA guideline 2r: the student-athlete with sickle cell trait. 2011-12 NCAA Sports Medicine Handbook, p. 86. Accessed November 25, 2011 at http://fs.ncaa.org/Docs/health_safety/2011_12_Sports_Medicine_Handbook.pdf.

86. Which of the following is true regarding the use of cryotherapy and heat in the treatment of athletic injuries?

    A. Cryotherapy and heat both decrease tissue metabolism
    B. Cryotherapy produces vasodilation and heat produces vasoconstriction
    C. Cryotherapy and heat can both decrease muscle spasm
    D. Cryotherapy and heat both increase soft tissue swelling
    E. Cryotherapy increases nerve conduction, and heat decreases nerve conduction

Correct Answer: C

Cryotherapy and heat are frequently used in the management of athletic injuries. Cryotherapy leads to vasoconstriction, decreased tissue metabolism, decreased inflammatory response, decreased pain, and decreased muscle spasm. Heat, on the other hand, leads to vasodilation, increased tissue metabolism, decreased pain, increased local circulation, and decreased muscle spasm.

1. Mac Auley DC. Ice therapy: how good is the evidence? Int J Sports Med 2001 Jul; 22(5):379-384.
2. Mayer JM, Mooney V, Matheson LN, Erasala GN, Verna JL, Udermann BE, et al. Continuous low-level heat wrap therapy for the prevention and early phase treatment of delayed-onset muscle soreness of the low back: a randomised conrolled trial. Arch Phys Med Rehabil 2006 Oct;87(10):1310-1317.

87. A right-hand-dominant 16-year-old female volleyball player has an x-ray in the emergency room showing an acute fracture of the middle third of her right clavicle. The distal fragment is displaced superiorly 0.8 cm with shortening of about 20 mm. Pulses and neuro exam are within normal limits. Management should include which of the following?

    A. Routine surgical fixation
    B. Immobilization in sling for four to six weeks
    C. Immobilization in figure-of-eight brace for four to six weeks
    D. Emergent surgical consultation

Correct Answer: A

Early studies showed that healing rates of clavicle fractures were very high. Newer studies have shown much higher nonunion rates of about 15% to 25% with higher rates of patient satisfaction with operative treatment. Although nonoperative treatment is a viable option, surgical fixation should be considered in patients with multiple risk factors. These include female sex, comminution, displacement, clavicle shortening (> 15 to 20 mm), older age, and greater levels of trauma. Therefore, Answer A of non-emergent surgical fixation is the best choice. Answers B and C are incorrect since immobilization in a female patient with displacement is not appropriate. Answer D is incorrect since this patient does not need emergent fixation as there is no neurovascular compromise.

1. Pecci M, Kreher JB. Clavicle fractures. Am Fam Physician 2008 Jan 1;77(1):65-70.
2. Rubino LJ. Clavicle fractures. Medscape. Accessed November 26, 2011 at http://emedicine.medscape.com/article/1260953.
3. Estephan A. Clavicle fracture in emergency medicine. Medscape. Accessed November 26, 2011 at http://emedicine.medscape.com/article/824564.

88. You are dealing with an athlete who just sustained a penetrating chest trauma from falling on a sharp object. The object was removed by a teammate and now you are concerned the victim has an open tension pneumothorax. Which of the following is the definitive method of treating this condition?

    A. Dressing affixed on three sides to create a flap valve
    B. Fully occlusive dressing
    C. Occlusive dressing with intercostal chest drain
    D. Intercostal chest drain with dressing affixed on three sides

Correct Answer: C

The definitive treatment is a chest tube with an occlusive dressing over the wound. There are considerations based on risk stratification for optimal treatment of pneumothorax. But, open tension pneumothorax has life-threatening potential, and definitive management includes chest tube placement. Additional measures include 100% oxygen via facemask and possibly intubation if adequate ventilation cannot be achieved. A three-sided dressing can be used in an emergency until transport to definitive care can be arranged. The theory is that it creates a flap valve to allow air to escape from the pneumothorax during expiration, but does not allow air in during inspiration.

1. Chest trauma pneumothorax—open. Trauma.org. Accessed November 26, 2011 at www.trauma.org/archive/thoracic/CHESTopen.html.
2. Bascom R. Pneumothorax treatment and management. Medscape. Accessed November 26, 2011 at http://emedicine.medscape.com/article/424547.

89. A soccer player presents with injury to the mandible from an elbow. You identify post-traumatic malocclusion, focal swelling, and tenderness over the mandible. On examination, you find defects of the dental occlusal surface, alveolar ridge disruptions, and anesthesia in the distribution of the anterior aspect of the chin and lower lip. You suspect a mandible fracture and injury to which of the following nerves?

    A. Anterior cutaneous nerve
    B. Mental nerve
    C. Infraorbital nerve
    D. Facial nerve
    E. Supratrochlear nerve

Correct Answer: B

Mandible fractures are common in soccer and martial arts. Anesthesia of the mental nerve, part of the mandibular branch of cranial nerve V (CNV3) distribution can occur. The mental nerve runs in a channel in the mandible. The anterior cutaneous nerve is from cervical nerve two. Infraorbital nerve is CNV2 and can be damaged with orbit fracture from a ball to the eye. The facial nerve (CNVII) provides a small amount of afferent innervation to the oropharynx above the palatine tonsil. Supratrochlear nerve (CNV1) can be injured by trauma to the inner portion of the eyebrow and supplies the forehead.

1. Maladière E, Bado F, Meningaud JP, Guilbert F, Bertrand JC. Aetiology and incidence of facial fractures sustained during sports: a prospective study of 140 patients. Int J Oral Maxillofac Surg 2001 Aug;30(4):291-295.
2. Cerulli G, Carboni A, Mercurio A, Perugini M, Becelli R. Soccer-related craniomaxillofacial injuries. J Craniofac Surg 2002 Sep;13(5):627-630.
3. Hwang K, You SH, Lee HS. Outcome analysis of sports-related multiple facial fractures. J Craniofac Surg 2009 May;20(3):825-829.

90. A 54-year-old male presents to your office, complaining of bilateral knee pain. He was diagnosed with osteoarthritis in both his knees after he was referred by his primary care provider to see an orthopedic surgeon. He was given a prescription for an anti-inflammatory medication and told that he may need knee replacement surgery some day. He does not like taking medications and has come to see you regarding non-pharmacologic treatment options. Which of the following statements regarding exercise and osteoarthritis is true?

A. Aerobic exercise should be encouraged because it may decrease the patient's pain
B. This patient's x-ray findings are moderate to severe, therefore, exercise is unlikely to be helpful
C. Strengthening exercises may be harmful and alter the disease progression
D. Aquatic exercise has not been shown to be beneficial for patients with osteoarthritis

Correct Answer: A

Answer A is correct. Improvements in muscle strength and proprioception gained from exercise programs may prevent and reduce the progression of osteoarthritis. For people with osteoarthritis, both high-intensity and low-intensity aerobic exercise have been shown to be effective in improving a patient's functional status, gait, pain, and aerobic capacity. Different exercise types have different effects; thus, an individualized approach to exercise prescription is recommended, based on presenting symptoms, problems, and the needs of the patient. For people with osteoarthritis of the knee, land-based therapeutic exercise has been shown to reduce pain and improve physical function. Optimal exercise type or dosage has not clearly been defined. Supervised exercise classes appeared to be as beneficial as treatments provided on a one-to-one basis. The effectiveness of exercise is independent of the severity of x-ray findings. There is evidence to support aquatic exercise for the treatment of knee osteoarthritis and/or hip, at least in the short term. Although no long-term effects have been documented (very few studies performed at this point), the short-term benefits make it a viable option for your patients.

1. Bartels EM, Lund H, Hagen KB, Dagfinrud H, Christensen R, Danneskiold-Samsøe B. Aquatic exercise for the treatment of knee and hip osteoarthritis. Cochrane Database Syst Rev 2007; Oct 17;(4):CD005523.
2. Roddy E, Zhang W, Doherty M, Arden NK, Barlow J, Birrell F, et al. Evidence-based recommendations for the role of exercise in the management of osteoarthritis of the hip or knee—the MOVE consensus. Rheumatology (Oxford) 2005 Jan;44(1):67-73.
3. Brosseau L, MacLeay L, Robinson V, Wells G, Tugwell P. Intensity of exercise for the treatment of osteoarthritis. Cochrane Database Syst Rev 2003;(2):CD004259.

91. A 19-year-old female basketball player tries to deflect a pass and sustains a proximal, interphalangeal (PIP) dorsal dislocation of her middle finger that you reduce on the sideline. Later, radiographs are negative for fracture and show good alignment. Which of the following is true for this injury?

    A. Delayed complications include Boutonniere deformity
    B. The injury can result in extension lag at the DIP joint
    C. Immediate orthopedic consult to prevent proximal migration of flexor profundus
    D. Delayed complications include swan neck deformity deformity

Correct Answer: D

This is a dorsal dislocation without fracture. The finger should be splinted in 20 to 30 degrees of flexion to allow the volar plate to heal. Delayed complications can include swan neck deformity (correct answer D) when the volar plate is lax: flexion at the DIP and hyperextension at the PIP. Boutonniere deformity is a delayed complication of tear at the central slip in volar dislocations. It is noted for flexion at PIP and extension at DIP, with inability to flex the DIP with the PIP extended. Migration of the profundus tendon occurs with jersey fingers. Extension lags at DIP can occur from mallet finger injuries.

1. Hodge DK, Safran MR. Sideline management of common dislocations. Curr Sports Med Rep 2002;1(3):149-155.
2. Leggit JC, Meko CJ. Acute finger injuries: part II. Fractures, dislocations, and thumb injuries. Am Fam Physician 2006 Mar 1;73(5):827-834.
3. Likes RL. Boutonniere deformity. Medscape. Accessed February 11, 2012 at http://emedicine.medscape.com/article/1238095.
4. Swan neck deformity. Wheeless' Textbook of Orthopaedics. Accessed February 11, 2012 at www.wheelessonline.com/ortho/swan_neck_deformity.

92. A 24-year-old female runner is being seen by you in your sports medicine clinic for two weeks of gradually worsening radial sided right wrist pain. She is six weeks post-partum after a normal spontaneous vaginal delivery of a relatively uncomplicated pregnancy. There has been no known trauma otherwise. Her pain is worse when she lifts her newborn, and she reports some wrist stiffness. Your examination reveals tenderness to palpation over the radial styloid and in the approximated soft tissues. There is a positive Finkelstein's test. The most likely involved structure(s) is (are) which of the following?

   A. The tenosynovial compartment associated with the abductor pollicis longus and extensor pollicis brevis
   B. The tenosynovial compartment associated with the extensor carpi radialis longus and extensor carpi radialis brevis
   C. The tenosynovial compartment associated with the extensor pollicis longus
   D. The tenosynovial compartment associated with the flexor carpi radialis
   E. The first carpal-metacarpal joint and its joint capsule

Correct Answer: A

The patient in this case has De Quervain syndrome. There are 12 extensor tendons in the dorsal wrist, running in extensor synovial sheaths, and arranged into six dorsal (extensor) compartments: first compartment-abductor pollicis longus and extensor pollicis brevis; second compartment-extensor carpi radialis longus and extensor carpi radialis brevis; third compartment-extensor pollicis longus; fourth compartment-extensor digitorum communis and extensor indicis proprius; fifth compartment-extensor digiti minimi (quinti); sixth compartment-extensor carpi ulnaris.

De Quervain syndrome (also known as De Quervain's tenosynovitis, De Quervain's disease, mother's wrist, and washerwoman's wrist) is a disease of the first dorsal compartment, which contains the abductor pollicis longus and extensor pollicis brevis tendons. There are multiple contributing risk factors and proposed causes for this condition, including a more prominent radial styloid, female sex, recent pregnancy, repetitive overuse, and other ergonomic factors. This disorder is commonly thought to be an inflammatory tenosynovitis, but this has become more controversial. Some authors have reported a lack of inflammatory changes in De Quervain syndrome, but rather myxoid deposition, fibrosis, and thickening more consistent with degenerative tendinosis. Finkelstein's test is often used to diagnose De Quervain syndrome, and this patient's test was positive for reproducible pain. While first carpal-metacarpal joint arthrosis may present with symptoms similar to De Quervain syndrome, it is less likely given this patient's age; although, a carpal-metacarpal grind test can help exclude this diagnosis. The number of other risk factors for De Quervain syndrome also makes this the most likely diagnosis. Treatment options include corticosteroid injection into the first dorsal (extensor) compartment, other anti-inflammatory medications, splinting, therapeutic exercises, hydro-dissection, and surgical release.

1. Daniels JM, Zook EG, Lynch JM. Hand and wrist injuries: Part I. Nonemergent evaluation. Am Fam Physician 2004 Apr 15;69(8):1941-1948.
2. Clarke MT, Lyall HA, Grant JW, Matthewson MH. The histopathology of De Quervain's disease. J Hand Surg Br 1998 Dec;23(6):732-734.
3. Lampe EW. Surgical anatomy of the hand with special reference to infections and trauma. Clin Symp 1969 Jul-Sep;21(3):66-109.

93. A 70-year-old unconditioned male comes into your office wanting to start working out again. He has a resting heart rate of 70 beats per minute, no medical problems, and takes a multivitamin every morning. His time is limited, so he wants to optimize his training. He has a heart monitor (exercise cardiotachometer), which consists of a wrist monitor that communicates with a strap that is placed around his chest. He wants to know what his heart rate range should be for cardiovascular fitness. You tell him that based on the ACSM guidelines, his range for target heart rate should be which of the following?

A. 60 to 70 beats per minute (bpm)
B. 75 to 90 bpm
C. 95 to 110 bpm
D. 115 to 130 bpm

Correct Answer: C

Based on the ACSM guidelines, there are two accepted methods for calculating target heart rates (HR), heart rate maximum (HRmax) and heart rate reserve (HRR):

HRmax = 220 – age
HRR = HRmax – resting heart rate

Initial training intensity is dictated by fitness level of the individual and based on a percentage of either of those two parameters. For an unconditioned individual, initial target HR is 60% to 70% of HRmax or 40% to 50% of HRR which is then added to the resting heart rate to arrive at a target HR. For intermediate (recreational athlete), the suggested initial training intensity is 70% to 80% of HRmax. For advanced fitness level patient, the suggested initial training intensity is 80% to 90% of HRmax or 60% to 80% of HRR. In the scenario above:

HRmax = 220 – 70 = 150 bpm
HRR = 150 bpm – 70 bpm = 80 bpm

Being unconditioned, his target HR is:

Using HRmax: 150 bpm x 0.60 to 0.70 = 90 to 105 bpm
Using HRR: 80 bpm x 0.40 to 0.50 = 32 to 40 bpm + 70 bpm = 102 to 110 bpm

Therefore, of the choices given, Answer C is the best response.

1. Anish EJ. The senior athlete. In: Mellion MB (ed). Team Physician's Handbook. 3rd ed. Philadelphia: Hanley and Belfus, 2002:100-104.
2. Latin RW. Preseason conditioning. In: Mellion MB, (ed). Team Physician's Handbook. 3rd ed. Philadelphia: Hanley and Belfus, 2002:116-117.
3. Suleman A. Exercise prescription. Medscape. Accessed November 26, 2011 at http://emedicine.medscape.com/article/88648.

94. A 16-year-old basketball player presents with eye pain after his teammate pokes him in the eye. You suspect he has a corneal abrasion and begin your discussion of antibiotic and non-steroidal drops while you examine him. The finding on exam that would cause you to send him to the emergency room for evaluation of possible globe injury is which of the following?

A. Abrasion of more than 50% of cornea surface
B. Abrasion related to a fractured contact lens
C. Multiple vertical abrasions
D. Abrasion with a positive Seidel's sign

Correct Answer: D

Corneal abrasions are common sporting injuries to the eye that involve a traumatic defect to the corneal epithelium from direct trauma, contact lens–related injury, or foreign body. An abrasion of more than 50% of corneal surface takes three to five days to heal and consideration should be given to an ophthalmology referral. Abrasions related to contact lens use should be evaluated on a daily basis to ensure healing and prompt referral to an ophthalmologist if an ulcer develops. Multiple vertical abrasions should evoke a thorough exam of the eye for a foreign body, including everting the eyelid. A Seidel's sign occurs when diluted fluorescein percolates from the eye, representing a penetrating injury to the globe. Any injury to the globe requires emergent ophthalmologic evaluation.

1. Seidel test. Family Practice Notebook. Accessed on November 26, 2011 at www.fpnotebook.com/Eye/Exam/SdlTst.htm.
2. Dargin JM, Lowenstein RA. The painful eye. Emerg Med Clin North Am 2008 Feb;26(1):199-216, viii.

95. Which of the following components of concussion assessment is the least sensitive in detecting a concussion?

    A. Anterograde amnesia
    B. Postural instability
    C. Retrograde amnesia
    D. Loss of consciousness
    E. Orientation

Correct Answer: E

Orientation questions regarding place and time are less sensitive in detecting concussion than recent memory questions. All the given components contribute to the team physician decision about return to play. Assessment of amnesia, loss of consciousness, and confusion are hallmarks for testing for concussion acutely, on the sidelines. Balance testing (force plate or BESS-balance error scorring system) have been shown to demonsrate postural deficits in stability up to 72 hours after concussion.

1. Whiteside JW. Management of head and neck injuries by the sideline physician. Am Fam Physician 2006 Oct 15;74(8):1357-1362.
2. Collins MW, Iverson GL, Lovell MR, McKeag DB, Norwig J, Maroon J. Onfield predictors of neuropsychological and symptom deficit following sports-related concussion. Clin J Sport Med 2003 Jul;13(4):222-229.
3. Reddy CC, Collins MW. Sports concussion: management and predictors of outcome. Curr Sports Med Rep 2009 Jan-Feb;8(1):10-15.
4. McCrory P, Meeuwisse W, Johnston K, Dvorak J, Aubry M, Molloy M, Cantu R. Consensus statement on cuncussion in sport—the 3rd International Conference on concussion in sport, held in Zurich, November 2008. J Clin Neurosci 2009 Jun;16(6):755-763.

96. The two types of bursitis that are associated with an infectious component and for which aspiration for culture and antibiotics should be considered as part of the management are the olecranon and which of the following?

    A. Trochanteric bursitis
    B. Prepatellar bursitis
    C. Subacromial bursitis
    D. Iliopsoas bursitis

Correct Answer: B

In a retrospective study of wrestlers with knee injuries, prepatellar bursitis had an infectious component in 2 out of 13 cases; the most common organism was staph aureus. In their experience, 50% of infectious prepatellar bursitis cases did not have any clinical evidence of infection. Therefore, the authors emphasized considering gram stain and culture of all prepatellar bursa aspirates. While there have been no similar studies regarding infectious etiology rates in trochanteric, subacromial, or iliopsoas bursits, it is not standard practice to send an aspirate for gram stain and culture in these conditions unless there are other clinical indications of infection.

1. Mysnyk MC, Wroble RR, Foster DT, Albright JP. Prepatellar bursitis in wrestlers. Am J Sports Med 1986 Jan-Feb;14(1):48-53.
2. Cardone DA, Tallia AF. Diagnostic and therapeutic injections of the hip and knee. Am Fam Physician 2003 May 15;67(10):2147-2152.
3. Cardone DA, Tallia AF. Diagnostic and therapeutic injections of the elbow region. Am Fam Physician 2002 Dec 1;66(11):2097-2100.

97. The most common activity associated with exercise-induced urticaria has been which of the following?

    A. Running
    B. Swimming
    C. Bicycling
    D. Weight lifting

Correct Answer: A

An episode may be precipitated by a variety of exercise activities at varying degrees of exertion. Most commonly, jogging and running have been described as the inciting activity.

1. Hosey RG, Carek PJ, Goo A. Exercise-induced anaphylaxis and urticaria. Am Fam Physician 2001 Oct 15;64(8):1367-1372.
2. Huynh PN. Exercise-induced anaphylaxis. Medscape. Accessed November 26, 2011 at http://emedicine.medscape.com/article/886641.

98. A nine-year-old overweight boy limps into your office with complaints of left knee pain for over three weeks. He does not participate in sports but plays computer strategy games for several hours a day. He denies any trauma to his knee, and his knee exam is normal. He has no fever or chills or night pain. Which of the following diagnostic tests do you order?

   A. Aspiration of knee joint for fluid analysis
   B. Erythrocyte sedimentation rate and CBC
   C. No further workup; tell his family that his knee is normal
   D. X-rays of his hips: AP and frog leg

Correct Answer: D

The most important tool in evaluating a child with the limp after the history is the exam. Look for gait changes. Evaluate range of motion; loss of internal and/or external rotation of the hip can be important. X-rays to look at the hip is the most appropriate diagnostic test at this point. Children who have knee pain may have problems with the knees or hips, so it is very important to examine both areas while present in the office. Lesions in the hips can often present as knee or anterior thigh pain. As this boy is limping, a more thorough exam is warranted beyond the general knee examination. Slipped capital femoral epiphysis and Legg-Calve-Perthes disease need to be ruled out by x-rays of the hips. Labs do not play a role at this time given no signs or history of infection or neoplasm.

1. Anderson SJ, Sullivan JA (eds). Care of the Young Athlete. Rosemont, IL: American Academy of Orthopaedic Surgeons and American Academy of Pediatrics, 2000.
2. Leet Al, Skaggs DL. Evaluation of the acutely limping child. Am Fam Physician 2000 Feb 15;61(4):1011-1018.

99. A college female lacrosse player comes to see you as she has been feeling tired more than usual the days after her games. Her history, physical, and lab work are otherwise unremarkable. She does tell you that she has been on a low carbohydrate diet to help lose weight. You tell her which of the following?

   A. Limiting her carbohydrates will help her fatigue and improve her physical and mental performance
   B. Her carbohydrate consumption should be 6 to 8 g/kg of body weight daily
   C. She should not eat after her games as this may upset her stomach and delay her recovery time
   D. Carbohydrates provide 9 calories per gram

Correct Answer: B

Achieving optimal carbohydrate nutrition is important to maintain the usual training intensity, to prevent hypoglycemia during exercise, to serve as fuel substrate for working muscles, and to assist in post-exercise recovery. Carbohydrate use increases with increased exercise intensity but decreases with increased exercise duration. The higher the initial glycogen stores, the longer an athlete can exercise at a given intensity level. The goal of carbohydrate feeding is to fill carbohydrate stores in the muscles and liver. Eating increases glycogen stores, whereas exercise depletes glycogen stores. Glycogen depletion can occur in sports requiring nearly maximal bursts of effort (such as lacrosse). Athletes may consume inadequate amounts of carbohydrate because of calorie restriction, avoidance of certain foods (e.g., sugar), fad diets, sporadic or infrequent meals, and poor nutrition knowledge of good carbohydrate sources versus marginal choices. Carbohydrates have 4 calories per gram.

The pre-exercise carbohydrate also elevates blood glucose levels to provide energy for the exercising muscles. Current guidelines recommend 1.8 g of carbohydrate per pound of body weight within three to four hours before exercise and 0.5 g per pound one hour before exercise.

   1. Sherman WM, Peden MC, Wright DA. Carbohydrate feeding one hour before exercise improves cycling performance. Am J Clin Nutr 1991 Nov;54(5):866-870.
   2. Jeukendrup AE. Carbohydrate intake during exercise and performance. Nutrition 2004 Jul-Aug;20(7-8):669-677.
   3. Shils ME, Skike M, Ross AC, Caballero B, Cousins RJ. Modern Nutrition in Health and Disease. 10th ed. Lippincott Williams & Wilkins, 2006.

100. Which of the following sports reports the highest incidence of incontinence during participation?

    A. Softball
    B. Gymnastics
    C. Golf
    D. Swimming

Correct Answer: B

Gymnasts report more than 67% incidence of incontinence while participating in the sport. Other sports with high incidences of incontinence include basketball at 66%, tennis at 50%, field hockey at 42%, and track at 29%. Swimming reported 10% incidence, while volleyball and softball reported incidences of 9% and 6%, respectively. Golf had no reports of incontinence in the study.

1. Nygaard IE, Thompson FL, Svengalis SL, Albright JP. Urinary incontinence in elite nulliparous athletes. Obstet Gynecol 1994 Aug;84(2):183-187.
2. Carls C. The prevalence of stress urinary incontinence in high school and college-age female athletes in the midwest: implications for education and prevention. Urol Nurs 2007 Feb;27(1):21-24, 39.

101. A 15-year-old high school basketball player is seeing you in the training room to look at her ankle. She suffered an inversion ankle injury two weeks ago that was confirmed on the game tape when reviewed by the athletic trainer. This is her fourth episode with this ankle in three years. The next-most recent sprain was three months ago. She says she was "nearly 100%" recovered from that episode when this one occurred. She also states that she is not progressing as well as she normally does when she "tweaks" this ankle. In particular, she states that there is no pain, but the ankle feels like it is giving out especially when jumping or cutting. Her anterior drawer and ankle inversion tests are definitely normal. The ankle hasn't been helped by the new active ankle brace the athletic trainer obtained to replace her old one that she has used since her last sprain. Current treatment has consisted of ice, rest, and gentle range of motion. Which of the following statements is true regarding her injury?

   A. Ankle instability should only be assessed with plain radiographs
   B. Aggressive early functional rehabilitation should be tried first
   C. The etiology of her recurrent injuries has to do with her age
   D. The primary ligament involved is the deltoid ligament
   E. Ankle instability cannot occur without increased mechanical laxity

Correct Answer: B

The history and physical exam clearly demonstrate functional instability. The history of giving way with jumping or cutting as well as the multiple injuries and incomplete recovery from the prior injury are key to understanding the functional instability. Mechanical instability was ruled out due to the clearly normal anterior drawer test. Answer A is incorrect because mechanical instability does not necessarily need evaluation with radiographs in the presence of a clearly normal exam. If you were going to perform radiographs, you would select stress views and not plain views. Ankle instability that is functional and not mechanical is best treated conservatively first with rehabilitation focusing on proprioception and strengthening, and is why Answer B is the best choice. Only after at least six weeks would one consider surgical repair. There is no clear evidence to support age as an etiological factor in ankle instability, so Answer C is incorrect. For Answer D to be correct, understanding that ankle instability primarily involves the ATFL and CFL is fundamental. And finally, Answer E is incorrect because mechanical laxity is not necessary for a person to have chronic ankle instability.

1. De Vries JS, Krips R, Sierevelt IN, Blankevoort L, Van Dijk CN. Interventions for treating chronic ankle instability. Cochrane Database Syst Rev 2011 Aug 10;(8):CD004124.
2. DiGiovanni BF, Partal G, Baumhauer JF. Acute ankle injury and chronic lateral instability in the athlete. Clin Sports Med 2004 Jan;23(1):1-19, v.
3. DiGiovanni CW, Brodsky A. Current concepts: lateral ankle instability. Foot Ankle Int 2006 Oct;27(10):854-866.

102. During pregnancy, which of the following components of the woman's respiratory system decreases during pregnancy?

    A. Tidal volume
    B. Vital capacity
    C. Minute ventilation
    D. Reserve volume

Correct Answer: D

Correct answer is D; reserve volume decreases during pregnancy. During pregnancy, both tidal volume and minute ventilation increase while reserve volumes decrease. As a result, the vital capacity remains unchanged. Physiologic changes in pregnancy affect the pulmonary function with a decrease in functional residual capacity (FRC) and 50% increase in minute ventilation.

1. Christian JS, Christian SS, Stamm CA, Mc Gregor JA. Pregnancy physiology and exercise. In: Ireland ML, Nattiv A (eds). The Female Athlete. Philadelphia: Saunders, 2002:186.
2. Gluck JC. The change of asthma course during pregnancy. Clin Rev Allergy Immunol 2004 Jun;26(3):171-180.
3. Camann WR, Ostheimer GW. Physiological adaptations during pregnancy. Int Anesthesiol Clin 1990 Winter;28(1):2-10.

103. A 45-year-old premenopausal African-American female comes into your office requesting a physical for initiation of an exercise program. She denies exertional symptoms of cough, headache, chest pain, reflux, dyspnea, near-syncope, or syncope. She is a non-smoker. Her BP is 124/84. Her BMI is 29.8. Physical exam is notable for lack of cardiovascular abnormalities or evidence of neurological injury. In regards to her exercise prescription, which of the following is the most appropriate initial step?

   A. Obtain an exercise stress test
   B. Obtain an electrocardiogram to rule out left ventricular hypertrophy or conduction abnormality
   C. Check for other major cardiovascular risk factors
   D. Rule out valvular disease with an echocardiogram
   E. Write a prescription using the FITT (frequency, intensity, time, and type) method

Correct Answer: C

The correct answer is to check for other major cardiovascular risk factors such as increased fasting glucose (for occult diabetes mellitus), increased plasma low-density lipoprotein (LDL) cholesterol, reduced high-density lipoprotein (HDL) cholesterol, and elevated triglycerides. Given her age and lack of hypertension or morbid obesity, the patient's cardiovascular disease risk is low and would not warrant exercise stress testing unless other risk factors were present. Electrocardiogram or echocardiograms are not indicated as screening methods in an otherwise asymptomatic individual with a normal clinical exam. The FITT (frequency, intensity, time, and type) method is an appropriate method to prescribe exercise once risk factors and need for exercise stress testing has been determined.

1. Fletcher GF, Balady GJ, Amsterdam EA, Chaitman B, Eckel R, Fleg J, et al. Exercise standards for testing and training: a statement for healthcare professionals from the American Heart Association. Circulation 2001 Oct 2;104(14):1694-1740.

104. Which of the following statements is true regarding the use of protective equipment?

    A. Requiring the use of protective equipment rarely changes the epidemiology of injury for a given sport
    B. Protective equipment may cause an increase in absolute numbers (e.g., injuries per 1,000 participants) of some injuries after adoption by a given sport
    C. Laws requiring use of protective equipment (e.g., bicycle helmet laws) have proven to be cost-effective, increasing protective equipment usage and decreasing sports-related injuries
    D. Athletes and coaches are usually eager to adopt the usage of protective equipment
    E. Health care providers should always campaign for the use of protective equipment

Correct Answer: B

The introduction of protective equipment usually changes the injury patterns of the sport. The decrease in certain injury types is usually the purpose of using a particular piece of protective equipment (e.g., drop in eye injuries with face mask use in hockey). However, often there is an absolute increase in other types of injuries as a consequence of the change in play style (e.g., use of helmets in hockey led to an increased incidence of cervical spine injuries and the use of wrist guards in in-line skating has caused an increase in proximal "splint-top" fractures). The use of laws requiring protective equipment for athletes has been controversial, and the effectiveness of such laws is still being debated. Professionals and elite athletes using protective equipment appears to be more effective than formal laws in the younger aged groups. Most athletes and coaches are initially resistant to the use of protective equipment, citing many concerns including cost, discomfort, and appearance. In summary, protective equipment can cause many changes in a sport, and these changes must be carefully weighed by sport-governing bodies and health care providers before requiring athletes to use them.

1. Robinson DL. Bicycle helmet legislation: can we reach a consensus? Accid Anal Prev 2007 Jan;39(1):86-93.
2. Daly PJ, Sim FH, Simonet WT. Ice hockey injuries. A review. Sports Med 1990 Aug;10(2):122-131.
3. Young CC, Seth A, Mark DH. In-line skating: Use of protective equipment, falling patterns, and injuries. Clin J Sports Med 1998 Apr;8(2):111-114.

105. A 16-year-old springboard diver complains of three weeks of lower back pain. The pain has progressed from activity-related pain now to pain at rest. X-rays of the lumbar spine are negative. You advise which of the following?

    A. Rest from diving and obtain CT scan
    B. Rest from diving and obtain MRI
    C. Continue diving
    D. Rest from diving

Correct Answer: A

Lower back pain in an athlete who competes in an extension-based sport (diving, gymnastics, and volleyball) is at high risk for spondylolysis. This condition is often not seen on x-rays. The next step is to rest the athlete from extension, and to obtain a CT scan to make a more definitive diagnosis to be able to give an accurate prognosis. MRI is not as accurate in terms of making this diagnosis and is not effective as a follow-up test to show healing. MRI is useful to rule out disc herniations, though. Continuing with diving would make the problem worse, and rest without a definitive diagnosis would not be helpful to the athlete. In this scenario, an athlete with hyperextension injury, often a SPECT scan can show subtle areas of involvement. SPECT scan has a false-positive rate of 15% when using CT scan.

1. Cassas K, Casseitari-Wayhs A. Childhood and adolescent sports-related overuse injuries. Am Fam Physician 2006 Mar 15;73(6):1014-1022.
2. Rothschild, BM. Lumbosacral spondylosis. Medscape. Accessed November 27, 2011 at http://emedicine.medscape.com/article/249036.

106. Which of the following statements about open and closed kinetic chain exercises is correct?

A. Open kinetic chain exercises occur when the distal aspect of the extremity is fixed and cannot move

B. Closed kinetic chain exercises typically involve functional weight-bearing and sport-specific activities

C. Knee extensions and straight leg raises are examples of closed kinetic chain exercises

D. During open kinetic chain exercises, motion occurs simultaneously at all joints comprising the kinetic chain

E. Closed kinetic chain exercises produce shearing forces, while open kinetic chain exercises produce compressive forces

Correct Answer: B

Open kinetic chain exercises involve free movement of the distal segment and are typically non-weight-bearing. Examples include knee extensions and straight leg raises. Conversely, closed kinetic chain exercises involve fixation of the distal aspect of the extremity, and they are important during functional weight-bearing activities (Answer B). Answer A is incorrect because the answer choice describes closed kinetic chain exercises. Answer C is incorrect because knee extensions and straight leg raises are examples of open kinetic chain exercises. Answer D is incorrect since simultaneous motion at all joints occurs during closed kinetic chain exercises. Answer E is incorrect because open chain exercises produce shearing forces, while closed chain exercises produce compressive forces.

1. McMahon PJ. Current Diagnosis and Treatment in Sports Medicine. New York: McGraw-Hill, 2007:272.
2. Fleming BC, Oksendahl H, Beynnon BD. Open- or closed-kinetic chain exercises after anterior cruciate ligament reconstruction? Exerc Sport Sci Rev 2005 Jul;33(3):134-140.

107. PIN syndrome involves a dysfunction of the posterior interosseus nerve branch of the radial nerve. A patient with PIN syndrome will report which of the following symptoms in the affected extremity?

    A. Altered sensation in the little and ring finger
    B. Decreased ability to make a fist
    C. Altered sensation of the dorsum of the wrist
    D. Decreased ability to extend the wrist

Correct Answer: D

The posterior interosseus nerve branch of the radial nerve has a pure motor function and allows wrist extension. In PIN syndrome, the patient will classically have intact sensation to the dorsum of the hand (a function of the radial nerve) but will have weakness or inability to extend the wrist. The ulnar nerve provides sensation to the little and ring finger. The median nerve contributes to the ability to make a fist.

1. Bencardino JT, Rosenberg ZS. Entrapment neuropathies of the shoulder and elbow in the athlete. Clin Sports Med 2006 Jul;25(3):465-487, vi-vii.
2. Regan WD, Morrey BF. Entrapment neuropathies about the elbow. In: DeLee JC, Drez D, Miller MD (eds). DeLee & Drez's Orthopaedic Sports Medicine. 3rd ed. Philadelphia: Saunders, 2003:1323-1334.

108. Which of the following biomechanical loading techniques, when done repetitively, is most effective in the treatment and management of patellar tendinopathy?

    A. Concentric
    B. Eccentric
    C. Isometric
    D. Isotonic

Correct Answer: B

Performing multiple repetitions of eccentric strengthening exercises has been shown to improve pain and functional scores in patients with patellar tendinopathy, thus eccentric is currently the loading technique of choice in the management of a patellar tendinopathy.

1. Visnes H, Bahr R. The evolution of eccentric training as treatment for patellar tendinopathy (jumper's knee): a critical review of exercise programmes. Br J Sports Med 2007 Apr;41(4):217-223.
2. Jonsson P, Alfredson H. Superior results with eccentric compared to concentric quadriceps training in patients with jumper's knee: a prospective randomised study. Br J Sports Med 2005 Nov;39(11):847-850.

109. You are performing a preparticipation exam on one of your patients who happens to be a student at the high school you cover. Which of the following items would require further evaluation?

    A. Mononucleosis three years ago
    B. Mildly enlarged liver
    C. Non-palpable spleen
    D. Small tattoo
    E. History of appendectomy

Correct Answer: B

Answers A, C, D, and E are frequently seen in the younger population. While noting the history of the appendectomy, no further workup is necessary. Remote history of mononucleosis that has resolved does not require reevaluation. Absence of splenomegaly is reassuring, and clearly does not need further inquiry. The small tattoo has no relevance to her suitability for athletics, unless it is somehow related to the enlarged liver or other medical problem. Answer B, the finding of any enlargement in the liver via exam, warrants further evaluation, including a history of tattoos, of course, and is the best answer.

1. Bernhardt D, Roberts W (eds). Preparticipation Physical Evaluation. 4th ed. McGraw-Hill, 2010:98-99.

110. When performing a preparticipation exam on a 14-year-old high school athlete trying out for football, a single testicle is detected. You must advise him and his mother about the implications of a single testicle and sports. Which of the following is correct?

    A. A protective cup eliminates the risk of loss of the testicle in contact collision sports
    B. Sperm banking is available and, while costly, is an option to preserve fertility if a single testicle is injured or lost later
    C. Athletes with an undescended testicle are managed the same as a player with a single testicle
    D. Due to the high risk in contact collision sports of losing a single testicle, the use of a cup is required

Correct Answer: B

Clearance is allowed with a single testicle for contact sports, but participation in sports becomes a secondary issue. Such clearance includes advising the athlete that risk of loss of the testicle is not eliminated and that if the athlete neglects the cup, then he increases the risk of loss. For an undescended testicle, an athlete must be informed of the increased risk of cancer in that testicle and referred to a consultant for evaluation. The incidence of injury or loss of a testicle is low in contact sports. But the athlete with a single testicle must be counseled on this risk and the implications of potential injury in contact sports. Athletic cup use is uncomfortable, frequently neglected by athletes, and not monitored closely.

1. Rice SG, American Academy of Pediatrics Council on Sports Medicine and Fitness. Medical conditions affecting sports participation. Pediatrics 2008 April;121(4):841-848.
2. McAleer IM, Kaplan GW, LoSasso BE. Renal and testis injuries in team sports. J Urol 2002 Oct;168:1805-1807.
3. Bernhardt D, Roberts W (eds). Preparticipation Physical Evaluation. 4th ed. McGraw-Hill, 2010:100.

111. A 40-year-old drummer presents with left wrist pain that developed one day after a four-hour concert. He has maximal tenderness 7 cm proximal to radial styloid with Finkelstein's test exacerbating pain at that location. There is also subtle swelling over the point of maximal tenderness. The most likely diagnosis is which of the following?

    A. De Quervain's tenosynovitis
    B. Carpal tunnel syndrome
    C. CMC arthritis
    D. Intersection syndrome
    E. Posterior interosseous nerve (PIN) entrapment

Correct Answer: D

Intersection syndrome can be easily confused with De Quervain's tenosynovitis. However, this question addresses the point of maximal tenderness that differentiates intersection syndrome from the other choices. Intersection syndrome is usually found to be 4 to 8 cm proximal to the radial styloid, the location where APL and EPB muscle bellies cross over the tendon sheath containing ECRL and ECRB. De Quervain's tenosynovitis has a point of maximal tenderness over the radial styloid and distal to it, as the APL and EPB pass together through the first dorsal compartment. Carpal tunnel syndrome and CMC arthritis also have distinct anatomical locations. PIN entrapment would not cause swelling.

1. Hanlon DP, Luellen JR. Intersection syndrome: a case report and review of the literature. J Emerg Med 1999 Nov-Dec;17(6):969-971.

112. Which of the following statements is true about herpes gladiatorum and herpes rubeiorum?

    A. Lesions are caused by herpes simplex virus type 2
    B. Return to play guidelines are lesions dry, crusted, covered, and antiviral treatment for 48 hours before competition
    C. No prodromal symptoms precede the painless clusters of small vesicles on an erythematous base
    D. Prophylaxis therapy in athletes with outbreaks in the past year is valacyclovir 500 mg twice daily

Correct Answer: D

Prophylaxis for athletes known to have had herpes gladiatorum within the past year is valacyclovir 500 mg twice daily. For athletes with a history of gladiatorum but no outbreaks in the past two years, valacyclovir 500 mg is effective prophylaxis. Skin lesions are caused by herpes simplex virus type 1. Infection may have a short prodrome before the outbreak of painful clusters of small vesicles on an erythematous base. Return to play guidelines are frequently revised but have moved toward treatment with antiviral medication for five days (120 hours) before competition along with all lesions being dry, crusted, and covered.

1. NCAA Sports Medicine Handbook. Accessed February 16, 2012 at http://fs.ncaa.org/Docs/health_safety/2011_12_Sports_Medicine_Handbook.pdf.
2. Bolin D. Dermatologic conditions in athletes. In: McKeag DB, Moeller JL (eds). ACSM's Primary Care Sports Medicine. 2nd ed. Philadelphia: Lippincott Williams & Wilkins, 2007:246.

113. You are seeing a 21-year-old football player in the athletic training room on Monday evening. He is complaining of a severe occipital headache with neck pain. He reports that he had a mild hyperextension injury in the game this past Saturday while making a tackle. His neck hurt for a brief instant and then it subsided, and he completed the game, as it was the fourth quarter. He denied loss of consciousness or other neurologic symptoms and reported nothing to the athletic trainer. His neck stiffness and headache started Sunday morning and have persisted. He has no migraine history. He takes no supplements, and his only medication has been Aleve for his headache. He denies fever, rash, cough, nausea, and photophobia. On examination, his range of motion is limited by pain with lateral flexion and rotation to the right, limiting his motion by 50%. He has a negative Spurling's test bilaterally. His neurological exam is grossly normal, but on further review he has a Horner's sign on the right. He is sent to the emergency room and cervical spine radiographs are normal. The most appropriate next step would be which of the following?

A. Lumbar puncture
B. Head CT
C. Neck CT
D. MRI of the brain
E. MRA of the neck

Correct Answer: E

Likely this scenario is that of vertebral artery dissection (VAD). The typical presentation of VAD is a young person with severe occipital headache and posterior nuchal pain following a recent, relatively minor, head or neck injury. The trauma is generally from a trivial mechanism but is associated with some degree of cervical distortion. Focal neurologic signs attributable to ischemia of the brain stem or cerebellum ultimately develop in 85% of patients; however, a latent period as long as three days between the onset of pain and the development of CNS sequelae is not uncommon. Delays of weeks and years also have been reported. Many patients only present at the onset of neurologic symptoms. Symptoms may include: ipsilateral facial dysesthesia (most common symptom), dysarthria or hoarseness (CN IX and X), contralateral loss of pain and temperature sensation in the trunk and limbs, ipsilateral loss of taste (nucleus and tractus solitarius), hiccups, vertigo, nausea and vomiting, diplopia or oscillopsia (image movement experienced with head motion), dysphagia (CN IX and X), disequilibrium, and unilateral hearing loss. The exam is often consistent with muscular strain with non-specific painful ROM. Other findings may include: limb or truncal ataxia, nystagmus, ipsilateral Horner syndrome in as many as one third of patients with VAD (i.e., impairment of descending sympathetic tract), ipsilateral hypogeusia or ageusia (i.e., diminished or absent sense of taste), ipsilateral impairment of fine touch and proprioception, contralateral impairment of pain and thermal sensation in the extremities (ie, spinothalamic tract), and lateral medullary syndrome. CT of the neck may be reasonable with a continuing suspicion for occult neck fracture, but less of a concern given the Horner's syndrome. Lumbar puncture may be considered to look for meningitis or signs of subarachnoid hemorrhage, but again those are less likely. Head CT and brain MRI are not indicated with the absence of any other cognitive deficits.

1. Lang ES. Vertebral artery dissection. Medscape. Accessed December 7, 2011 at http://emedicine.medscape.com/article/761451.

2. Karimi M, Razavi M, Fattal D. Rubral lateropulsion due to vertebral artery dissection in a patient with Klippel-Feil syndrome. Arch Neurol 2004 Apr;61(4):583-585.

114. A 21-year-old male golfer comes to you for his preparticipation physical exam. He denies having any previous cardiac symptoms or difficulty working out with his teammates. The only finding on exam is a systolic ejection murmur that increases with standing and lessens with laying down. Which of the following is not considered a major risk factor for sudden cardiac death in this athlete?

A. Sudden death in his younger brother
B. Nonsustained ventricular tachycardia during ambulatory ECG monitoring
C. Maximal wall thickness > 30 mm
D. Genotype assessment in genetic testing
E. Drop in systolic blood pressure > 15 mm HG from peak recorded to end of exercise on treadmill stress test

Correct Answer: D

This athlete has physical findings concerning for hypertrophic cardiomyopathy. In an asymptomatic patient with hypertrophic cardiomyopathy (HCM), many potential predictors of sudden death have been described. The most widely recognized major risk factors for sudden cardiac death (SCD) are: marked LVH (> 30 mm), resuscitation from sudden death, multiple sudden deaths in the kindred, non-sustained ventricular tachycardia, syncopal episodes especially with or after exercise, and either a drop in systolic blood pressure > 15 mm HG or an increase in systolic blood pressure < 25 mm Hg from peak recorded to end of exercise on treadmill stress test in those under 40 years of age. Some more recent studies looking at risk factors and predictive value summarized not very promising results. But the trend is to globally assess risk burden. For example, the ACC/ESC guidelines for prevention of SCD recommend ICD implantation in those with a history of sustained ventricular arrhythmia and in patients with one or more of the recommended risk factors. There is some indication that the degree of left outflow track obstruction may also play a part in predicting SCD.

While earlier studies demonstrated that genotype in genetic testing, especially the MYH7 and TNNT2 genes, may be predictive, later and larger studies demonstrated that HCM shows too much homogeneity to be helpful in a predictive role.

1. Christiaans I, van Engelen K, van Langen IM, Birnie EB, Bonsel GJ, Elliott PM, et al. Risk stratification for sudden cardiac death in hypertrophic cardiomyopathy: systematic review of clinical risk markers. Europace 2010 12(3):313-321.
2. Frenneaux MP. Assessing the risk of sudden cardiac death in a patient with hypertrophic cardiomyopathy. Heart 2004 May;90(5):570-575.
3. Beckerman J, Wang P, Hlatky M. Cardiovascular screening of athletes. Clin J Sport Med 2004 May;14(3):127-133.
4. Maron BJ. Sudden death in young athletes. N Engl J Med 2003 Sep 11;349(11):1064-1075.
5. Pelliccia A, Maron BJ, De Luca R, Di Paolo FM, Spataro A, Culasso F. Remodeling of left ventricular hypertrophy in elite athletes after long-term deconditioning. Circulation 2002 Feb;105(8):944-949.

115. Which of the following may reduce lower limb soft tissue injuries in runners?

   A. Stretching
   B. Long, gradual increase in training program for novice runners
   C. Patellofemoral (PFPS) type braces for anterior knee pain
   D. Running shoes fitted for foot type
   E. Not using insoles as opposed to using custom biomechanical insoles

Correct Answer: C

In a recent Cochrane review, 25 trials of over 30,000 participants were reviewed. The majority of the studies involved military recruits, but also three included runners from the general population—one from soccer referees and two were conducted in prisons. They looked at four interventions: exercises, modification of training regimen, use of orthoses, and footwear-socks. Trials looked at stretching the muscles of the lower leg on injury prevention. Other trials looked at various types of custom-made biomechanical orthoses and also knee braces for preventing (PFPS) anterior knee pain. Other interventions included modifying training schedule utilizing graduated running programs, utilizing the no more than 10% increase rule and also modified weight-loaded walking program compared to a running program. Lastly, use of prescribed running shoes for foot type and also double sock, padded polyester sock versus. standard issue sock in recruits.

Overall, the only studies reviewed that showed significant interventional reduction of lower leg soft tissue injuries in runners were: knee braces preventing PFPS anterior knee pain; and custom biomechanical orthoses did reduce shin splints (but not other soft tissue injuries in the lower extremities).

1. Yeung SS, Yeung EW, Gillespie LD. Interventions for preventing lower limb soft-tissue running injuries. Cochrane Database Syst Rev 2011 Jul 6;(7):CD001256.

116. A college football player jumps up to catch a high pass and is hit hard and tackled from behind. He plays several more downs before leaving the field, complaining of right flank and back pain. Which of the following is true regarding his probable injury?

    A. His injury has clearly identifiable signs and symptoms
    B. Renovascular hypertension is a frequent complication of this injury
    C. The degree of hematuria is indicative of the severity and extent of injury
    D. CT scan with contrast is the procedure of choice in identifying the full extent of urologic injury
    E. Athletes with solitary kidney are at high risk for kidney loss in contact sports

Correct Answer: D

CT scan with contrast is the procedure of choice in identifying the full extent of renal injury. Renal injuries do not have clearly identifiable signs and symptoms, though mechanism and location of pain may be helpful. Renovascular hypertension is a rare complication of this injury. The degree of hematuria is not indicative of the degree of injury. An athlete with shock and microscopic hematuria may likely have a more significant renal injury. Athletes with a solitary kidney are at a low risk of kidney loss in both contact and non-contact sports.

1. Schneider RE. Genitourinary system. In: Marx JA, Hockberger RS, Walls RM (eds). Rosen's Emergency Medicine Concepts and Clinical Practice. 6th ed. Philadelphia: Mosby-Elsevier, 2006:526-529.
2. Bernard JJ. Renal trauma: evaluation, management, and return to play. Curr Sports Med Rep 2009 Mar-Apr;8(2):98-103.

117. Pronation of the subtalar joint is an important part of the biomechanics of the walking and running gait. Which of the following accurately describes the component motions of pronation?

    A. Forefoot abduction, hindfoot inversion, and plantarflexion
    B. Forefoot adduction, hindfoot eversion, and plantarflexion
    C. Forefoot abduction, hindfoot eversion, and dorsiflexion
    D. Forefoot adduction, hindfoot inversion, and dorsiflexion
    E. Forefoot abduction, hindfoot inversion, and plantarflexion

Correct Answer: C

This is a definition. Pronation is defined as abduction of the forefoot, eversion of the hindfoot, and dorsiflexion. Supination is defined as adduction, inversion, and plantarflexion.

1. Brukner P, Khan K. Clinical Sports Medicine. 3rd ed. Sydney: McGraw-Hill, 2007.
2. Pronation of the foot. Wheeless' Textbook of Orthopaedics. Accessed December 7, 2011 at www.wheelessonline.com/ortho/supination_and_pronation_of_foot.

118. A 35-year-old male aerobics instructor is seen in your clinic because he has had several months of lower abdominal and groin pain. He reports that over the past two months the pain has increased, exacerbated by coughing or laughing. He reports no acute injury and no prior muscle strains. He stopped all physical activity for the past four weeks. An inguinal hernia is not appreciated on physical exam. Plain films, MRI, and bone scan do not show any bony anomalies. Which of the following would be considered the best initial treatment plan for this athlete?

A. Corticosteroid injection to the conjoined tendon sheath
B. Reassurance and rest
C. Non-weight-bearing and crutches for six weeks given patient may have occult stress fracture
D. Conservative treatment with a comprehensive rehabilitation program to improve core strengthening and posterior abdominal wall weakness

Correct Answer: D

Conservative treatment with a comprehensive rehabilitation program to improve core strengthening and posterior abdominal wall weakness is first-line treatment. This athlete most likely has a sports hernia, which is a disruption of the inguinal canal characterized by a torn external oblique aponeurosis, a torn conjoined tendon and a dehiscence between the torn conjoined tendon and inguinal ligament. A corticosteroid injection has not been shown to be an effective treatment for this problem. The patient has had symptoms for several months including four weeks of rest without any improvement; thus, Answer B is incorrect. Placing the patient on crutches is not indicated since his radiologic studies and clinical exam do not support a bony injury requiring him to be non-weight-bearing.

1. Morrelli V, Smith V. Groin injuries in athletes. Am Fam Physician 2001 Oct 15;64(8):1405-1414.
2. Housner, JA. Sports hernia. In: Puffer JC (ed). 20 Common Problems Sports Medicine. New York: McGraw-Hill, 2002:148-149.

119. A female cyclist presents to you for $\dot{V}O_2$max testing. She has heard that a high $\dot{V}O_2$max is predictive of aerobic fitness. You know that $\dot{V}O_2$max is determined by measuring pulmonary ventilation and the difference in directly measured fraction of oxygen in expired and inspired air: $\dot{V}O_2 = V_e (FiO_2 - FeO_2)$. The pulmonary ventilation is increased primarily during exercise by increases in the respiratory rate and increase in which of the following?

    A. Total lung capacity
    B. Residual volume
    C. Functional residual capacity
    D. Vital capacity
    E. Tidal volume

Correct Answer: E

The minute ventilation can increase 20 to 30 times over resting airflow values. The tidal volume increase five- to seven-fold, and oxygen consumption increases 20- to 25-fold over resting values. These are substantial changes that allow exercise to occur. Total lung capacity does not change with exercise. The functional residual capacity and residual volume are the area the amount of space available in the lung after a breath and a maximal breath and do not increase with exercise. Vital capacity is a fixed number that represents the maximum amount of air a person can expel from the lungs after first filling the lungs to its maximum extent.

1. Hopkins SR. The lung at maximal exercise: insights from comparative physiology. Clin Chest Med 2005 Sep;26(3):459-468, vi.
2. Dempsey JA, McKenzie DC, Haverkamp HC, Eldridge MW. Update in the understanding of respiratory limitations to exercise performance in fit, active adults. Chest 2008 Sep;134(3):613-622.
3. Lovering AT, Haverkamp HC, Eldridge MW. Responses and limitations of the respiratory system to exercise. Clin Chest Med 2005 Sep;26(3):439-457, vi.

120. A female cross country runner presents early in the season, complaining of heel pain. She states the pain has been present for two weeks. Initially, the pain only occurred with long runs, but now it hurts most of the time. On exam, pain is elicited by squeezing the heel. X-rays are initially unremarkable. Repeat x-rays obtained two weeks later, however, confirm the diagnosis. Which of the following statements about this condition is true?

     A. Surgical intervention is required
     B. Patient should be counseled that healing is expected to take 10 to 12 weeks and may end her season
     C. Patient is at increased risk of plantar fascia rupture
     D. Patient can expect to return to activity in four to six weeks
     E. Patient's body habitus is not a factor in this diagnosis

Correct Answer: D

Calcaneal stress fractures are not considered a high-risk injury. They typically heal four to six weeks after injury with activity modification, including crutches with weight-bearing as tolerated. Surgery is usually not required, and most patients improve prior to season's end. Patient has a positive squeeze test, suggesting bony rather than soft tissue pathology. Low weights, as often seen in cross country runners, can increase the risk of stress fractures.

1. Calcaneal stress fractures. Wheeless' Textbook of Orthopaedics. Accessed February 12, 2012 at www.wheelessonline.com/ortho/calcaneus_fatigue_fractures.
2. Aldridge T. Diagnosing heel pain in adults. Am Fam Physician 2004 Jul;70(2):332-338.
3. Calcaneal stress fracture. Accessed February 11, 2012 at www.learningradiology.com/archives2011/COW%20470-Stress%20Fx-Calcaneous/stressfxcorrect.htm.
4. Pfeffer GB. Plantar heel pain. Instr Course Lect 2001;50:521-531
5. Coris EE, Lombardo JA. Tarsal navicular stress fractures. Am Fam Physician 2003 Jan 1;67(1):85-90.

121. A 45-year-old construction worker presents to see you regarding right-sided neck pain. The pain began five days ago, and has not improved. He does describe regular physical labor at work most recently working in a small space, which has caused him to maintain some awkward positions. He has been unable to work since the injury. He has tried some Tylenol with little relief. He has rare radiating pain into the top of his shoulder on the right but otherwise no numbness or weakness. He had a minor MVA with neck pain five years ago, but that resolved in one week without any long-term issues. Exam reveals limited range of motion to flexion and lateral bending to the left, a negative neurologic exam and a Spurling's test which reproduces pain in right paraspinal area without radiation. He has some palpable muscle spasm along the right cervical paraspinal musculature. Which of the following is the best diagnostic/treatment option?

    A. Request plain x-rays including oblique views
    B. Place him in a cervical collar, and give him a note off of work for 14 days
    C. Prescribe ibuprofen 600 mg TID, which has been shown to be effective for acute neck pain
    D. Discuss the benefits of early mobilization, and refer to physical therapy

Correct Answer: D

This patient has findings consistent with a cervical strain. In uncomplicated neck pain without neurologic deficits, randomized control trials have demonstrated that active physical therapy reduces pain compared with passive treatment. There is insufficient evidence to suggest any medications—including NSAIDs, analgesics, or muscle relaxants—are of benefit. There is also no evidence to suggest that soft collars are of benefit. There is no role for x-ray in acute uncomplicated atraumatic neck pain.

1. Binder A. Neck pain. Clin Evid 2004 Jun;(11):1534-1550.
2. Hunter OK. Cervical sprain and strain. Medscape. Accessed December 10, 2011 at http://emedicine.medscape.com/article/306176.

122. The primary prophylactic medical treatment for prevention of acute mountain sickness is which of the following?

    A. Dexamethasone
    B. Calcium carbasalate
    C. Acetazolamide
    D. Scopolamine patch
    E. Nifedipine

Correct Answer: C

Acetatozolamide remains the mainstay in prophylactic medical treatment for prevention of acute mountain sickness. Calcium carbasalate and scopolamine have no place in the prevention of acute mountain sickness. Nifedipine is used in the treatment of high-altitude pulmonary edema. While dexamethasone may be used, rebound can occur if it is stopped at altitude prior to acclimatization.

1. Basnyat B, Gertsch JH, Holck PS, Johnson EW, Luks AM, Donham BP, et al. Acetazolamide 125 mg BD is not significantly different from 375 mg BD in the prevention of acute mountain sickness: the prophylactic acetazolamide dosage comparison for efficacy (PACE) trial. High Alt Med Biol 2006 Spring;7(1):17-27.
2. Altitude illness. Centers for Disease Control and Prevention. Accessed December 7, 2011 at wwwnc.cdc.gov/travel/yellowbook/2012/chapter-2-the-pre-travel-consultation/altitude-illness.htm.

123. At the finish line of the local marathon, a runner stops by your medical station, having completed the race and then stands to get his picture taken. He states he is lightheaded, and doesn't feel like he can walk to his car. You subsequently determine he has exercise-associated collapse (EAC), and in your management you remember that EAC is due to which of the following?

   A. Depletion of muscle glycogen, commonly known as "hitting the wall"
   B. Pooling of venous return in the lower extremities contributing to postural hypotension
   C. Altered cerebral circulatory autoregulation
   D. Common premature atrial contractions that reduce systemic filling pressure
   E. Reduced glomerular filtration rate (GFR)

Correct Answer: B

The treatment for a collapsed runner after the finish line begins with evaluation of the patient in the Trendelenburg position. After cessation of prolonged exercise, inactivation of the calf muscle pump produces lower extremity blood pooling, which ultimately leads decreased cardiac filling pressure and poor cerebral blood flow. By simply placing the patient in a position that aids venous return to the heart and providing oral rehydration, most of the collapsed runners will recover spontaneously. While depletion of muscle glycogen can affect performance, it doesn't result in EAC or syncope. Premature atrial contractions can result in decreased cardiac output and lightheadedness, but are not recognized as a cause of exercise-associated collapse. Cerebral autoregulation occurs with changes in systemic blood pressure, but has not been implicated in collapse of endurance athletes. Reduced GFR is a physiologic occurrence during endurance events, but not a cause of collapse.

   1. Jaworski, CA. Medical concerns of marathons. Curr Sports Med Rep 2005 Jun;4(3):137-143.
   2. Roberts, WO. Exercise-associated collapse care matrix in the marathon. Sports Med 2007;37(4-5):431-435.

124. Shoulder abductors can be paralyzed due to a lesion, affecting which of the following pairs of nerves?

    A. Axillary/musculocutaneous
    B. Thoracodorsal/upper subscapular
    C. Suprascapular/axillary
    D. Radial/lower subscapular
    E. Suprascapular/dorsal scapular

Correct Answer: C

The supraspinatus muscle originates from the anterosuperior part of the scapula above the spine and runs along the upper surface of the glenoid above the shoulder joint, where it becomes a tendon that inserts on the greater tuberosity lateral on the humeral head. It functions as a shoulder abductor. It is innervated by the suprascapular nerve. The deltoid muscle originates anterior from the lateral part of the clavicle and from the anterior, lateral, and posterior border of the acromion. It inserts on the lateral upper third of the humeral shaft and is an important and forceful abductor and flexor of the shoulder. It is innervated by the axillary nerve that comes from the quadrangular space posterior and runs on the undersurface of the muscle.

1. Suprascapular nerve entrapment. Wheeless' Textbook of Orthopaedics. Accessed December 7, 2011 at www.wheelessonline.com/ortho/suprascapular_nerve.
2. Axillary nerve entrapment. Wheeless' Textbook of Orthopaedics. Accessed December 7, 2011 at www.wheelessonline.com/ortho/axillary_nerve.

125. A 40-year-old female presents to your first-aid station during a 20-mile fundraising walk, complaining of confusion, lethargy, and dizziness. She says that she has been drinking water regularly and eating energy bars along the walk and has used the portable toilets at each scheduled rest stop. Which of the following is the most likely cause of her symptoms?

    A. Dehydration
    B. Hypoglycemia
    C. Hypokalemia
    D. Hyponatremia
    E. Hypernatremia

Correct Answer: D

This patient has symptoms of hyponatremia. Hyponatremia can occur during endurance events as a result of sodium loss through urination, respiration, and sweating coupled with inadequate sodium replacement. Her symptoms could also be caused by dehydration, but she gives a history of adequate fluid replacement and calorie supplementation. Hypokalemia (fatigue, cramping, nausea), hypoglycemia (trembling, clammy skin, hunger), and hypernatremia (restless, muscle weakness extreme thirst) do not present with these symptoms.

1. Cosca DD, Navazio F. Common problems in endurance athletes. Am Fam Physician 2007 July 15;76(2):237-244.
2. Shapiro SA, Ejaz AA, Osborne MD, Taylor WC. Moderate exercise induced hyponatremia. Clin J Sport Med 2006 Jan;16(1):72-73.

126. Which of the following findings should always be considered pathologic on a screening ECG of an asymptomatic athlete?

    A. First-degree A-V block
    B. Sinus bradycarida
    C. QTc of > 460 ms in a male
    D. Left ventricular hypertrophy
    E. Sinus arrhythmia

Correct Answer: C

Athletes can have many findings on their ECGs including sinus bradycardia, sinus arrythmia, first-degree A-V block, incomplete right bundle branch block, right or left ventricular hypertrophy, and some repolarization changes that may be physiologic variations due to conditioning. However, a prolonged QTc of greater than 460 ms should be considered pathologic and raise concern for long QT syndrome.

1. Corrado D, Pelliccia A, Bjørnstad HH, Vanhees L, Biffi A, Borjesson M, et al. Cardiovascular pre-participation screening of young competitive athletes for prevention of sudden death: proposal for a common European protocol. Consensus Statement of the Study Group of Sport Cardiology of the Working Group of Cardiac Rehabilitation and Exercise Physiology and the Working Group of Myocardial and Pericardial Diseases of the European Society of Cardiology. Eur Heart J 2005 Mar;26(5):516-524.

2. Wu J, Stork TL, Perron AD, Brady WJ. The athlete's electrocardiogram. Am J Emerg Med 2006 Jan;24(1):77-86.

127. You are at a high school football game, evaluating your starting running back. Earlier in the game, he was tackled from behind and ended up lying over the football at the bottom of a pile of tacklers. He is now complaining of abdominal pain and left shoulder pain. You are concerned about which of the following?

    A. Myocardial infarction
    B. Liver laceration
    C. Sickle cell crisis
    D. Shoulder dislocation
    E. Splenic injury

Correct Answer: E

Splenic injury is the most commonly injured abdominal organ from blunt abdominal trauma and the most frequent cause of death due to abdominal injury in sport. Splenic injury typically presents initially with sharp pain in the left upper abdomen, then becomes a dull, left-sided flank pain that may be accompanied by abdominal distention and Kehr's sign, which is left shoulder pain from free intraperitoneal blood irritation of the diaphragm, or Seagasser's sign, which is neck pain from phrenic nerve irritation.

1. Chang CJ, Graves DW. Athletic injuries of the thorax and abdomen. In: Mellion MB, Walsh WM, Madden C, Putukian M, Shelton GL (eds). Team Physician's Handbook. 3rd ed. Philadelphia: Hanley and Belfus, 2002:441-459.
2. Gannon EH, Howard T. Splenic injuries in athletes: a review. Curr Sports Med Rep 2010 Mar-Apr;9(2):111-114.

128. Which of the following statements is correct when referring to athletes with spinal cord injury?

   A. There is decreased incidence of overuse injuries above the spinal cord lesion
   B. Spinal-cord-injured patients have a normal ability to maintain body temperature in cold environments but not in hot environments
   C. There is a potential for reduced perception of exertion due to nociceptive input below the spinal cord lesion
   D. There is increased sweating below the spinal cord lesion
   E. There is normal bone mineral density in lower extremity

Correct Answer: C

Autonomic dysreflexia can be a life-threatening condition in spinal cord injured athletes. It occurs when nociceptive input below the level of the spinal cord lesion—say, from an ingrown toenail, kidney stones, constipation, or a blocked urinary catheter, causing bladder distention—results in inappropriate noradrenalin (norepinephrine) secretion. This may lead to hypertension, headache, sweating, skin blotching, and sometimes a reduced perception of exertion. This reduced perception of exertion has been used as an ergogenic effect by some spinal-cord-injured athletes and is termed "boosting." Since case reports have described hypertension from this condition as causing cerebral hemorrhage and death, autonomic dysreflexia is a medical emergency, and measures to remove the nociceptive stimulus and decrease the blood pressure must be urgently performed. Pre-competition blood pressure measurements may be helpful in preventing this condition. Overuse injuries of the shoulders are very common in wheelchair athletes.

The spinal-cord-injured athlete has difficulty regulating body temperature in both cold and warm environments. In cold environments, this is due to lack of sensory input and shivering response. In warm environments, this is due to reduced sweating below the lesion. Bone mineral density typically decreases below the level of injury due to disuse. The spinal-cord-injured athlete is, thus, at increased risk of fracture from minimal trauma or impact collisions in a wheelchair.

1. Webborn N. The disabled athlete. In: Brukner P, Khan K (eds). Clinical Sports Medicine. 3rd ed. New York: McGraw-Hill, 2006:780-781.
2. Klenck C, Gebke K. Practical management: common medical problems in disabled athletes. Clin J Sport Med 2007 Jan;17(1):55-60.

129. A 16-year-old African-American basketball player with hypertrophic cardiomyopathy and an implantable cardiac defibrillator (ICD) is cleared by cardiology to play. While providing medical coverage for a game where you have an automated external defibrillator (AED), this athlete collapses while running. You begin an assessment and find he is not breathing and has no pulse. You should do which of the following?

A. Wait to see if the ICD will fire
B. Place an AED on the chest to get a rhythm analysis, and shock if advised
C. Begin CPR and await EMS. An AED is contraindicated in a collapsed athlete with an ICD
D. Avoid doing CPR because the ICD may shock you

Correct Answer: B

Collapsed athletes with sudden cardiac arrest should be managed by standard BLS/ACLS protocols, whether they have an ICD or not. An ICD may not fire if a lead is fractured or the device malfunctions. The athlete, in this case, has hypertrophic cardiomyopathy, which is associated with ventricular arrhythmias, and he likely has a ventricular arrhythmia as the cause of his collapse. An AED can defibrillate ventricular arrhythmias and be life-saving. An AED can be used in an athlete with ICD but the external electrodes should not be placed directly over the ICD because of potential damage to the ICD. A person performing CPR can be shocked by an ICD, and it is recommended that they wear gloves. However, the amplitude of the shock is not enough to defibrillate the person doing CPR.

1. Stevenson WG, Chaitman BR, Ellenbogen KA, Epstein AE, Gross WL, Hayes DL, et al. Clinical assessment and management of patients with implantable cardioverter-defibrillators presenting to nonelectrophysiologists. Circulation 2004 Dec 21;110(25):3866-3869.

2. Drezner JA, Courson RW, Roberts WO, Mosesso VN, Link MS, Maron BJ. Inter-association task force recommendations on emergency preparedness and management of sudden cardiac arrest in high school and college athletic programs: a consensus statement. Clin J Sport Med 2007 Mar;17(2):87-103.

130. You are performing a preparticipation physical on a 15-year-old high school freshman, accompanied by his mother, who is trying out for the football team. During the history, you find the student had a brief syncopal event during conditioning drills one year ago. He says he got light-headed and passed out for a few seconds, but with some rest was able to continue the workout. You ask the mother about family history of syncope, and she tells you that there are several people in her extended family that pass out all the time, but it is "no big deal." You obtain an ECG on the student that shows a prolonged QTc interval. He wants to be able to participate in some form of athletic activity. Based on the findings of the ECG, which of the following sports (if any) would you clear him to play this year?

A. Basketball
B. Golf
C. Wrestling
D. Table tennis
E. He is not clear to participate in any organized sports

Correct Answer: B

The 36th Bethesda Conference Guidelines state: "Regardless of QTc or underlying genotype, all competitive sports, except those in class 1A category should be restricted in a patient who has previously experienced either: an out-of-hospital cardiac arrest, or a suspected LQTS-precipitated syncopal episode." Class 1A sports include: billiards, bowling, cricket, curling, golf, riflery. Basketball is a class 2C. Wrestling is class 3B. Table tennis is class 1B.

1. 36th Bethesda Conference. Eligibility recommendations for competitive athletes with cardiovascular abnormalities. Accessed December 8, 2011 at www.csmfoundation. org/36th_Bethesda_Conference_-_Eligibility_Recommendations_for_Athletes_with_Cardiac_Abnormalities.pdf.

131. Repetitive valgus extension overload to the medial epicondyle can lead to medial epicondylitis. Which of the following are involved in this injury?

    A. Origins of the pronator teres, palmaris longus, flexor carpi ulnaris
    B. Biceps brachii, flexor carpi ulnaris, pronator teres
    C. Origin of pronator teres, extensor carpi ulnaris
    D. Insertion of pronator teres and flexor carpi ulnaris

Correct Answer: A

Medial epicondylitis involves primarily the flexor-pronator muscles (i.e., pronator teres, flexor carpi radialis, palmaris longus) at their origin on the anterior medial epicondyle not the insertion (Answer D). Less often, medial epicondylitis affects the flexor carpi ulnaris and flexor digitorum superficialis but not the extensors (Answer C). The biceps brachii (Answer B) is not involved. Repetitive valgus overload stresses at the musculotendinous junction, and its origin at the epicondyle leads to tenosynovitis in its most acute form and to tendinosis in its more chronic form.

1. Wheeless CR. Medial epicondylitis. Wheeless' Textbook of Orthopaedics. Accessed December 8, 2011 at www.wheelessonline.com/ortho/medial_epicondylitis.
2. Gibbs SJ, Dauber KS. Medial epicondylitis. Medscape. Accessed December 8, 2011 at http://emedicine.medscape.com/article.
3. Hosey RG. Upper extremity problems. In: Puffer JC (ed). 20 Common Problems in Sports Medicine. New York: McGraw-Hill, 2002:58-59.

132. According to the *Preparticipation Physical Evaluation* (4th ed.), which of the following is a "yes, may participate" as opposed to a "qualified yes"?

    A. Kidney, absence of one
    B. Liver, enlarged
    C. Ovary, absence of one
    D. Spleen, enlarged
    E. Eye, loss of one

Correct Answer: C

The *Preparticipation Physical Evaluation* (4th ed.) states the risk of a severe injury to a remaining, solitary ovary is minimal, so the athlete may participate. The other conditions all require some continued assessment and may have limiting factors, depending on the participating sport.

1. Bernhardt D, Roberts W (eds). Preparticipation Physical Evaluation. 4th ed. McGraw-Hill, 2010:76.

133. Ankle dislocations at the tibiotalar joint mortise without fracture occur with motor vehicle accidents, falls, and sports injuries. The most common position at the time of dislocation is which of the following?

    A. Maximal dorsiflexion with an external rotation force
    B. Maximal plantar flexion with an external rotation force
    C. Maximal plantar flexion with an axial load and forced inversion
    D. Maximal dorsiflexion with an axial load and forced inversion
    E. Neutral position with a direct medial to lateral blow to the tibia

Correct Answer: C

Maximal plantar flexion with an axial load and forced inversion of the foot appears to place the ankle at risk of dislocation. The talus has a rhomboidal shape when viewed from the superior aspect, and the posterior aspect is narrower than the anterior aspect. Plantar flexion places the narrowest portion of the talus in the mortise—the most unstable position. An inversion force then causes ligamentous and capsular failure and the potential for ankle dislocation.

1. Tranovich M. Ankle dislocation without fracture. Phys Sportsmed 2003 May;31(5):42-44.

2. Keany JE. Ankle dislocation in emergency medicine. Medscape. Accessed December 10, 2011 at http://emedicine.medscape.com/article/823087.

134. A 15-year-old student-athlete presents prior to a high school track meet with symptoms of a viral upper respiratory illness accompanied by a temperature of 101 degrees Fahrenheit (38 degrees Celsius). Which of the following recommendations should you give to the athlete?

   A. If he has no respiratory compromise, he can participate in the meet
   B. Body effects of his elevated temperature are independent of the effect of environmental temperature
   C. Cardiac output and aerobic capacity are adversely affected in febrile athletes, and he should not participate
   D. There is no risk for orthostatic hypotension when exercising while febrile
   E. Fever has no effect on endurance or strength

Correct Answer: C

Effects of fever on exercise include decreases in strength, aerobic capacity, endurance, coordination, and concentration. The effects of fever are additive to those of ambient environmental temperature, causing additive decreases in cardiac output and aerobic capacity. In addition, dehydration magnifies the effects of fever and can precipitate an episode of heat illness. Finally, fever may accompany myocarditis or other severe illness that would make athletic participation dangerous.

1. Martin TJ. Infections in athletes. In: Mellion MB, Walsh MW, Madden C, Putukian M, Shelton GL (eds). Team Physician's Handbook. 3rd ed. Philadelphia: Hanley and Belfus, 2002:225.

135. Which of the following is not consistent with a diagnosis of complex regional pain syndrome?

    A. Focal increased activity on bone scan
    B. Diffuse increased activity with juxta-articular accentuation uptake on delayed images
    C. Pain out of proportion to physical findings
    D. Transient cyanosis and skin mottling in the affected limb

Correct Answer: A

Triple phase bone scan may be helpful particularly in the early phases (< 20 weeks) of CRPS. Increased uptake is seen in 60% of adult patients with CRPS; it is usually diffuse but can be seen on delayed images the best. Phases 1 and 2 were less specific and sensitive for CRPS. In these patients, with diffuse findings on bone scan, they predicted which responded best to steroid treatment. Focal increased activity is not consistent with CRPS. Marked pain out of proportion to the physical exam or history is common with CPRS. Intermittent skin color changes, felt to be sympathetically mediated, are also a common finding.

1. Singh MK. Physical medicine and rehabilitation for complex regional pain syndromes. Medscape. Accessed December 8, 2011 at http://emedicine.medscape.com/article/328054.
2. Hughes DE. Complex regional pain. In: Domino FJ (ed). The 5-Minute Clinical Consult. 20th ed. Philadelphia: Lippincott Williams & Wilkins, 2003:258-259
3. Harden RN, Bruehl S, Stanton-Hicks M, Wilson PR. Proposed criteria for complex regional pain syndrome. Pain Med 2007 May-Jun;8(4):326-331.

136. A 58-year-old female golfer presents with pain in the lumbar spine after a particular swing. She has point tenderness over L1 and limited range of motion. She does not have sensory or motor deficits on exam. A radiograph shows a compression fracture of L1 with approximately 50% loss of height. A CT scan should be ordered to rule out which of the following types of fracture?

    A. Compression fracture
    B. Middle column and burst fractures
    C. Spondylolysis
    D. Spondylolisthesis

Correct Answer: B

All patients with wedge fractures with more than 50% loss of height of the vertebral body should undergo CT scanning to rule out middle column and burst fractures. Up to 25% of fractures initially diagnosed as wedge fractures were found to be burst fractures on further imaging. A CT scan will allow for better visualization of a spondylolytic defect; however, in this patient, it is more important to rule out the middle column and burst fracture. Lateral flexion and extension studies, standing if possible, can be helpful to look for gross instability seen with spondylolisthesis.

1. Sherman AL. Lumbar compression fractures. Medscape. Accessed December 8, 2011 at http://emedicine.medscape.com/article/309615.

137. A 54-year-old male former football player presents to your office complaining of low back pain. He has a prior history of acute low back pain due to "a herniated disc" four years ago, which was successfully treated with a short course of oral corticosteroids, physical therapy, and a home exercise program. Your patient had been doing well until about six months before seeing you, when he began to experience a vague, poorly localized low back pain, radiating to both his thighs. He reports that these symptoms are constant although he has "good days and bad days." His symptoms do seem to be worse after prolonged sitting. Which of the following clinical features is most consistent with a correct diagnosis of lumbar spinal stenosis?

A. A positive Hoover's test
B. Low back pain worse with lumbar forward flexion than with lumbar extension
C. Low back pain alleviated when leaning over an object while standing
D. Leg and calf pain that recurs predictably after walking four city blocks
E. Low back pain worse with walking uphill than with walking downhill

Correct Answer: C

It has been estimated that complaints of low back pain make up over 12 million physician visits a year; about 4% of these patients will have spinal stenosis. Risk factors for lumbar spinal stenosis include a prior history of herniated nucleus pulposus, chronic low back pain, spinal surgery, and age greater than 55 years old. It has been estimated that 95% of patients with spinal stenosis have back pain, and 71% may complain of vague lower extremity complaints such as pain, burning, cramping, numbness, tingling, or fatigue. These complaints are often bilateral, and about 15% will localize these peripheral symptoms to the thighs only. Leg weakness occurs in about 33% of spinal stenosis patients. While 94% of patients will have neurogenic or pseudo-claudication, true claudication—with leg pain consistently and predictably occurring after a given walking distance, resolving with cessation of ambulation—is more consistent with peripheral vascular disease and is uncommon in cases of isolated lumbar spinal stenosis.

Overall, the patient may report that symptoms are exacerbated with lumbar extension and relieved by flexion-biased activities, such as sitting, lying supine, or assuming a simian posture (stooped over while standing with loss of lumbar lordosis; the so-called "shopping cart sign"). Ambulating up an incline is flexion-biased and would be better tolerated by a patient with lumbar spinal stenosis that ambulating down an incline, which is more extension-biased. The Hoover's test is one of a collection of examination maneuvers for distinguishing non-organic from organic causes of low back pain; a positive Hoover's test would not favor a diagnosis of lumbar spinal stenosis.

1. Amundsen T, Weber H, Lilleås F, Nordal HJ, Abdelnoor M, Magnaes B. Lumbar spinal stenosis. Clinical and radiologic features. Spine 1995;20:1178-1186.
2. Alvarez JA, Hardy RH Jr. Lumbar spine stenosis: a common cause of back and leg pain. Am Fam Physician 1998 Apr 15;57(8):1825-1834, 1839-1840.
3. North American Spine Society (NASS). Diagnosis and Treatment of Degenerative Lumbar Spinal Stenosis. Burr Ridge, IL: North American Spine Society (NASS), 2007.

138. An 18-year-old first semester college soccer player with type 1 diabetes mellitus uses an insulin pump to control her glucose. Since she plays a contact sport, she removes her pump prior to exercise. She notices that she is very high (300 finger stick glucose) after practice but acceptable (110) prior to practice. She monitors her glucose every 30 minutes in practice. In order to help her with this problem of elevated post-exercise glucose, you recommend which of the following?

A. She should increase her pre-exercise insulin rate by 50% for an hour prior to exercise
B. She should stop playing soccer and participate in a sport in which she can wear her pump at all times
C. She should increase her food intake prior to exercise
D. She should look for the onset of glucose increase and give herself 50% of basal rate bolus
E. She should avoid all sugar prior to and during exercise

Correct Answer: D

Normal response to exercise is a lowering of insulin levels in the body with increase catecholamine production. This is accomplished with the discontinuation of the pump. Eventually, with prolonged practices over one hour, the insulin levels will drop too low and the glucose levels will start to rise because of a relative low insulin state. Therefore, a 50% basal rate bolus is indicated. Pre-exercise rate increase will increase the chance of hypoglycemia, and the later low insulin state will still occur. Increasing food intake will not prevent the hyperglycemia. She should be able to play soccer safely and would not have to change sports with proper medical care. Avoiding all sugar prior to and during exercise will affect performance, deplete glycogen stores over time, and will not correct the low insulin state later in practice.

1. Macknight JM, Mistry DJ, Pastors JG, Holmes V, Rynders CA. The daily management of athletes with diabetes. Clin Sports Med 2009 Jul;28(3):479-495.
2. Chansky ME, Corbett JG, Cohen E. Hyperglycemic emergencies in athletes. Clin Sports Med 2009 Jul;28(3):469-478.
3. Lisle DK, Trojian TH. Managing the athlete with type 1 diabetes. Curr Sports Med Rep 2006 Apr;5(2):93-98.

139. You are admitting a 28-year-old male after being hit by a car while cycling. Among his other bumps and bruises, he has an unstable hip fracture. While the orthopedic surgeon is preparing for an open reduction internal fixation of the patient's hip, you want to start the patient on prophylaxis against deep venous thromboembolism and pulmonary embolism. Which of the following is the best regimen to begin along with intermittent pneumatic compression devices?

A. Unfractionated heparin daily
B. Low molecular weight heparin daily
C. 325 mg aspirin daily
D. Warfarin daily
E. No anti-coagulation is necessary

Correct Answer: B

Hip fracture patients are at a very high risk of venous thromboembolism and pulmonary embolism. The rate of fatal pulmonary embolism after hip fracture surgery is 2% to 7%, which is higher than hip or knee replacement. Patients are at risk because of advanced age, delayed surgery, positioning during surgery, decreased ambulation after surgery, intimal injury secondary to trauma and surgery, and possible hypercoagulability due to the release of tissue factors. Along with intermittent compression devices, medical therapy is recommended for prophylaxis. Unfractionated heparin twice daily and low molecular weight heparin daily have been found to be equivalent to each other and superior to aspirin. Also low molecular weight heparin has a lower risk of thrombocytopenia than unfractionated heparin. Low molecular weight heparin was found to be superior to warfarin and the monitoring of INR with warfarin was another possible drawback.

1. Geerts WH, Berrgvist D, Pineo GF, Heit JA, Samama CM, Lassen MR, et al. Prevention of venous thromboembolism: American College of Chest Physicians Evidence-Based Clinical Practice Guidelines (8th Edition). Chest 2008 Jun;133(6 Suppl):381S-453S.

140. If an athletic event is suspended or postponed due to lightning activity, it is important to establish criteria for resumption of activities. Which of the following is a reasonable guideline for when it is generally safe to resume activity?

A. If the sky is blue and there is no rain, it is fine to resume activities no matter how long it has been from the last lightning or thunder
B. Activity may be resumed when flash activity in the area is slowing down
C. Wait at least 30 minutes after the last lightning flash or sound of thunder
D. Wait until the storm is at least five miles from your location
E. Indoor pool activities may continue despite thunder and lightning activity outside the building

Correct Answer: C

This is a portion of the 30-30 rule. Waiting at least 30 minutes after the last lightning flash or sound of thunder is recommended. A typical thunderstorm moves at a rate of approximately 25 miles per hour. Experts believe that 30 minutes allow the thunderstorm to be about 10 to 12 miles from the area, minimizing the probability of a nearby—and, therefore, dangerous—lightning strike. Using this rule means the storm should be at least 10 miles away and using the flash-to-bang rule (30 seconds from lightning to associated thunder divided by 5 miles), the storm should be at least six miles away, so Answer D is not the right choice.

Blue sky in the local area or lack of rainfall are not adequate reasons to breach the 30-minute return-to-play rule. Lightning can strike far from where it is raining, even when the clouds begin to clear and show evidence of blue sky. This is often called a "bolt out of the blue." Researchers have found that the end of the storm is just as deadly as the middle of the storm. Following the 30-minute rule will help in the situation when the storm is slowing down. An indoor swimming pool can be a dangerous location during thunderstorms. The current can be propagated through plumbing and electric connections via the underwater lights and drains of most swimming pools.

1. Walsh KM, Bennett B, Cooper MA, Holle RL, Kithi R, Lopez RE. National Athletic Trainers' Association position statement: lightning safety for athletics and recreation. J Athl Train 2000 Oct;35(4):471-477.
2. NCAA guideline 1d: lightning safety. 2009-10 NCAA Sports Medicine Handbook. 20th ed. Indianapolis, IN: National Collegiate Athletic Association, July 2009:13-15.

141. Which phase of the throwing motion is characterized by hyper-external rotation of the shoulder, eccentric stresses on internal rotators and shoulder adductors, and leads to the subscapularis activating to begin internal rotation of the shoulder?

    A. Windup
    B. Early cocking
    C. Late cocking
    D. Acceleration
    E. Follow-through

Correct Answer: C

The biomechanics of the pitching windup are complex and describe the body's attempt to convert gravitational, chemical, and elastic potential energy to kinetic energy and impart it to a thrown object. During windup, the body rotates so that the hips and shoulders are perpendicular to the target and flexion of the lead hip raises the center of gravity. During this phase, the shoulder muscles are relatively inactive. During the early and late cocking motions, potential elastic energy is stored in order to be used during the acceleration phase. Late cocking involves terminal external rotation of the shoulder with eccentric stressing of internal rotators and mild stretching of the anterior capsule. Late cocking ends with the planting of the lead foot. Acceleration thus begins, and the subscapularis internally rotates the shoulder to begin propelling the ball forward. When the ball is released, deceleration and the follow-through dissipate leftover energy and results in the pitcher in a fielding position.

1. Kibler B. Upper limb biomechanics. In: Brukner P, Khan K (eds). Clinical Sports Medicine. 2nd ed. Sydney: McGraw-Hill, 2007:66.
2. Meister K. Injuries to the shoulder in the throwing athlete. Am J Sports Med. 2000;28:265-275.

142. A 16-year-old recreational snowboarder presents with a history of a fall on an outstretched hand, which occurred one day prior to presentation. He was seen in the emergency room and radiographs demonstrate a 1.5 mm displaced fracture at the proximal anatomic section of the scaphoid. On examination, he has mild swelling and scaphoid tenderness on the affected side. Which of the following is the most appropriate next step in management?

   A. Strict immobilization in a well-molded short arm thumb spica cast
   B. Strict immobilization in a well-molded long arm thumb spica cast
   C. Application of a short arm thumb spica splint and re-image in two weeks
   D. Referral for screw fixation by an orthopedic hand specialist
   E. Referral for MRI evaluation of the affected wrist

Correct Answer: D

Nondisplaced distal anatomic section fractures heal well with strict immobilization in a well-molded short arm thumb spica cast. Controversy exists over whether to use a long arm or a short arm cast. This patient presents with displacement of the proximal anatomic section of the scaphoid. Because the proximal portion of the scaphoid has poor blood supply, nonunion is an important complication of scaphoid fracture. There is no need to re-image since the fracture is evident on plain radiographs and exceeds 1 mm of displacement. Fractures with greater than 1 mm displacement are prone to nonunion, and operative treatment is recommended. Although a meta-analysis review in JBJS showed surgical treatment for nondisplaced or minimally displaced scaphoid fractures had better outcomes in measurements of patient satisfaction, grip strength, shorter time to union, and earlier return to work, there were no significant differences in outcomes between conservative and surgical fixation in terms of pain, rate of nonunion, infection, and total cost of treatment. But, the surgical group had more complications, such as osteoarthritis and complex regional pain syndrome, or required another surgery. As the fracture line moves proximally, there is a greater risk of displacement and nonunion; therefore, splinting and orthopedic consultation are indicated in this case. Magnetic resonance imaging and bone scintigraphy are accurate methods for detecting occult scaphoid fractures, but the fracture has already been identified with standard radiographs.

1. Phillips TG, Reibach AM, Slomiany WP. Diagnosis and management of scaphoid fractures. Am Fam Physician 2004 Sep 1;70(5):879-884.
2. Buijze GA, Doornberg JN, Ham JS, Ring D, Bhandari M, Poolman RW. Surgical compared with conservative treatment for acute nondisplaced or minimally displaced scaphoid fractures: a systemic review and meta-analysis of random controlled trials. J Bone Joint Surg Am 2010 Jun;92(6):1534-1544.
3. Fowler C, Sullivan B, Williams LA, McCarthy G, Savage R, Palmer A. A comparison of bone scintigraphy and MRI in the early diagnosis of the occult scaphoid wrist fracture. Skeletal Radiol 1998 Dec;27(12):683-687.

143. A female softball pitcher is hit in the left chest with a line drive. She is initially gasping for air due to the sudden impact but regains her breath and does not lose consciousness. On exam, she is noted to have tenderness, ecchymosis, and unilateral enlargement of the left breast. Which of the following studies is (are) always indicated in this situation?

    A. None needed if she has no further shortness of breath
    B. Mammogram
    C. Chest x-ray
    D. ECG
    E. Chest x-ray and ECG

Correct Answer: E

Chest contusions are common in softball, baseball, hockey, and basketball. They may cause resultant bleeding and swelling to the breast or chest. Ice, NSAIDs, and proper support and padding are usually adequate treatment. Occasionally, hematoma may require aspiration. Any chest contusion to the left side of the chest needs to be evaluated for commotio cordis or heart irregularities that are stimulated by the contusion with the heart. The athlete's shortness of breath should prompt an ECG immediately. A chest x-ray is used to rule out rib fractures with resulting hematoma as a cause of the shortness of breath and breast swelling. Mammograms are not indicated in this setting, and evaluation early in the acute phase may be difficult to differentiate between fat necrosis and fibrocystic changes from the injury and carcinoma.

1. Chang CJ, Graves DW. Athletic injuries of the thorax and abdomen. In: Mellion MB, Walsh MW, Madden C, Putukian M, Shelton GL (eds). Team Physician's Handbook. 3rd ed. Philadelphia: Hanley and Belfus, 2002:441-459.
2. Mancini MC. Blunt chest trauma. Medscape. Accessed December 8, 2011 at http://emedicine.medscape.com/article/428723.

144. Which of the following drugs would be an appropriate choice as initial first line medication for long-term asthma control in a patient with persistent asthma?

    A. Inhaled albuterol
    B. Inhaled salmeterol
    C. Oral theophylline
    D. Inhaled fluticasone
    E. Oral montelukast

Correct Answer: D

Current guidelines for the treatment of persistent asthma advise institution of an inhaled corticosteroid as first line therapy for long-term treatment. Fluticasone is the only inhaled steroid among the options listed. Albuterol, a short acting beta-agonist, though used for acute exacerbations is not an appropriate agent for long-term control of asthma. Salmeterol, a long acting beta-agonist, is not considered an appropriate choice for first line control of persistent asthma. Though used as a controller medication in the treatment of asthma, theophylline is not an appropriate first choice. Montelukast is not considered a first line agent for asthma control.

1. Pollart S, Elward KS. Overview of changes to asthma guidelines: diagnosis and screening. Am Fam Physician 2009 May 1;79(9):761-767.

145. Patients with fibromyalgia may benefit from exercise programs. Which of the following types of programs would help improve physical capacity the most?

    A. Aerobic exercise
    B. Strength training exercises
    C. Muscle lengthening exercises
    D. Flexibility training exercises
    E. Resistance training

Correct Answer: A

Several high-quality aerobic training studies reported significantly greater improvements in the exercise groups versus control groups in aerobic performance and improvements in pain. Aerobic exercise training has beneficial effects on physical capacity and FMS (fibromyalgia syndrome) symptoms. Strength training may also have benefits on some FMS symptoms. Further studies on muscle strengthening and flexibility are needed. Research on the long-term benefit of exercise for FMS is needed.

1. Busch AJ, Barber KA, Overend TJ, Peloso PM, Schachter CL. Exercise for treating fibromyalgia syndrome. Cochrane Database Syst Rev 2007 Oct 17;(4):CD003786.
2. Busch AJ, Schachter CL, Overend TJ, Peloso PM, Barber KA. Exercise for fibromyalgia: a systematic review. J Rheumatol 2008 Jun;35(6):1130-1144.
3. Busch AJ, Webber SC, Brachaniec M, Bidonde J, Bello-Haas VD, Danyliw AD, et al. Exercise therapy for fibromyalgia. Curr Pain Headache Rep 2011 Oct;15(5):358-367.

146. A high-mileage competitive runner presents with complaints of posterior lateral knee pain. His pain has gradually progressed from an occasional irritant to a persistent pain while running. He denies pain at rest and reports no history of trauma. His recent training history includes an increase in mileage and a significant increase in the amount of running on hilly terrain. You have previously diagnosed the patient as an overpronator. Examination demonstrates tenderness to palpation of the area just anterior and posterior to the lateral collateral ligament with the patient sitting in a cross-legged (figure-of-four) position. Which of the following is the most likely diagnosis?

   A. Medial meniscus tear
   B. Medial collateral ligament injury
   C. Popliteal cyst
   D. Posterior tibialis tendonopathy
   E. Popliteus tendonopathy

Correct Answer: E

The popliteus muscle has three origins, the strongest of which is from the lateral femoral condyle, just anterior and inferior to the LCL origin. A second origin is from the fibula, and the third from the posterior horn of the lateral meniscus. The femoral and fibular origins form the arms of an oblique Y-shaped ligament, the arcuate ligament.

The insertion site is the posterior surface of the tibia above the soleal or popliteal line. The popliteus tendon runs deep to LCL and passes through a hiatus in the coronary ligament to attach to the femur at a point anterior and distal to the femoral attachment of the LCL. The origin can best be examined by palpation with the patient in a cross-legged position. The popliteus tendon is responsible for medial tibial rotation and assistance in initiating knee flexion. Due to this action, it resists external rotation of the tibia that occurs in overpronators and in downhill running. The medial meniscus, medial collateral ligament, and the posterior tibialis tendon are located medially on the lower extremity. A popliteal cyst if palpated would be located much more posterior than described and does not correlate with the history given.

   1. Popliteus Tendon. Wheeless' Textbook of Orthopaedics. Accessed December 8, 2011 at www.wheelessonline.com/ortho/popliteus_muscle.

147. A 22-year-old male senior soccer player presents to your office with a two-year history of right hip pain. The pain is not present during activities of daily living but is becoming increasingly more painful and limiting with running, kicking, jumping, and cutting movements. He points to the area of pain as the right groin. There is occasional painful clicking but no low back pain or paresthesias. Exam shows pain deep to the anterior groin that is non-palpable but present with internal log roll and with flexion, adduction, and internal rotation motions. Hip flexion strength is good, and no pain is reported with manual testing. There is no pain with flexibility testing, and flexibility is good during the Thomas test. There is no palpable pain over the trochanter. Standard AP pelvis/cross-table lateral radiographs show a normal head-neck junction of the femur, no degenerative joint disease, but a large crossover sign (figure-of-eight sign). The most likely diagnosis for this patient is which of the following?

A. Hip flexor strain
B. Cam impingement
C. Pincer impingement
D. Trochanteric bursitis

Correct Answer: C

This athlete has the classic history for femoroacetabular impingement (FAI). There are two types of FAI with a third type being a combination of the first two or a mixed pattern. On standard radiographic examination, the anteroposterior (AP) radiograph shows the acetabulum. The normal acetabulum should cover the femoral head, with the anterior and posterior walls meeting at the lateral edge. In cases of acetabular retroversion, the anterior and posterior walls of the acetabulum cross over the femoral head, forming the crossover or figure-of-eight sign. This is called pincer impingement. The other form of impingement is called cam impingement. This is best visualized on the standard cross-table lateral x-ray. On the x-ray, the femoral head is aspherical with a reduced femoral head-neck offset or bump. This is not trochanteric bursitis as palpation is non-tender, and this should not cause deep pain into the groin but pain over the trochanter. This is not a hip flexor strain as it has been progressive over two years and on exam, the strength and flexibility of the hip flexors are good, and these tests are painless.

1. Beaulé PE, O'Neill M, Rakhra K. Acetabular labral tears. J Bone Joint Surg Am 2009 Mar 1;91(3):701-710.

2. Clohisy JC, Beaulé PE, O'Malley A, Safran MR, Schoenecker P. AOA symposium. Hip disease in the young adult: current concepts of etiology and surgical treatment. J Bone Joint Surg Am 2008 Oct;90(10):2267-2281.

3. Keogh MJ, Batt ME. A review of femoroacetabular impingement in athletes. Sports Med 2008;38(10):863-878.

148. A mother of a post-puberty female athlete wants to discuss Vitamin D with you. She is interested in the benefits and dangers of Vitamin D. You explain that Vitamin D does which of the following?

    A. With calcium supplementation, it has been shown to reduce stress fractures
    B. It can be toxic and should not be taken in doses higher than 1,000 IU per day
    C. It is rarely (< 5%) deficient in adolescent females in the United States of America
    D. Deficiency in Vitamin D has not been linked to increases in the risk of autoimmune diseases and nonskeletal chronic diseases like diabetes
    E. It is commonly found in foods that are eaten in United States of America and can replace lack of sun exposure

Correct Answer: A

A study of Navy recruits found that 2,000 mg calcium and 800 IU vitamin D per day supplementation had a 20% lower incidence of stress fractures than the control group. In a Finnish study, people with low Vitamin D 25 (OH) level had higher rate of stress fractures, Studies have shown that Vitamin D deficiency is a problem in adolescent females, with approximately 25% being deficient. Vitamin D toxicity does not occur with 1,000 IU per day. 50,000 IU orally weekly is often used to replace Vitamin D deficiency without toxicity. There is association between low Vitamin D levels and autoimmune diseases, diabetes, and non-skin cancers. Studies have shown that diet alone does not replace the Vitamin D levels.

1. Ruohola JP, Laaksi I, Ylikomi T, Haataja R, Mattila VM, Sahi T, et al. Association between serum 25(OH)D concentrations and bone stress fractures in Finnish young men. J Bone Miner Res 2006 Sep;21(9):1483-1488.
2. Stoffman N, Gordon CM. Vitamin D and adolescents: what do we know? Curr Opin Pediatr 2009 Aug;21(4):465-471.
3. Lappe J, Cullen D, Haynatzki G, Recker R, Ahlf R, Thompson K. Calcium and vitamin d supplementation decreases incidence of stress fractures in female navy recruits. J Bone Miner Res 2008 May;23(5):741-749.
4. Willis KS, Peterson NJ, Larson-Meyer DE. Should we be concerned about the vitamin D status of athletes? Int J Sport Nutr Exerc Metab 2008 Apr;18(2):204-224.

149. You are the team physician for the Paralympic wheelchair basketball team. One of the new players comes to you asking about "boosting" that he heard another team talking about. Which of the following describes a form of "boosting"?

    A. Wearing tight leg straps to increase sympathetic tone
    B. Taking 10 grams of carbohydrates every 30 minutes during exercise
    C. Emptying his bladder and bowels before each workout
    D. Using caffeine in excess to boost the metabolism

Correct Answer: A

Emptying the bowel and bladder refers to prevention of autonomic dysreflexia, a medical emergency. Autonomic dysreflexia is caused by increased sympathetic input from the splanchnic nerves, caused by noxious stimuli. The majority of cases are caused by a distended bladder (90%) or bowel (9%). Prevention includes bowel and bladder maintenance and skin care.

Wearing tight leg straps to induce autonomic dysreflexia (a practice known as "boosting") is illegal in Paralympics sports. The practice aids the spinal-cord-injured athlete to boost blood pressure and flow and, hence, performance—with the risk of intracranial hemorrhage and death. Carbohydrate intake is a recommendation for a type 1 diabetic. Caffeine is an ergogenic aid that may have some benefit in endurance sports, but has no relation to the practice of boosting in Paralympic sports.

1. Scuderi GR, McCann PD (eds). Sports Medicine: A Comprehensive Approach. 2nd ed. Philadelphia: Mosby, 2005:725-737.
2. Klenk C, Gebke K. Practice management: common medical problems in disabled athletes. Clin J Sport Med 2007 Jan;17(1):55-60.
3. Autonomic dysreflexia and boosting: lessons from an athlete survey. Bhambhani Y, Mactavish J, Warren S, Thompson WR, Webborn AN, Bressan E, et al. Accessed January 28, 2012 at www.paralympic.org/export/sites/default/Science_Education/Science/Conferences/Thompson_Autonomic_Dysreflexia_and_Boosting.pdf.

150. Which of the following symptoms or findings is most suggestive of ankylosing spondylitis in a patient with two-year history of back pain?

A. Prominent morning back stiffness
B. Presence of HLA-B27
C. Recurrent sciatic pain
D. Symmetric peripheral arthropathy
E. Presence of rheumatoid factor

Correct Answer: A

Morning back stiffness and night-time pain relieved by activity are the most suggestive findings of ankylosing spondylitis. Presence of HLA-B27 is nonspecific, and rheumatoid factor is generally negative in these patients. Peripheral arthritis does occur, but is most typically asymmetric. Recurrent sciatic pain would suggest other causes of back pain.

1. Kataria RK, Brent LH. Spondyloarthropathies. Am Fam Physician 2004 Jun 15;69(12):2853-2860.

151. Which of the following is an example of a modifiable internal risk factor for musculoskeletal injury?

A. A snow-covered natural grass field
B. An athlete's gender
C. An athlete's prior history of musculoskeletal injury
D. An athlete's joint range of motion

Correct Answer: D

There are two main categories of risk factors for musculoskeletal injury. They are internal and external. The internal risk factors are also known as intrinsic or athlete-related risk factors, whereas the external risk factors are also known as extrinsic or environmental risk factors. In addition, the risk factors can be divided into modifiable and non-modifiable. Examples of non-modifiable risk factors include the participant's age and gender. Examples of risk factors that are modifiable through physical training or behavioral approaches include strength, balance, and flexibility. In the choices given, a snow-covered natural grass field is an external risk factor; an athlete's gender and prior history of musculoskeletal injury are non-modifiable internal risk factor; and the athlete's joint range of motion is a modifiable internal risk factor—the correct answer.

1. Bahr R, Holme I. Risk factors for sports injuries—a methodological approach. Br J Sports Med 2003;37(5):384-392.

152. A 35-year-old high-level female marathoner presents to your office with complaint of four to six weeks of left heel pain. She reports that her pain started gradually while increasing her mileage in preparation to run the Boston Marathon. She notes that she recently started using new running shoes about six to eight weeks ago. Training includes both indoor and outdoor surfaces. She also notes in her history that she is a paralegal who wear high heels to work at least four days a week. She locates most of her pain to the posterior ankle and denies any subsequent numbness or tingling. She has increased pain with walking uphill or upstairs. On physical examination, there is soft tissue swelling of the distal portion and attachment of the Achilles tendon. There is severe tenderness to palpation of this swelling as well as pain with both plantar and dorsiflexion. The patient has significant pain with toe-raising. X-rays of the left ankle show a retrocalcaneal exostosis. Which of the following is the most appropriate diagnosis?

A. Posterior impingement-type syndrome
B. Sever's disease
C. Tarsal tunnel syndrome
D. Haglund's syndrome

Correct Answer: D

This high-level marathoner has developed both an Achilles tendonitis along with a retrocalcaneal bursitis from her continued running and poorly fitting shoes (i.e., high heels). Her x-ray findings are consistent with a Haglund's deformity (exostosis of the posterolateral calcaneus). Together, these findings make the diagnosis of Haglund's syndrome. Posterior impingement-type syndrome or os trigonum syndrome is associated with an accessory ossicle at the posterior talus. Usually seen in athletes who participate in sports that cause extreme plantar flexion with an axial load or distal load to the foot (e.g., female ballet dancers (en pointe), downhill runners, and soccer players). Sever's disease is an apophysitis of the posterior calcaneous and usually occurs in males, 8 to 13 years of age. Pain is usually bilateral and self-limiting. X-rays are usually not helpful in the diagnosis. With regards to tarsal tunnel syndrome, patients tend to have pain in the midfoot rather than the heel. Nocturnal symptoms are worse than those during the day and paresthesias/numbness usually accompany the pain.

1. Jayanthi N. Lower leg and ankle. In: Moeller JL, McKeag DB (eds). ACSM's Primary Care Sports Medicine. 2nd ed. Philadelphia: Lippincott Williams & Wilkins, 2007:499.
2. Haglund's deformity. Wheeless' Texbook of Orthopaedics. Accessed December 7, 2011 at www.wheelessonline.com/ortho/haglunds_deformity.

153. A college fullback is struck on the anteromedial knee. He has difficulty walking but is able to bear weight. He is unable to continue playing in the game, and you are asked to evaluate his knee in the training room after the game. The player reports that his knee is sore laterally, that he has mild swelling, and that he feels that his foot his weak. The most likely diagnosis is which of the following?

    A. Lateral collateral ligament injury
    B. Isolated popliteus strain
    C. Lateral meniscus injury
    D. Posterolateral corner injury
    E. Anterior cruciate ligament tear

Correct Answer: D

His symptoms are consistent with an injury to the posterolateral aspect of his knee. Given that the peroneal nerve is involved, it requires assessment of the posterolateral corner, which, if significantly disrupted, can require surgery. Testing can include (after isolated testing of ACL, PCL, LCL, MCL): dial test, reverse pivot shift, and external rotation test. 15% of posterolateral corner injuries are associated with injury to the peroneal nerve.

1. Examination for posterolateral rotary instability of the knee. Wheeless' Textbook of Orthopaedics. Accessed December 7, 2011 at www.wheelessonline.com/ortho/ examination_for_posterolateral_rotary_instability_of_the_knee.
2. Ho SSW. Lateral collateral knee injury. Medscape. Accessed December 7, 2011 at http:// emedicine.medscape.com/article/89819.

154. A 50-year-old left-hand-dominant female patient with a history of diabetes had an insidious onset of left shoulder pain that has been progressively worsening over three months. She can no longer comb her hair and wash her back with the left arm. She has no neck pain, paresthesias, or radiating pain. Pain is deep in her shoulder and worsens with any motion. There are no mechanical symptoms. Active and passive range of motion is limited in both flexion and external rotation. Plain films radiographs were normal. Which of the following is the next step?

   A. An MRI is needed with intra-articular gadolinium to evaluate for a labral tear
   B. This condition often will resolve on its own in the next few months
   C. Anti-inflammatory medications shorten the overall length of the symptoms by altering the pathophysiologic process
   D. This condition is much more common among diabetics
   E. Scapular strengthening should be the focus of rehabilitation for this problem

Correct Answer: D

This is a case of classic adhesive capsulitis. Adhesive capsulitis has an incidence of 3% to 5% in the general population, and up to 20% in diabetics. An MRI is not needed to make the diagnosis, as it is a clinical diagnosis once osteoarthritis has been ruled out by a standard XR. The patient will have loss of both active in particular passive ROM. When a patient has severely limited active and passive ROM, diagnosis of adhesive capsulitis should be considered (SORT C).

Adhesive capsulitis presentation is generally broken into three distinct stages. The first stage that is described is called the freezing or painful stage, Patients may not present during this stage because they think that eventually the pain will resolve if self-treated. As the symptoms progress, pain worsens and both active and passive ROM becomes more restricted, eventually resulting in the patient seeking medical consultation. This phase typically lasts between three and nine months and is characterized by an acute synovitis of the glenohumeral joint. Most patients will progress to the second stage, the frozen or transitional stage. During this stage, shoulder pain does not necessarily worsen. Because of pain at end ROM, use of the arm may be limited, causing muscular disuse. The frozen stage lasts anywhere from 4 to 12 months. The common capsular pattern of limitation has historically been described as diminishing motions with external shoulder rotation being the most limited, followed closely by shoulder flexion, and internal rotation. There eventually becomes a point in the frozen stage that pain does not occur at the end of ROM. The third stage begins when ROM begins to improve. This third stage is termed the thawing stage. This stage lasts anywhere from 12 to 42 months and is defined by a gradual return of shoulder mobility. Anti-inflammatory medications are used to relieve symptoms, but there is no evidence that inflammation is part of the pathophysiology of this condition, and there is no evidence that they alter the natural course of the disease process.

1. Burbank KM, Stevenson JH, Czarnecki GR, Dorfman J. Chronic shoulder pain: part I. Evaluation and diagnosis. Am Fam Physician 2008 Feb 15;77(4):453-460.

2. Burbank KM, Stevenson JH, Czarnecki GR, Dorfman J. Chronic shoulder pain: part II. Treatment. Am Fam Physician 2008 Feb 15;77(4):493-497.

3. Manske R, Prohaska D. Diagnosis and management of adhesive capsulitis. Curr Rev Musculoskeletal Med 2008 Dec;1(3-4):180-189.

155. Which of the following statements is true for epidemiology of collegiate women's soccer injuries?

   A. Rate of injury is higher in practices compared to games
   B. Concussion is the most common injury in both games and practices
   C. The majority of game injuries involve non-contact mechanisms
   D. The majority of practice injuries involve non-contact mechanisms
   E. ACL injury is the most common injury in both games and practices

Correct Answer: D

Women's soccer rate of injury is three times greater in games versus practices. Game injuries are more often related to player-to-player contact (54%), while practice injuries are most often noncontact (only 20% player-to-player contact injury). Ankle is the most common injury during games (18.3%) and is the second-most common during practice (15.3%), second only to upper leg muscle tendon strains (21.3%). ACL injuries and concussions are the second- and third-most common injuries (15.6% and 8.9%, respectively) seen in the game setting, and are less common still in practices (ACL 7.7%).

1. Dick R, Putukian M, Agel J, Evans TA, Marshall SW. Descriptive epidemiology of collegiate women's soccer injuries: National Collegiate Athletic Association Injury Surveillance System, 1988-1989 through 2002-2003. J Athl Train 2007 Apr-Jun;42(2):278-285.

156. A seven-year-old female soccer player presents to your office with pain in her left knee. The pain began during a soccer practice, and she was unable to walk after onset. On examination, she is acutely tender on the inferior aspect of her patella. She is unable to perform a straight-leg raise. Which of the following is the most likely diagnosis in this patient?

A. Traction apophysitis of the tibial tubercle (Osgood-Schlatter's disease)
B. Traction apophysitis of the distal patellar pole (Sindig-Larsen-Johansson disease)
C. Patellofemoral dysfunction
D. Patellar sleeve fracture
E. "Growing pains"

Correct Answer: D

A patellar sleeve fracture should be considered in children with open growth plates that present with acute onset of patellar pain during activity. The injury occurs due to excessive traction on the patellar apophysis and can be distinguished from Sindig-Larsen-Johansson disease by the inability of the patient to perform straight leg raising (due to disruption of the knee extensor mechanism). Because the process occurs mainly through cartilage, there may be little radiographic evidence of injury, so diagnosis is made on a clinical basis. Children with patellar sleeve fractures will require surgical repair by open reduction and internal fixation. In contrast, treatment of the more common traction apophysitis is conservative, with increased activity as tolerated. In addition, all of the other listed causes of knee pain in children tend to be more insidious in onset.

1. Chang D, Mandelbaum BR, Weiss JM. Special considerations in the pediatric and adolescent athlete. In: Frontera WR, Micheli LJ, Herring SA, Silver JK (eds). Clinical Sports Medicine: Medical Management and Rehabilitation. Philadelphia: Elsevier, 2006:82-83.
2. Pediatric patellar avulsion frx (sleeve fracture). Wheeless' Textbook of Orthopaedics. Accessed December 7, 2011 at www.wheelessonline.com/ortho/pediatric_patellar_avulsion_frx_sleeve_fracture.

157. A high school freshman with office-spirometry-confirmed exercise-induced asthma comes into the office, complaining of shortness of breath 10 minutes after she starts running in gym class. She feels as if she cannot get air into her lungs. She is using her albuterol inhaler 30 minutes prior to gym class. She uses the albuterol again when the shortness of breath starts, but has no response. Gym class is the only time that she gets short of breath. The shortness of breath started two weeks ago when she had an asthma attack in gym class after forgetting her albuterol inhaler that day. Which of the following is the appropriate treatment of the shortness of breath?

   A. Repeat the office spirometry testing with an exercise challenge; continue the albuterol as needed for shortness of breath and 30 minutes prior to gym class; reassess in one week

   B. Refer the patient to a pulmonologist for pulmonary function tests; add a long-acting bronchodilator and corticosteroid combination for better control of her asthma; continue the albuterol 30 minutes prior to gym class; reassess in one week

   C. Continue albuterol 30 minutes prior to gym class; teach the patient relaxation and slowed breathing techniques for when the attack happens; reassure her that her asthma is controlled with the albuterol; reassess in one week

   D. Repeat the office spirometry with an exercise challenge; add a long-acting broncholdilator, and continue albuterol 30 minutes prior to gym class and as needed for shortness of breath; reassess in one week

Correct Answer: C

The patient is suffering from vocal cord dysfunction after having suffered an asthma attack two weeks ago. She is worried that she will have another asthma attack. The treatment of vocal cord dysfunction involves breathing techniques and psychologic management as needed. In this patient, start with reassurance and breathing techniques and reassess to see if a referral to a speech pathologist or psychiatrist is needed. Answer A is not correct because it has not addressed the patient's new systems of vocal cord dysfunction. Answer B and D are not correct because the shortness of breath is not due to worsening asthma and the treatment has not addressed the vocal cord dysfunction.

1. Chiang WC, Goh A, Ho L, Tang JP, Chay OM. Paradoxical vocal cord dysfunction: when a wheeze is not asthma. Singapore Med J 2008 Apr;49(4):e110-112.
2. Reed TS, Gregore DR. Vocal cord dysfunction. Athl Ther Today 2007 Sep;12(5):38-39.

158. The sport with highest overall number of catastrophic cervical spine injuries is which of the following?

    A. Ice hockey
    B. Gymnastics
    C. Equestrian sports
    D. Football
    E. Snowboarding

Correct Answer: D

Sports injuries are the fourth-most common cause of spinal cord injury behind motor vehicle accidents, violence, and falls. Although football has a lower rate of catastrophic cervical spine injuries (per 100,000 players) than ice hockey or gymnastics, the large number of participants in the United States has resulted in football being associated with the largest overall number of catastrophic cervical spine injuries.

1. Banerjee R, Palumbo MA, Fadale PD. Catastrophic cervical spine injuries in the collision sport athlete, part 1: epidemiology, functional anatomy, and diagnosis. Am J Sports Med 2004 Jun;32(4):1077-1087.

159. Which of the following are correct about testicular torsion?

    A. Prehn's sign is a reliable way of distinguishing testicular torsion from epididymitis
    B. A painless swollen testicle is common as an early finding
    C. Cremasteric reflex is absent on affected side
    D. Radionuclide imaging is the imaging modality of choice

Correct Answer: C

Cremasteric reflex is absent on the affected side. Testicular torsion is a urological emergency. Ischemia leading to necrosis and permanent loss of a testis occurs if prompt diagnosis and treatment is not achieved. Ideally, surgery should occur in less than four to six hours after onset of symptoms. Evidence indicates cooling the scrotal contents may buy some time.

Testicular torsion has a bimodal peak: first year of life (extravaginal involves processus vaginalis, spermatic cord rotates above testes) and early puberty (intravaginal, occurs within the tunica vaginalis, where it attaches high on the spermatic cord, allowing the testes to dangle below the bell clapper deformity). Torsion can occur at any age with most cases occurring between 5 months and 41 years.

The hallmark is sudden testicular pain. The patient may also present with nonspecific abdominal pain, which can occur at rest or may be associated with nausea and vomiting. 41% may have had a prior episode which spontaneously resolved. The scrotal skin will become red and edematous with loss of the cremasteric reflex on the ipsilateral side. Prehn's sign (elevation of the scrotum relieving pain) is not reliable enough to exclude torsion, but it can represent epididymitis if present. The finding of urethral discharge or an abnormal CBC and urinalysis helps rule out torsion.

The study of choice is Doppler ultrasound due to improved specificity, availability and speed of getting results. The radionuclide imaging is effective; however, it should not be performed prior to urology consult as it may delay diagnosis.

Treatment of choice is urgent surgical detorsion to save the testis. Manual detorsion can be attempted if surgical consultation is not immediately available.

1. Rupp TJ. Testicular torsion in emergency medicine. Medscape. Accessed December 7, 2011 at http://emedicine.medscape.com/article/778086.
2. Burroughs KE, Hilts MJ. Renal and genitourinary problems. In: Mellion MB, Walsh MW, Madden C, Putukian M, Shelton GL (eds). Team Physician's Handbook. 3rd ed. Philadelphia: Hanley and Belfus, 2002:258-259.

160. If the lateral tubercle of the posterior talus ossifies separately, which of the following bones is formed?

 A. Fabella
 B. Os vesalianum
 C. Os trigonum
 D. Os calcis

Correct Answer: C

The fabella is a sesamoid bone in the lateral head of the gastrocnemius near the knee. The os vesalianum is an accessory bone located at the base of the fifth metatarsal in the peroneus brevis. The os calcis is another name for the calcaneus bone. The os trigonum is the accessory bone formed from the posterior talus if the lateral process does not fuse to the body. Typically, it unites between 8 and 11 years of age. If it does not unite, it will undergo fibrous or cartilaginous union. Conditions such as fracture or posterior ankle impingement arise when an individual repeatedly places the ankle in extreme plantar flexion, such as with dancing or kicking sports.

1. Foot and ankle. In: DeLee JC, Drez D, Miller MD (eds). DeLee & Drez's Orthopaedic Sports Medicine. 3rd ed. Philadelphia: Saunders, 2003:2019, 2031, 2168, 2213, 2615.
2. Accessory bones of the foot. Wheeless' Textbook of Orthopaedics. Accessed December 7, 2011 at www.wheelessonline.com/ortho/accessory_bones_of_the_foot.

161. The current American College of Sports Medicine (ACSM) and Centers for Disease Control and Prevention (CDC) guidelines for adult physical activity are which of the following?

     A. 20 minutes of physical activity at 80% to 90% of maximal heart rate most days of the week
     B. 30 minutes of low-intensity physical activity three days per week
     C. 30 minutes or more of moderate-intensity, physical activity on most if not all days of the week
     D. 20 to 50 minutes of vigorous-intensity physical activity on all days of the week

Correct Answer: C

It has been well established that increases in physical activity and cardiorespiratory fitness are associated with a reduced risk of death from coronary heart disease as well as all causes. In 1995, the CDC and the ACSM suggested that the focus of prevention should be broadened to include physical activity. The guidelines created state that every U.S. adult should accumulate 30 minutes of moderate-intensity physical activity on most, preferably all, days of the week.

1. Pate R, Pratt M, Blair SN, Haskell WL, Macera CA, Bouchard C, et al. Physical activity and public health. A recommendation from the Centers for Disease Control and Prevention and the American College of Sports Medicine. JAMA 1995 Feb 1;273(5):402-407.

162. You see a high school football player in the training room for an injury, which occurred yesterday morning. He says his dog bit him on the arm. On exam, there is a 4 cm long laceration. The wound is fairly deep but you see no injury to bone, muscle, or tendon. There is minimal erythema or swelling. He believes he had a tetanus shot within the last five years. The best initial management to prevent infection is which of the following?

    A. Suture the wound
    B. Use a cyanoacrylate tissue adhesive to close the wound
    C. Irrigate and debride
    D. Give a Td booster

Correct Answer: C

The best initial management of bite wounds or lacerations is to irrigate and debride with a minimum of 200 ml of normal saline. Wound closure can be considered for lacerations that have been open less than 12 hours, but not in this case since it has been a full day. Contraindications to laceration repair are wounds more than 12 hours old, animal bites (except on face), and puncture wounds. Tissue adhesives may be used to close certain lacerations but are also contraindicated for animal bites, puncture wounds, and contaminated wounds. A tetanus booster should also be considered if this patient has had less than three doses lifetime or the last dose was over five years ago. Antibiotic treatment with Augmentin® should also be considered for dog and cat bites to prevent infection of Pasteurella multocida, but does not replace irrigation as the best initial management.

1. Usatine RU, Coates WC. Laceration and incision repair. In: Pfenninger J, Fowler GC (eds). Pfenninger & Fowler's Procedures For Primary Care. 3rd ed. St. Louis, MO: Mosby, 2010:157-170.
2. Hollander JE, Singer AJ. Laceration management. Ann Emerg Med 1999 Sep;34(3):356-367.
3. Bruns TB, Worthington JM. Using tissue adhesive for wound repair: a practical guide to dermabond. Am Fam Physician 2000 Mar 1;61(5):1383-1388.

163. A collegiate gymnast has a chronic history of biceps femoris muscle strain in his left leg, which has precluded him from participating in three consecutive meets. He is concerned because the league meet is four weeks away, and he wants to be healthy for that event. Which of the following statements is true regarding the most effective timing for stretching?

    A. It is most effective during the warm-up phase of the exercise regimen
    B. It is most effective during the workout phase of the exercise regimen
    C. It is most effective during the cool-down phase of the exercise regimen
    D. Stretching is most effective between workouts

Correct Answer: C

The most effective stretching occurs while the muscle temperature is elevated and evolving through a cooling process. With systematic reviews of the literature, it has been shown that stretching before exercise does not prevent injuries. There are some studies lacking in quality that have suggested this, but these studies have not held up to more rigorous review. Furthermore, stretching prior to activity is different in terms of muscle properties (compliance, etc.) compared with stretching at other times. And, it is possible—better quality studies need to be done—that regular stretching not done pre-exercise may prevent injury.

1. Blanke D. Preseason conditioning. In: Mellion MB, Walsh MW, Madden C, Putukian M, Shelton GL (eds). Team Physician's Handbook. 3rd ed. Philadelphia: Hanley and Belfus, 2002:128.
2. Shrier I. Does stretching help prevent injuries. In: MacAuley D, Best TM (eds). Evidence-Based Medicine. 2nd ed. Malden, MA: Blackwell Publishing, 2007:36-68.

164. With regard to the Good Samaritan laws and being a team physician, one should understand which of the following?

    A. Good Samaritan laws exist throughout all 50 states and will protect the physician covering any event
    B. Good Samaritan laws apply only if receiving nominal financial compensation
    C. No matter what the Good Samaritan laws are in your area, it is best to clearly define responsibility and level of coverage in written form
    D. Compensation for event coverage is based on absolute dollar amounts
    E. Documentation of medical care is not required if the physician is acting solely as a Good Samaritan

Correct Answer: C

A team physician should execute a written contract or memorandum defining the physician's responsibilities and clarifying the level of coverage expected no matter what the Good Samaritan laws state. Most Good Samaritan laws apply only if a physician is receiving no compensation for the medical care provided, but in some states compensation may be considered as little as being given a shirt to wear while covering the event. Proper and thorough documentation of medical care should always be done.

1. Ranney CB, Beutler AI, Wilckens JH. The team physician. In: O'Connor FG, Sallis RE, Wilder RP, St. Pierre P (eds). Sports Medicine: Just the Facts. New York: McGraw-Hill, 2005:1-3.

165. You are consulted on a female track athlete with a known seizure disorder. Her favorite events are in the middle distances, and she has never had a seizure training or in competition. She has not had a seizure in three years and has not changed medications. The school is concerned about whether she should be allowed to compete due to her medical condition. Refraining from which of the following sports is most appropriate for this patient?

    A. Track
    B. Cycling
    C. Singles ice skating
    D. Football
    E. Gymnastic uneven parallel bars

Correct Answer: E

Answer A is not correct. There are no specific prohibitions. Aerobic activities such as track occasionally cause seizure exacerbations. However, on average, aerobic exercise decreases frequency. In the rare reports where seizures are triggered, patients readily identify the triggers. Medication can be adjusted for altered pharmacokinetics in aerobically conditioned athletes. Additionally, seizing during the activity (running) does not pose life-threatening scenarios for other competitors as in pistol shooting or automobile racing, and does not pose a life-threatening scenario for the athlete as in sky diving or SCUBA diving, where a seizure may put the patient at risk for death. Aerobically trained athletes do not have a lower seizure threshold during activity. Answers B and C are not correct. Cycling and ice skating can be encouraged since they are aerobic activities with same principles already stated. Answer D is incorrect. There is no epidemiological evidence that mild head injuries of up to 30 minutes of unconsciousness result in an increased risk of developing epilepsy. The occasional post-concussive convulsions are not true seizures. Answer E is correct. The prohibition for a patient with a seizure disorder would be from events such as uneven bars where a seizure could be life-threatening due to the nature of the activity. Other gymnastic activities would not be discouraged.

1. Fountain NB, May AC. Epilepsy and athletics. Clin Sports Med 2003 Jul;22(3):605-616, x-xi.
2. Matheson GO, Boyajian-ONeill LA, Cardone D, Dexter W, DiFiori J, Fields KB, et al. Preparticipation Physical Evaluation. 3rd ed. Minneapolis: McGraw-Hill, 2005:28-29, 74-75.

166. A 72-year-old physically active man presents to your clinic for a regular check-up. He enjoys golf, walking, light jogs, and tennis. He is generally healthy, he states "I want to stay that way," and he seeks your expertise about exercise in the older person. Your advice for him is which of the following?

A. Strength trained older athletes maintain muscle fiber type distribution similar to their younger counterparts
B. Maximum heart rate declines with age and aerobic training does not slow its decline
C. VO_2max declines with age, and aerobic training does not slow its decline
D. Masters athletes who already participate in high intensity training programs can maintain that intensity for at least a decade
E. Weight training in older athletes does not result in muscle hypertrophy

Correct Answer: A

Aging causes a decline in aerobic fitness, resting metabolism, muscle mass, insulin sensitivity, joint mobility, bone density, and sense of well-being. The elderly experience increased blood and body fat and elevated blood pressure. Exercise can improve these parameters. Aging decreases age-adjusted maximum heart rate due to longer relaxation phase in the cardiac cycle (decrease in sarcoplasmic reticulum calcium ATPase) and longer contraction time (shift to slower isoform of myosin). Training can slow the decline, but cannot increase the heart rate (Answer B is incorrect). Maximum aerobic capacity declines as well with age due to both the cardiovascular and musculoskeletal system. Along with maximum heart rate, stroke volume declines. Training can slow the decline of VO_2max (Answer C is incorrect), but a majority of masters athletes decrease the intensity of their exercise over time. It is difficult to assess the main reason. It could be due to age-related physiologic changes or a result of athletes modifying a longstanding activity program. But in either respect, it has been observed that most master athletes do not continue with high-intensity training program for more than 10 years (Answer D is incorrect). With aging, loss of both types I (slow twitch) and type II (fast twitch) muscle fibers occur. Older athletes preferentially choose activities that support type I activities. Training can build type II fibers in an elderly population in a similar fashion to younger athletes. Their muscles can hypertrophy with an increase size in both type I and II (Answer E is incorrect). Strength trained older athletes maintained fiber distribution pattern similar to a younger control group, whereas endurance runners and swimmers who were not strength trained appeared to have a relative loss of type II fibers (Answer A is correct).

1. Powell AP. Issues unique to the masters athlete. Curr Sports Med Rep 2005 Dec;4(6):335-340.
2. DeJong AA, Franklin BA. Prescribing exercise for the elderly: current research and recommendation. Curr Sports Med Rep 2004 Dec;3(6):337-343.

167. A 22-year-old vegetarian female runner presents with increasing fatigue over the past three to four months. She denies changes in her exercise routine, but has noted that her times have increased over that period and that her recovery times have increased as well. On examination, you notice pale conjunctivae. Her laboratory studies reveal a microcytic, hypochromic anemia. Which of the following is the most likely underlying etiology for her anemia?

   A. Foot strike hemolysis
   B. Vitamin B12 deficiency
   C. Folate deficiency
   D. Iron deficiency anemia
   E. G6PD deficiency

Correct Answer: D

This patient has classic historical and physical exam findings of anemia, and her laboratory findings confirm the diagnosis. By far, the most common of the microcytic, hypochromic anemias is iron deficiency anemia, and this patient has a number of reasons to have such a disorder. Iron deficiency anemia is commonly seen in menstruating females, especially those at risk for decreased iron in their diet, such as vegetarians. Although foot strike hemolysis can be present in distance runners (as well as in swimmers and rowers), it is more likely to tip a patient over the edge into symptomatic anemia, rather than serve as a primary cause of the anemia. This patient may also have dietary vitamin B12 or folate deficiency, but these are causes of macrocytic, rather than microcytic, anemia. G6PD deficiency can result in anemia, but such an anemia is generally a normochromic, normocytic anemia when present with normal iron stores.

   1. Harper JL. Iron deficiency anemia. Medscape. Accessed December 7, 2011 at http://emedicine.medscape.com/article/202333.
   2. Blood diseases, anemias: iron deficiency anemia. University of Maryland Medical Center. Accessed December 7, 2011 at www.umm.edu/blood/aneiron.htm.

168. An 18-year-old soccer player presents to the training room with left elbow and forearm pain, with swelling and obvious deformity. While running during practice, she was accidentally pushed by another player and sustained a FOOSH (fall on outstretched hand) injury. Her neurovascular exam is intact. Fluoroscopy in the training room reveals a fracture of the proximal third of the ulna with dislocation of the radial head. Which of the following is the correct diagnosis?

    A. Nightstick fracture
    B. Greenstick fracture
    C. Monteggia's fracture
    D. Galeazzi's fracture
    E. Rolando's fracture

Correct Answer: C

Monteggia's fractures are uncommon fractures and usually occur with a fall on an outstretched hand in forced pronation. It is very important to check neurovascular status in this injury, especially of the radial nerve, which wraps around the radial head before diving into the supinator muscle. It is important to obtain prompt reduction of the radial head. In adults, these fractures are usually managed on an elective basis with ORIF, whereas most often children are managed in a closed fashion. A nightstick fracture refers to a fracture of the ulnar shaft. Greenstick fracture refers to an incomplete, angulated fracture in children. Galeazzi's fracture is a fracture of the middle to distal third of the radius with subluxation of the distal ulna. Rolando's fracture is a Y-shaped, intra-articular fracture at the base of the first metacarpal.

1. Putigna F. Monteggia fracture. Medscape. Accessed December 7, 2011 at http://emedicine.medscape.com/article/1231438.
2. Monteggia fracture. Wheeless' Textbook of Orthopaedics. Accessed December 7, 2011 at www.wheelessonline.com/ortho/monteggias_fracture.
3. Magnes SA. Orthopedic sports medicine terminology. In: O'Connor FG, Sallis RE, Wilder RP, St. Pierre P (eds). Sports Medicine: Just the Facts. New York: McGraw-Hill, 2005:32-33.

169. A 22-year-old male football player suffers a hyperpronation injury of the right forearm and this results in a first-time dorsal-ulnar dislocation of the distal radioulnar joint (DRUJ). Radiographs rule out fracture and adequate closed reduction is achieved. How should this injury be managed?

    A. Thumb spica splint for two weeks
    B. Short arm cast for four weeks
    C. Long arm cast for six weeks
    D. Orthopedic referral for arthrodesis
    E. Ulnar gutter splint

Correct Answer: C

The long arm cast for six weeks is the correct management for a distal radioulnar joint dislocation without fracture. The thumb spica, gutter splint and short arm cast would not provide the correct immobilization of supination and pronation of the forearm that is necessary. Orthopedic referral for arthrodesis is incorrect, as this can be treated conservatively since there is no evidence of chronic instability, fracture, or complications. There is some evidence that percutaneous pin fixation may help maintain the reduction better, but not with arthrodesis.

1. Radial ulnar joint instability. Wheeless' Textbook of Orthopaedics. Accessed December 12, 2011 at www.wheelessonline.com/ortho/radial_ulnar_joint_instability.
2. Garrigues GE, Aldridge JM III. Acute irreducible distal radioulnar joint dislocation. A case report. J Bone Joint Surg Am 2007 Jul;89(7):1594-1597.
3. Ozer K, Luis R, Scheker LR. Distal radioulnar joint problems and treatment options. Orthopedics 2006 Jan;29(1):38-49.

170. A 36-year-old female athletic trainer comes in with a two-day history of severe low back pain. This started after she lifted a water cooler from the ground and felt a "pop" before a football game the previous day. She reports that the pain goes down to her buttocks and posterior thigh with any type of movement. The exam today is limited because of pain, although she is positive for straight leg raise, both sitting and supine. Plain films are negative. An MRI shows lumbar disc herniation. She wants to get back to working as soon as possible because of the upcoming games. Which of the following is the most appropriate next step to get her back to activity?

A. Epidural steroid/analgesic injection
B. Soft lumbar bracing and analgesics as needed, go back to regular activity
C. Bed rest as needed with early mobilization and NSAIDs/analgesics, reevaluate
D. Microsurgical discectomy
E. Traction therapy

Correct Answer: C

Initial management of lumbar disc herniation should include relative rest as needed, with encouragement to activity as tolerated, anti-inflammatory medications, and one can consider medications to relieve muscle spasm—often at night. Current evidence does not consistently support the use of injection therapy in the management of acute low back pain. Surgery is reserved when conservative measures fail, or a large fragment causes progressive loss. Traction has not been shown to be helpful in the management of acute back pain.

1. Dillin W, Eismont F, Kitchel S. Thoracolumbar injuries. In: DeLee JC, Drez D, Miller MD (eds). DeLee & Drez's Orthopaedic Sports Medicine. 3rd ed. Philadelphia: Saunders, 2003:714.
2. Perina GC. Mechanical back pain. Medscape. Accessed December 7, 2011 at http://emedicine.medscape.com/article/822462.
3. Knight CL, Deyo RA, Staiger TO, Wipf JE. Treatment of acute back pain. UpToDate. Accessed December 7, 2011 at www.uptodate.com.

171. Which of the following is a criterion for x-ray, according to the Ottawa Ankle Rules or Ottawa Foot Rules?

    A. Pain over the talus
    B. Positive anterior drawer sign
    C. Positive Talar tilt test
    D. Inability to bear weight for four steps either immediately or in the emergency room
    E. Pain over the shaft of the fifth metatarsal

Correct Answer: D

According to the Ottawa Ankle Rules, ankle x-rays are required only in the following circumstances: the presence of bone tenderness at the posterior edge of the distal 6 cm or tip of either maleolus. The patient is unable to weight-bear for at least four steps immediately after injury and at the time of evaluation. Foot x-rays are also indicated where: there is bone tenderness at the base of the fifth metatarsal or at the navicular. The patient is unable to weight-bear for at least four steps immediately after injury and at the time of evaluation. The Ottawa Ankle Rules have been found to have a sensitivity of almost 100%, but they are intended in cases where intoxication, head injuries, multiple trauma, or sensory deficits are present.

1. Steill IG, McKnight D, Greenberg GH, McDowell I, Nair RC, Wells GA, et al. Implementation of the Ottawa ankle rules. JAMA 1994 Mar;271(11):827-832.
2. Bachman LM, Kolb E, Koller MT, Steurer, Ter Riet G. Accuracy of Ottawa ankle rules to exclude fractures of the ankle and mid-foot: systematic review. BMJ 2003 Feb 22;326(7386):417.

172. A 16-year-old high school linebacker misses his tackle and receives a knee to the right side of his helmet. He loses consciousness for a few seconds but then is able to get up by himself and walk toward the sideline. He complains of a headache and blurry vision. After an initial medical evaluation onsite using standard emergency management principles, he sits on the bench for the rest of the first half. During halftime, he is reevaluated and states that he has no more symptoms and would like to return to play. Your sideline evaluation at that time does not show any significant neurological deficiencies. According to the recent consensus guidelines from the Zurich conference in 2008, what is the minimum time frame that has to pass before he can return to the game unrestricted?

    A. Seven days with return to game play on the eighth day if he remains asymptomatic
    B. Five days with return to game play on the sixth day if he remains asymptomatic
    C. Three days with return to game play on the fourth day if he remains asymptomatic
    D. The next day if he is still asymptomatic
    E. Second half if he is still asymptomatic

Correct Answer: B

According to the Zurich guidelines about safe return to play, a gradual return to physical activity is recommended. This is true in particular for youth/adolescent players. The following step-by-step program with a minimum duration of 24 hours per step is advised:

- Day 1: No activity
- Day 2: Light aerobic exercise
- Day 3: Sport-specific exercise
- Day 4: Non-contact training
- Day 5: Full contact practice
- Day 6: Return to play

If any post-concussion symptoms occur while in the stepwise program, then the patient should drop back to the previous asymptomatic level and try to progress again after a further 24-hour period of rest has passed.

1. McCrory P, Meeuwisse W, Johnston K, Dvorak J, Aubry M, Molloy M, et al. Consensus statement on concussion in Sport: the 3rd International Conference on Concussion in Sport held in Zurich, November 2008. J Athl Train 2009 Jul-Aug;44(4):434-448.

173. You are covering a college football game and are called to the field to evaluate a running back that has remained on the ground after a fumble recovery. A number of players had piled on him, and he is lying on his back, complaining of severe pain at the right sternoclavicular joint. You note exquisite tenderness at the joint and a non-palpable medial head of the clavicle. There is evidence of jugular venous congestion on that side, and he is noted to have stridorous respirations. You diagnose a posterior dislocation of the clavicle. The next-most appropriate step in management would be which of the following?

   A. Ice to the area and a sling for the right arm
   B. Figure-of-eight splint and relocation in the emergency room at the end of the game
   C. Transport by ambulance to the nearest emergency room with cervical spine immobilization
   D. Attempt emergent sideline reduction of the dislocation because of vascular and airway compromise

Correct Answer: D

Posterior dislocations of the clavicle at the sternoclavicular joint can be medical emergencies because of compression on the trachea and the great vessels at that location. Often, these injuries are caused by compression and rolling forward of the shoulder as can happen in a piling on injury during a football game. Closed reduction is the treatment of choice for this injury, and the presentation described makes this a medical emergency. Answers A and B are incorrect because the reduction needs to happen immediately and cannot wait for the end of the game. Answer C is incorrect because it also does not address the emergent airway and vascular compromise. Transportation by ambulance is not incorrect, but sideline attempt at reduction is the most appropriate first step in management. Reduction is accomplished by abduction of the shoulder and applying anterior traction to the clavicle with fingers or even a towel clamp if needed. If a towel clamp is used, appropriate sterile technique needs to be followed.

1. Roipal CE, Wirth MA, Da Silva Leitao IC, Rockwood CA. Section B injuries to the sternoclavicular joint in the adult and child. DeLee JC, Drez D, Miller MD (eds). DeLee & Drez's Orthopaedic Sports Medicine. 3rd ed. Philadelphia: Saunders, 2003:791-825.
2. Honig K, McMarty E. Shoulder injuries. In: Madden C, Putukian M, Young C, McCarty E (eds). Netter's Sports Medicine. Philadelphia: Saunders, 2010:355-356.

174. A 22-year-old track athlete presents to you for a follow-up visit after a grade 2 ankle sprain. Which of the following modules should be added to her rehabilitation in the intermediate stage, after she successfully had early rehabilitation measures?

   A. Range of motion exercises
   B. Isometric strength training
   C. Isotonic strength training
   D. Proprioceptive training

Correct Answer: D

Early functional rehabilitation of the ankle should include range-of-motion exercises and isometric and isotonic strength training exercises. In the intermediate stage of rehabilitation, a progression to proprioception training exercises should be incorporated. Advanced rehabilitation should focus on sport-specific activities to prepare the athlete for return to competition. Although it is important to individualize each rehabilitation program, this well-structured template for ankle rehabilitation can be adapted as needed.

1. Noehren BJ. Lower leg ankle and foot rehabilitation. In: Andrews JR, Harrelson GL, Wilk K (eds). Physical Rehabilitation of the Injured Athlete. 4th ed. Philadelphia: WB Saunders. 2012:Chapter 20.
2. Mattacola C, Dwyer M. Rehabilitation of the ankle after acute sprain or chronic instability. J Athl Train 2002 Dec;37(4):413-429.

175. A 16-year-old male patient presents for his preparticipation evaluation. He has no significant medical problems and a normal physical examination. Which of the following are currently recommended as part of his screen?

   A. Complete blood count
   B. Electrocardiogram
   C. Screening echocardiogram
   D. Urinalysis
   E. No additional testing is generally required

Correct Answer: E

There is no evidence that additional screening beyond a preparticipation history and physical examination will positively affect outcomes. Because of this, no additional testing is generally required in an asymptomatic normal patient with no significant family history.

1. Moeller JL, McKeag DB. Preparticipation screening. In: Moeller JL, McKeag DB (eds). ACSM's Primary Care Sports Medicine. 2nd ed. Philadelphia: Lippincott Williams & Wilkins, 2007:55.

176. A 35-year-old female long-distance runner who is training for a marathon by running 50 to 70 miles per week presents with a one-month history of right anterior hip and groin pain. The pain develops after two miles of running and is alleviated by stopping. Her exam demonstrates right anterior groin tenderness to palpation over the pubic ramus and pain with hopping on the affected leg. Which of the following statements is correct in regards to the diagnosis of a pubic ramus stress fracture?

A. Men are more susceptible to pubic rami stress fractures than women
B. A positive radionuclide bone scan definitively confirms the diagnosis of a pubic ramus stress fracture
C. A small avulsion fracture off the inferior pubic ramus is pathognomonic of a pubic ramus stress fracture
D. Pubic rami stress fractures are caused by the adductor and gracilus muscles pulling on the lateral aspect of the pubic ramus
E. "Flamingo view" plain radiographs are useful in the diagnosis of a pubic ramus stress fracture

Correct Answer: D

Pubic rami stress fractures are relatively rare, only 1.25% of all stress fractures. They are more commonly seen in military recruits and female runners. An increase in the incidence of pubic rami stress fractures corresponds to the increase in female participation in marathon running. Women are more susceptible to pubic rami stress fractures than men. The reason that women are more susceptible to pubic stress fractures is unknown, but may be related to the different anatomical configuration of the female pelvis or differences in gait. Although highly sensitive in the detection of stress fractures, radionuclide bone scintigraphy lacks specificity and provides poor anatomical detail. It has been reported to be falsely positive in as high as 32% of patients presenting with hip or groin pain. This is presumably due to high osteoblastic activity in the area because of high stress loads and constant remodeling. Periosteitis, adductor tendonitis, and avulsion fractures are other causes of a positive bones scan. An MRI has both sensitivity and specificity for detecting pubic rami stress fractures as well as those arising from the femoral neck, acetabulum and sacrum.

A fatigue fracture of traumatic etiology, involving the bony attachment of the gracilis muscle to the pubic ramus, is termed the gracilis syndrome. This results in an avulsion fracture of the tendinous insertion of the gracilis muscle at the anterior edge of the inferior pubic ramus. Pubic rami stress fractures differ from other sites as being caused by a response to tensile forces rather than compressive forces. The tensile forces are produced by muscular forces of the adductor and gracilis muscles pulling on the lateral aspect of the pubic ramus and ischium during hip extension. Radiographic evaluation with plain films has shown limited usefulness in the diagnosis of pelvic and femoral neck stress fractures. Bony changes typically lag behind onset of symptoms by two to four weeks and 50% of patients who have stress fractures never exhibit changes on plain films. "Flamingo view" plain films are useful in diagnosing osteitis pubis. These views are performed anteroposteriorly with alternating unilateral lower extremity weight bearing. Instability of the pubic symphysis, which is characteristic of osteitis pubis, is suggested when the symphysis is widened more than 7 mm or when the top surfaces of the superior pubic rami move more than 2 mm.

1. Morelli V, Espinoza L. Groin injuries and groin pain in athletes: part 2. Prim Care 2005 Mar;32(1):185-200.
2. Thorne DA, Datz FL. Pelvic stress fractures in female runners. Clin Nucl Med 1986 Dec;11(12):828-829.
3. Nelson EN, Kassarjian A, Palmer WE. MR imaging of sports-related groin pain. Magn Reson Imaging Clin N Am 2005 Nov;13(4):727-742.
4. Wiley JJ. Traumatic osteitis pubis: the gracilis syndrome. Am J Sports Med 1983;(5):360-363.

177. You are approached by parents of one of your patients, a 17-year-old male with Down syndrome. They are interested in exploring the possibility of his participation in Special Olympics sporting activities. Which of the following are important considerations regarding Special Olympics participation?

    A. There are no special considerations for his participation, and he can be cleared after a routine preparticipation evaluation
    B. Because of the increased incidence of atlantoaxial instability in Down syndrome patients, he should have cervical spine radiographs prior to participating in sports activities
    C. Epidemiologic studies have shown increased incidence of injury in Down syndrome patients who participate in winter sports
    D. Eye problems are an unusual finding among Special Olympics participants
    E. Although there is an increased incidence of seizures among Special Olympics participants, no special precautions are taken around water sports venues

Correct Answer: B

The Special Olympics movement has become one of the largest participation events worldwide for special populations athletes. Because of open inclusion and stratification of participation by age, sex, and ability, many young people with mental retardation are able to compete in a meaningful way in a wide variety of sports at the regional, national, and international levels. Among the largest groups of individual participating in Special Olympics activities are those with Down syndrome, consisting of 14% of Special Olympics participants. Along with cardiac anomalies, gastrointestinal defects, and increased joint laxity, individuals with Down syndrome have an increased incidence of atlantoaxial instability, which places them at increased risk for catastrophic injury when participating in sports requiring hyperextension or flexion of the neck or direct pressure on the head and spine. Therefore, all Down syndrome patients should have a screening cervical radiograph prior to participation. If the screening radiograph is abnormal, they should be referred for neurosurgical evaluation. Before participating in Special Olympics activities, athletes are required to complete a careful and thorough history and physical examination. In a recent epidemiologic analysis, Down syndrome patients were no more likely than other athletes to suffer injury when participating in winter sports. Eye problems, including cataracts, are the most common findings on physical examination of Special Olympics athletes. Finally, seizures around water venues are considered to be among the most serious problems at Special Olympics events, and extra seizure precautions are taken at those sites.

1. McCormick DP. Medical coverage for Special Olympics games. In: Mellion MB, Walsh MW, Madden C, Putukian M, Shelton GL (eds). Team Physician's Handbook. 3rd ed. Philadephia: Hanley and Belfus, 2002:108-111.

178. With respect to the normal gait cycle, which of the following statements is true?

    A. There is one step in each gait cycle
    B. The faster the walking speed, the more time one will have in the swing phase
    C. The stance to swing ratio is stable when moving from walking to running
    D. The gait cycle has one double-support phase
    E. Cadence is the number of steps over distance

Correct Answer: B

A step is defined as the time measured from an event in one foot to the same event in the opposite foot (usually initial contact of one foot to the initial contact of the other foot). A gait cycle is defined as an entire sequence of functions by one limb (usually initial contact to initial contact). You need two steps to complete an entire sequence; therefore, there are two steps per gait cycle. A gait cycle is sometimes known as a stride.

Cadence is the stride of step frequency (steps/minute). For Answer C, the statement should read "...reverses when moving from walking to running." This is really is a reflection of the distribution stance: swing phase when walking is 60:40, and decreases as one increases speed. Running generally consumes 66% of the cycle in swing phase. The faster one walks, the less time one is in stance and the more time one is in the swing phase so that the ratio essentially reverses when running. For Answer D, the gait cycle has two double-support phases. This occurs when both feet are simultaneously on the ground and is the transfer of weight from one side to the other.

1. Braddom RL, Buschbacher RM, Chan L. Physical Medicine and Rehabilitation. 3rd ed. Philadelphia: Elsevier Saunders, 2006:94-95.
2. Kerrigan DC, Della Croce U. Gait analysis. In: O'Connor FG, Sallis RE, Wilder RP, St. Pierre P (eds). Sports Medicine: Just the Facts. New York: McGraw-Hill, 2005:126.

179. Injection for a carpal tunnel syndrome is best done in which manner?

    A. At a site just ulnar to the palmaris longus tendon and at the proximal wrist crease

    B. At a site just radial to the palmaris longus tendon and at the proximal wrist crease

    C. Volar side of the forearm 4 cm proximal to the wrist crease between the tendons of the flexor carpi radialis and flexor carpi ulnaris

    D. Volar side of the forearm 4 cm proximal to the wrist crease between the tendon of the flexor carpi ulnaris and the palmaris longus tendon

Correct Answer: A

The injection is performed at a site just ulnar to the palmaris longus tendon and at the proximal wrist crease. For those few patients without a palmaris longus tendon, the needle is inserted just ulnar to the midline of the wrist. The needle is inserted at a 30-degree angle and directed toward the ring finger. If the needle meets obstruction or if the patient experiences paresthesias, the needle should be withdrawn and redirected in a more ulnar fashion. Another injection site is at the volar side of the forearm, 4 cm proximal to the wrist crease between the tendons of the radial flexor muscle and the palmaris longus muscle. In this approach, the angle of insertion is between 10 and 20 degrees, depending on the thickness of the wrist. As with any injection, aspirate to ensure that the needle has not been placed in a blood vessel. Inject slowly, but with consistent pressure.

1. Tallia AF, Cardone DA. Diagnostic and therapeutic injection of the wrist and hand region. Am Fam Physician 2003 Feb 15;67(4):745-750.

180. Children are a population at risk for heat-related injuries because of which of the following?

    A. Children sweat more and thus are at increased risk for dehydration
    B. Children have a lower surface area to body mass ratio and consequently they dissipate heat less efficiently
    C. Children produce higher temperature elevations because they tend to generate more heat secondarily to higher percentage of adipose tissue
    D. Children have higher surface area to body mass ratio, which may cause higher absorption from ambient environment

Correct Answer: D

Children have higher surface volume to body mass ratios, which generally works to their benefit, when the temperatures and humidity are high, children absorb relatively more heat from the environment. Generally, higher surface area to body mass ratio allows for heat dissipation. Children sweat less, require greater core temperature increases to trigger sweating, acclimatize more slowly, and produce more metabolic heat per mass unit than adults. Children also may lack adequate blood flow for both muscles and cooling needs because cardiac output at a given metabolic rate is lower.

1. American Academy of Pediatrics Committee on Sports Medicine and Fitness. Climatic heat stress and the exercising child and adolescent. Pediatrics 2000 Jul;106(1 Pt 1):158-159.

181. The recurrence rate after a primary, traumatic glenohumeral dislocation in an athlete less than 20 years old with non-surgical management is which of the following?

    A. 10%
    B. Less than 30%
    C. 50%
    D. Greater than 60%

Correct Answer: D

The risk of recurrent anterior glenohumeral dislocation is higher in younger athletes. The risk of recurrent dislocation after conservative therapy in young athletes has been reported as 66% in one study and as high as 90% to 95% in others.

1. Dunlap J. Shoulder dislocations. In: Puffer J (ed). 20 Common Problems in Sports Medicine. New York: McGraw-Hill, 2002:29-43.
2. Welsh S. Shoulder dislocation surgery treatment and management. Medscape. Accessed December 6, 2011 at http://emedicine.medscape.com/article/1261802-treatment.

182. A 32-year-old male recreational squash player is seen in your sports medicine clinic for a one-week history of right volar wrist pain with associated numbness and tingling along the volar aspect of the radial half of the hand. He spends a significant amount of time working at a computer, using a mouse without a wrist pad, and takes a "smoke break" about every three hours. He recalls an injury involving a fall onto his outstretched right hand the day prior to the onset of symptoms. Your examination reveals nonspecific tenderness in multiple areas of the right wrist, and a positive Tinel's sign over an area that approximates the median nerve. The best next step in the management of this case would be which of the following?

A. Recommend night wrist splints, occupational therapy, and ergonomic precautions such as the use of gel wrist pads at work

B. Perform a corticosteroid injection into the carpal tunnel

C. Obtain electrodiagnostic studies of the upper extremity, including a complete electromyogram and nerve conduction studies

D. Obtain a complete set of point-of-care plain film radiographs including a clenched fist and carpal tunnel views

E. Obtain a workup for metabolic causes for peripheral neuropathies

Correct Answer: D

Carpal tunnel syndrome is usually an occupational, ergonomic, degenerative, or overuse phenomenon. Encroachment, restriction, and resulting irritation of the median nerve usually results in a gradual onset and progression of symptoms, including numbness, tingling, clumsiness, and motor weakness in the innervated sensory and muscular structures. Less commonly, median nerve symptoms may be an early manifestation of a variety of metabolic peripheral neuropathies. However, perilunate dislocations may present with acute carpal tunnel syndrome, and a high index of suspicion should be maintained for this often-missed diagnosis, especially since early operative treatment provides better outcomes.

Perilunate dislocations commonly occur after a fall onto the outstretched dorsiflexed hand with enough force to cause severe ligamentous disruption, bony fractures of the scaphoid or triquetrum, or a combination thereof, resulting in dissociation of the distal carpal row from the lunate. The different types of perilunate dislocations include transscaphoid-perilunate, perilunar, transscaphoid-transcapitate-perilunate, and transradial-styloid types. In severe cases, the lunate may be dislocated into the carpal tunnel, causing symptoms consistent with carpal tunnel syndrome. Plain film radiographs (the correct answer)—including a clenched-fist stress view, carpal tunnel view, scaphoid views, and oblique views—may aid in making this diagnosis, facilitating early recognition and appropriate surgical intervention. Electrodiagnostic studies are often unrevealing this early in the disease process, and a corticosteroid injection would be inappropriate for this injury. The other answer options are less favorable choices, as they may delay the diagnosis and result in a poorer clinical outcome, such as avascular necrosis.

1. Daniels JM II, Zook EG, Lynch JM. Hand and wrist injuries: part I. Nonemergent evaluation. Am Fam Physician 2004 Apr 15;69(8):1941-1948.

2. Dumontier C, Meyer zu Reckendorf G, Sautet A, Lenoble E, Saffar P, Allieu Y. Radiocarpal dislocations: classification and proposal for treatment. A review of twenty-seven cases. J Bone Joint Surg Am 2001 Feb;83-A(2):212-218.

3. Taleisnik J. Current concepts review. Carpal instability. J Bone Joint Surg Am 1988 Sep;70(8):1262-1268.

183. A 23-year-old cross-country runner is complaining of a generalized papular itchy rash that occurs only during exercise. You would recommend that he do which of the following?

    A. Use sunscreen with PABA (para-aminobenzoic acid) at least 20 minutes prior to exercise

    B. Use topical steroids on the rash during exercise

    C. Take a hot shower the night before a long run, or try an antihistamine tablet one hour prior to exercise

    D. Desensitize with PUVA (psoralen + UVA)

Correct Answer: C

This athlete has cholinergic urticaria, which is characterized by papular wheals with surrounding erythema occurring during and after heat exposure or exercise. A hot shower prior to a long run may deplete histamine and provide a refractory period for the athlete. H1 antihistamines are effective when taken one hour prior to activity. Sunscreen with PABA or PUVA has no effect on cholinergic urticaria.

1. Brown DL, Haight DD, Brown LL. Allergic diseases in athletes. In: O'Connor FG, Sallis RE, Wilder RP, St. Pierre P (eds). Sports Medicine: Just the Facts. New York: McGraw-Hill, 2005:220.

2. Schwarts RA. Cholinergic urticaria. Medscape. Accessed December 6, 2011 at http://emedicine.medscape.com/article/1049978.

3. Batts KB. Dermatology. In: O'Connor F, Sallis RE, Wilder RP, St. Pierre P (eds). Sports Medicine: Just the Facts. New York: McGraw-Hill, 2005:152.

4. Hosey RG, Carek PJ, Goo A. Exercise-induced anaphylaxis and urticaria. Am Fam Physician 2001 Oct 15;64(8):1367-1372.

184. According to most recently published studies, there is general agreement that repetitive heading of a soccer ball can demonstrate which of the following?

    A. Evidence of lasting neurocognitive deficits in well-controlled studies
    B. Ball type and size not important in epidemiology of head injuries
    C. Protective headgear not helpful in reducing ball impact to the head
    D. No evidence of gender differences in contact type and incidence of injuries

Correct Answer: C

Study of various types of headgear did not show any evidence that protective headgear attenuated ball impact to the head. Most likely because of the plasticity of the ball in terms of surface area being greater than what protection the headgear could provide. They may provide some protection from injuries sustained from head to head contact, but not ball to head.

The earlier studies linking cognitive deficits in former soccer players were not controlled; there was no pre-injury data, there was selection bias, failure to control for acute head injuries, and lack of observer blinding. Also, the findings of cognitive deficits that were noted could be explained by alcohol-related brain impairment, which was not controlled in these studies.

Current literature supports that purposeful heading is safe and concussion in soccer is most likely due to incidental contact with another opponent (head to head in females, and head to upper extremities in males). Other articles have looked at biomechanical properties in soccer heading and noted that ball mass, pressure, and construction can reduce the impact severity to the head and neck.

1. Zetterberg H, Jonsson M, Rasulzada A, Popa C, Styrud E, Hietala MA, et al. No neurochemical evidence for brain injury caused by heading in soccer. Br J Sports Med 2007 Sep;41(9):574-577.
2. Dvorak J, McCrory P, Kirkendall PT. Head injuries in the female football [soccer] player: incidence, mechanisms, risk factors and management Br J Sports Med 2007 Aug;41(Suppl 1):i44-46.
3. Shewchenko N, Withnall C, Keown M, Gittens R, Dvorak J. Heading in football [soccer]. Part 1: development of biomechanical methods to investigate head response. Br J Sports Med 2005 Aug;39(Suppl 1):i10-25.
4. Shewchenko N, Withnall C, Keown M, Gittens R, Dvorak J. Heading in football [soccer]. Part 2: biomechanics of ball heading and head response. Br J Sports Med 2005 Aug;39(Suppl 1):i26-32.
5. Tysvaer AT, Løchen EA. Soccer injuries to the brain. A neuropsychologic study of former soccer players. Am J Sports Med 1991 Jan-Feb;19(1):56-60.

185. Examples of appropriate activities to improve cardiorespiratory endurance include which of the following?

   A. Jogging and cycling
   B. Wind sprints and weight lifting
   C. Power lifting
   D. Handheld video games
   E. Pilates

Correct Answer: A

The best improvements in cardiorespiratory endurance occur when large muscle groups are engaged in rhythmic aerobic activity. Wind sprints, weight lifting, and Pilates require short bursts of anaerobic activity. Handheld video games to not provide activity of large muscle groups.

1. Pollock ML, Gaesser G, Butcher JD, Despres JP, Dishman RK, Franklin BA, et al. American College of Sports Medicine position stand. The recommended quantity and quality of exercise for developing and maintaining cardiorespiratory and muscular fitness, and flexibility in healthy adults. Med Sci Sports Exerc 1998 Jun;30(6):975-991.

186. At a local collegiate football game, a player on the sidelines presents to you after he felt an insect sting. He feels like his throat is tightening, and you notice that it is becoming increasingly difficult for him to breath. The drug of choice to be administered first to this patient would be which of the following?

    A. Diphenhydramine
    B. Epinephrine
    C. Ranitidine
    D. Loratadine
    E. Nebulized beta-2 agonist

Correct Answer: B

In 2008, the World Allergy Association published a position statement reporting that epinephrine is currently underutilized and often dosed improperly to treat anaphylaxis, is underprescribed for potential future self-administration, that most of the reasons proposed to withhold its clinical use are flawed, and that the therapeutic benefits of epinephrine exceed the risk when given in appropriate IM doses. The recommended doses: aqueous epinephrine 1:1000 dilution (1 mg in 1 ml), 0.2 to 0.5 mg (0.01 mg/kg in children, maximum dose, 0.3 mg) administered intramuscularly every 5 to 15 minutes or as necessary, depending on the severity. Diphenhydramine (Answer A), ranitidine (Answer C) and beta-2 agonists (Answer E) may all be considered but should occur after epinephrine has been administered. Other measures to consider after epinephrine injections, where appropriate: consider epinephrine infusion, systemic corticosteroids, vasopressor (e.g., dopamine). Consider glucagon for a patient taking beta blocker. Consider atropine for symptomatic bradycardia and transportation to an emergency department or an intensive care facility, for cardiopulmonary arrest during anaphylaxis, high-dose epinephrine and prolonged resuscitation efforts are encouraged. Loratadine should not be considered a treatment option.

1. Kemp SF, Lockey RF, Simons FE. World Allergy Organization ad hoc Committee on Epinephrine in Anaphylaxis. Epinephrine: the drug of choice for anaphylaxis. A statement of the World Allergy Organization. Allergy 2008 Aug;63(8):1061-1070.
2. Tang AW. A practical guide to anaphylaxis. Am Fam Physician 2003 Oct 1;68(7):1325-1332.

187. A 17-year-old basketball player visits her school's training room complaining of a 10-day history of insidious onset right-sided chest pain that is constant but worse with adduction of the right shoulder. There was no antecedent trauma. She is otherwise well and denies any medical problems and takes no medications. On exam, the athlete is in no distress. Heart rate is 72 bpm, BP 110/84 mm Hg in the right arm, and respiratory rate 16 breaths/minute. Inspection of the chest reveals no abnormalities. Palpation of the chest elicits tenderness over the cartilaginous articulations of the second through fifth ribs. There is no warmth or swelling. Auscultation of the lungs and precordium are normal. The most likely diagnosis is which of the following?

A. Costochondritis
B. Epidemic myalgia
C. Pulmonary catch syndrome
D. Slipping rib syndrome
E. Tietze's syndrome

Correct Answer: A

Musculoskeletal chest wall pain is a common complaint among athletes. The history and physical exam of the patient in the vignette support a diagnosis of costochondritis. Costochondritis is a benign, self-limited condition of unknown etiology that usually involves the second through fifth costochondral articulations. Imaging is usually nondiagnostic. Symptoms usually last days to weeks, but may persist for months and relapses are not uncommon. Treatment is conservative and usually involves NSAIDs and activity modification. Epidemic myalgia is described as chest pain associated with an acute viral infection, most frequently Coxsackie viruses. Sharp pains are felt in the lateral chest or upper abdomen following a viral prodrome. The patient in the vignette denied recent illness. Tietze's syndrome is differentiated from costochondritis by the presence of non-suppurative swelling and warmth of the involved costochondral joints, which are absent in the patient in the vignette. As with costochondritis, the etiology is poorly understood. Slipping rib syndrome is characterized by hypermobility of the costal cartilage of the false (eighth through tenth) ribs. The floating (eleventh and twelfth) ribs have also been implicated in some reports. The condition causes sharp subcostal pain associated with the sensation of a rib slipping or popping sensation, which is absent in the patient in this vignette.

1. Gregory PL, Biswas AC, Batt ME. Musculoskeletal problems of the chest wall in athletes. Sports Med 2002:32(4);235-250.

188. A 12-year-old swimmer is evaluated at the poolside during a water polo match after kicking another player's foot. She has a gross deformity of the fourth toe, and the clinical exam suggests a fracture. She would like to continue competing in this event. As pertaining to fractures of the phalanges, you explain that if pain permits, she can buddy tape the injured toe to an adjacent toe and continue competing. Regarding fractures of the phalanges, which of the following is true?

A. Overall, most toe fractures require referral and specialist management
B. Referral is usually not recommended for first toe fracture-dislocations, displaced intra-articular fractures, and children with first-toe fractures involving the physis because they may require internal fixation
C. Circulatory compromise and open fractures do not warrant orthopedic referral
D. Children with nondisplaced Salter-Harris types I and II fractures do not warrant an orthopedic referral
E. Unstable, displaced fractures can be treated with splinting and a rigid-sole shoe to prevent joint movement

Correct Answer: D

Nondisplaced Salter-Harris type I and II fractures can be managed by a sports medicine physician, though referral should be considered for other fractures involving the physis.

Most toe fractures can be managed with splinting an immobilization and do not require orthopedic referral. First toe fracture-dislocations, displaced intra-articular fractures and pediatric first toe fractures involving the physis require consultation.

1. Eiff M, Hatch RL, Calmbach WL. Toe fractures. Fracture Management for Primary Care. 2nd ed. Philadelphia: E.B. Saunders, 2003:353.
2. Hatch RL, Hacking S. Evaluation and management of toe fractures. Am Fam Physician 2003 Dec 15;68(12):2413-2418.

189. During coverage of a cross country ski meet, an athlete presents to the medical team after she finished the race. She is shivering and slow to respond to your questions. You suspect hypothermia and quickly determine her rectal temperature to be 91.4 degrees Fahrenheit (33 degrees Celsius). Which of the following warming strategies should be considered first?

   A. Encouraging the athlete to move as much as possible to generate body heat
   B. Administration of warmed IV fluids
   C. Extracorporeal blood rewarming using cardiopulmonary bypass
   D. Removal of all wet clothing followed by application of warm blankets

Correct Answer: D

Classification of hypothermia is: mild = 89.6 to 95 degrees Fahrenheit (32 to 35 degrees Celsius), moderate = 82.4 to 89.6 degrees Fahrenheit (28 to 32 degrees Celsius), and severe = less than 82.4 degrees Fahrenheit (28 degrees Celsius). This patient has mild hypothermia as defined by a rectal temperature greater than 90 degrees Fahrenheit (32 degrees Celsius). With few exceptions, an otherwise healthy athlete can be treated on the spot. Passive rewarming should be attempted first, as most patients will safely respond to this method. Wet clothes should be removed and replaced with warm dry blankets or allow the patient to shiver within a sleeping bag within a warm shelter. Answer A is incorrect, as the athlete should be instructed to remain inactive, refraining from any movement to avoid triggering ventricular fibrillation. Answer B is incorrect. Warmed IV fluids may be considered if the initial passive attempts to rewarm are unsuccessful. Answer C is incorrect; extracorporeal blood rewarming has been shown to be the fastest method to rewarm a hypothermic patient. For mild hypothermia, it is not indicated; however, it has been used to resuscitate patients successfully with cardiopulmonary arrest due to very low body temperatures.

1. McCullough L, Arora S. Diagnosis and treatment of hypothermia. Am Fam Physician 2004 Dec 15;70(12):2325-2332.
2. Bowman WD. Safe exercise in the cold and cold injuries. In: Mellion MB, Walsh MW, Madden C, Putukian M, Shelton GL (eds). Team Physician's Handbook. 3rd ed. Philadelphia: Hanley and Belfus, 2002:148-150.
3. Edelstein JA. Hypothermia. Medscape. Accessed February 17, 2012 at http://emedicine. medscape.com/article/770542.

190. Correct fit of a road bicycle is critical for optimal performance and reduction of overuse injuries. Which of the following factors is most important when fitting a bike?

    A. Forward/back saddle adjustment: This adjustment is made with the pedals at 3 and 9 o'clock or parallel to the ground, correct position is reached when the forward knee is in front of the corresponding pedal spindle/ball of the foot
    B. Saddle height: When seated on the bike with one pedal at the 6 o'clock position, the seat height is adjusted so the knee is flexed < 30 degrees
    C. The handlebar position should always be higher than the seat height when viewed from the side
    D. Bicycle frame size should be as tall as possible (longer seat tube length), optimizing power output per stroke

Correct Answer: B

Correct saddle placement causes the knee to be directly over the pedal spindle, using a plumb line from the distal patella. If the forward knee is in front of the pedal stem below, the saddle is too far forward. This causes in excessive knee flexion and anterior overuse pain. If the seat is too far back, reaching for the pedals results, predisposing to ilio-tibial band pain and hamstring overuse irritation. Seat height may be the most common adjustment error, especially in novices and casual cyclists. Adjusting the seat too high results in rocking of the pelvis across the seat, causing friction and perineal and ischial pain. More commonly, a seat that's too low results in excess knee flexion in excess of 30 degrees. This predisposes to patello-femoral pain, especially if cadence is low (more PF pressure per cm square per pedal stroke). Biomechanically optimal aerodynamics improves training, efficiency, and speed. Wind resistance moving forward is determined by frontal profile. A more upright position (as many beginning riders prefer) increases wind resistance and work while decreasing efficiency. For training and fitness, handlebar height should always be lower than saddle height. As riders become more proficient and flexible, they will gradually be able lower the handlebar height as tolerated. Biomechanically, the smallest frame size that fits results in the smallest frontal profile, least wind resistance, and best efficiency. Frame size that is too large can produce many problems, including saddle discomfort and perineal trauma if unable to straddle the top bar while standing over it when coming to a stop.

1. Silberman MR, Webner D, Collina S, Shiple BJ. Road bicycle fit. Clin J Sport Med 2005 Jul;15(4):271-276.
2. Asplund C. Bicycling injuries. In: O'Connor FG, Sallis RE, Wilder RP, St. Pierre P (eds). Sports Medicine: Just the Facts. New York: McGraw-Hill, 2005:480-485.
3. Bicycle fit. Colorado Cyclist. Accessed December 6, 2011 at www.coloradocyclist.com/bikefit.

191. The pathology on the radiograph shown is indicative of which of the following injuries?

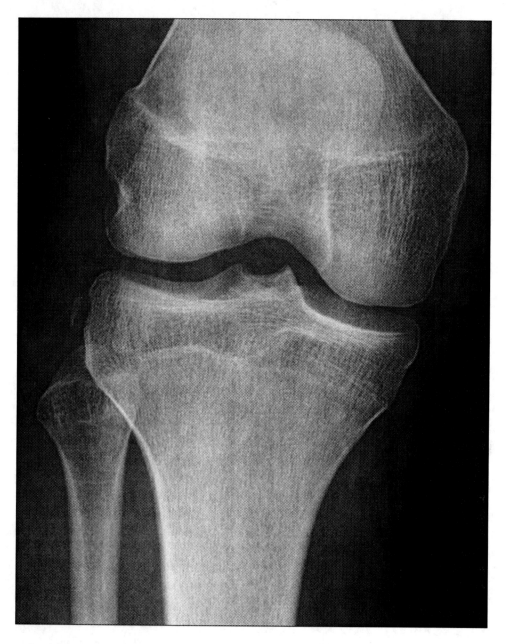

A. ACL tear

B. MCL tear

C. PCL tear

D. LCL tear

Correct Answer: A

The image shows a Segond fracture. This is a capsular avulsion fracture of the anterolateral tibial plateau at the attachment of the lateral capsular ligament. This fracture correlates highly with a tear of the ACL.

1. Friedberg RP. Anterior cruciate ligament injury. UpToDate. Accessed December 7, 2011 at www.uptodate.com.
2. Sanders TG, Miller MD. A systematic approach to magnetic resonance imaging interpretation of sports medicine injuries of the knee. Am J Sports Med 2005 Jan;33(1):131-148.
3. Shearman CM, El-Khoury GY. Pitfalls in the radiologic evaluation of extremity trauma: Part II. The lower extremity. Am Fam Physician 1998 Mar 15;57(6)1314-1322.

192. Identify which of the following dermatomes of the upper extremity is *not* appropriately matched with its corresponding nerve root supply?

    A. Lateral upper arm: C5
    B. Axilla: C7
    C. Lateral forearm: C6
    D. Medial upper arm: T1
    E. Medial forearm: C8

Correct Answer: B

The nerve root from T2 supplies the axilla. Nerve roots from C5 supply the lateral upper arm. Nerve roots from C6 supply the lateral forearm. Nerve roots from T1 supply the medial upper arm. Nerve roots from C8 supply the medial forearm.

1. Hoppenfeld S. Physical Examination of the Spine and Extremities. East Norwalk, CT: Prentice Hall, 1976:105-132.

193. A 13-year-old softball player is struck in the right eye with a batted ball. Upon ophthalmological evaluation at the local emergency room, a fluid level is visible in the lower third of child's anterior chamber, and there is a slight drop in visual acuity when compared to the non-traumatized eye. The remainder of the eye exam is unremarkable. Therapy will be directed to avoid which of the following complications?

    A. Hemosiderin lens staining
    B. Rebleeding
    C. Further deterioration of visual acuity
    D. Clot formation in the anterior chamber
    E. Retinal hemorrhage

Correct Answer: B

In the management of acute traumatic hyphema, the two greatest concerns to the practitioner are acute elevation of intraocular pressure (IOP), and subsequent rebleeding. The source of bleeding in traumatic hyphema is the fragile network of vessels surrounding the iris and the angle. Rebleeding is a poor prognostic indicator. These may be disrupted with a direct blow of sufficient force. Bloodstaining of the cornea is also concerning, and is a criterion for surgical referral, as is continuously elevated IOP > 35 and complete filling of the anterior chamber by blood (grade 4 hyphema). Once hemorrhage has completed, there should be no further deterioration of visual acuity.

1. Olson DE, Sikka RS, Pulling T, Broton M. Eye injuries in sports. In: Madden C, Putukian M, Young CC, McCarty EC (eds). Netter's Sports Medicine. Philadelphia: Saunders, 2010:337.
2. Sheppard JD. Hyphema. Medscape Accessed December 6, 2011 at http://emedicine.medscape.com/article/1190165.

194. Which of the following is true of resistance training during childhood and adolescence?

    A. Strength gains are not lost during detraining
    B. Growth in height and weight of pre-adolescents can be influenced by resistance training
    C. Resistance training can result in increased strength without muscle hypertrophy or changes in body composition
    D. Resistance training is generally discouraged in children and adolescents due to safety concerns

Correct Answer: C

Resistance training in children and adolescents has been shown to increase muscular strength significantly, and this is independent of body composition changes or muscle hypertrophy. Strength gains are lost with detraining. Growth (height or weight) is not influenced by resistance training. Resistance training is generally thought to be safe when properly supervised.

1. Malina RM. Weight training in youth-growth, maturation, and safety: an evidence-based review. Clin J Sport Med 2006 Nov;16(6):478-487.
2. Faigenbaum AD. Youth resistance training. President's Council on Physical Fitness and Sports Research Digest 2003 Sep;4(3). Accessed December 6, 2011 at www.fitness.gov/Reading_Room/Digests/september2003digest.pdf.

195. Which of the following carpal bones is at highest risk for avascular necrosis?

    A. Trapezium
    B. Triquetrium
    C. Lunate
    D. Pisiform

Correct Answer: C

The wrist is supplied by the radial and ulnar arteries. These arteries create the three pairs of transverse arches, which permit excellent collateral flow. However, the tortuous nature of the vasculature also results in retrograde flow distal to proximal. Thus, the scaphoid, capitate, and 20% of lunate depend on this retrograde flow and consequently are at risk for avascular necrosis and non-union if fractured.

1. Blood supply to the wrist. Wheeless' Textbook of Orthopaedics. Accessed December 6, 2011 at www.wheelessonline.com/ortho/blood_supply_to_the_wrist.
2. Morhart M. Wrist fractures and dislocations. Medscape. Accessed December 6, 2011 at http://emedicine.medscape.com/article/1285825.
3. Cohen PH, Aish B. The acutely injured wrist. In: Puffer J (ed). 20 Common Problems in Sports Medicine. New York: McGraw-Hill, 2002:76-78.

196. After what time period does evaluation of microscopic hematuria after an intense run in an under-40-year-old warrant further investigation?

    A. 12 hours
    B. 24 hours
    C. 36 hours
    D. 48 hours
    E. 96 hours

Correct Answer: D

After 48 to 72 hours of persistent microscopic hematuria after an intense exercise activity in an under-40-year-old, a more complete workup is indicated. This could include repeat microscopic urinalysis with culture and sensitivity, renal function tests, and cystoscopy. Also bleeding disorders, ingested foods, and medications should be reviewed. Imaging can include ultrasound, intravenous pyelography, urography, and KUB. In those older than 50, diagnostic workup should start earlier.

1. Siegel AJ, Hennekens CH, Solomon HS, Van Boeckel B. Exercise-related hematuria. Findings in a group of marathon runners. JAMA 1979 Jan 26;241(4):391-392.
2. Mercieri A. Exercise-induced hematuria. UpToDate. Accessed December 6, 2011 at www.uptodate.com/contents/exercise-induced-hematuria.
3. Thallere TR, Wang LP. Evaluation of asymptomatic microscopic hematuria in adults. Am Fam Physician 1999 Sep 15;60(4):1143-1152, 1154.
4. Webb CW, White CT. Hematuria. In: Bracker MD (ed). The 5-Minute Sports Medicine Consult. 2nd ed. Philadelphia: Lippincott Williams & Wilkins, 2011:298-299.

197. A 42-year-old male is interested in beginning an exercise program. Which of the following is true regarding cardiovascular health and exercise?

    A. Arterial compliance increases with normal aging
    B. Aerobic exercise increases arterial compliance
    C. Resistance training increases arterial compliance
    D. Once resistance training is stopped, arterial resistance will increase

Correct Answer: C

Arterial compliance is the ability of an artery to distend in response to change in pressure. Compliance decreases with age due to a variety of different changes at the molecular level. Several studies have shown that regular aerobic exercise can slow or even stop this decrease in compliance. There have also been studies that show resistance training can increase arterial resistance even after a short time. After a period of no resistance training, the compliance will return to baseline. It is postulated that by increasing arterial compliance, there will be a subsequent decrease in cardiovascular disease.

1. Gate PE, Seals DR. Decline in large elastic artery compliance with age: a therapeutic target for habitual exercise. Br J Sports Med 2006 Nov;40(11):897-899.
2. Joyner MJ. Effect of exercise on arterial compliance. Circulation 2000 Sep 12;102(11):1214-1215.

198. A 17-year-old male is playing a casual soccer game with his friends after school. He plants his right foot, and as he cuts sharply, he feels a pop on the outside of his ankle. He is not able to bear weight and has radiographs at the local urgent care facility that shows soft tissue swelling, closed physis, and a small fleck of bone lateral to the lateral malleolus at the level of the mortise. He is placed in a posterior splint, and he is seen in clinic two weeks later. The maneuver most likely to reproduce his symptoms is which of the following?

 A. Anterior drawer
 B. Syndesmosis squeeze
 C. Peroneal subluxation test
 D. Inversion stress test
 E. Passive dorsiflexion and external rotation of the foot

Correct Answer: C

The scenario is the description of a peroneal subluxation with a loud pop, pain, and the radiographic findings. The provocative maneuver that will reproduce the pain and the pop of the peroneus brevis subluxating out of the fibular tunnel and out past the injured retinaculum is the peroneal subluxation test. Lateral ankle sprain may produce instability sensation and pain with the anterior drawer or inversion stress test. High ankle sprain with syndesmosis injury may have widened clear space on mortise views and pain reproduced with the syndesmosis squeeze or passive dorsiflexion/external rotation.

1. Maffulli N, Ferran NA, Oliva F, Testa V. Recurrent subluxation of the peroneal tendons. Am J Sports Med 2006 Jun;34(6):986-992.
2. Peroneal tendon dislocation. Wheeless' Textbook of Orthopaedics. Accessed December 6, 2011 at: www.wheelessonline.com/ortho/peroneal_tendon_dislocation.

Test 2 Answers, Critiques, and References

199. An athlete travels from sea level to a city at 3,000 m altitude in anticipation of a competition. Which of the following is a true physiological adaptation that occurs in this setting?

    A. Mild hyperventilation induces respiratory alkalosis
    B. Mild hypoxia increases stage 3 and stage 4 sleep
    C. Decreased diuresis and increased plasma volume
    D. Increased red blood cell mass in two to four days due to increased erythropoietin secretion
    E. Pulmonary arterial vasodilation to increase PaO_2 (alveolar partial pressure of oxygen)

Correct Answer: A

The first physiological adaptation to occur at altitude is that of increased respiratory rate. This induces a mild alkalosis by blowing off excess alveolar CO_2, which in turn lowers the alveolar partial pressure of CO_2. This allows the partial pressure of oxygen to rise in the alveolus, which maintains oxyhemoglobin levels. Alkalosis increases the periodic breathing and fragments sleep with increased nighttime awakenings and more stage 1 and 2 sleep, and less stage 3 and 4 sleep. There is a mild altitude diuresis that occurs to athletes approaching 10,000 feet (3,000 m). Increased numbers of nucleated red blood cells (nRBC) are seen in the circulation in days, but it takes weeks to months for a rise in the RBC mass. Pulmonary artery vasoconstriction leads to elevated pulmonary arterial pressures that may approach systemic levels at extreme altitude. The response of pulmonary vasculature to hypoxia is constriction, not dilation.

1. Koehle MS. Exercise at the extremes of cold and altitude. In: Brukner P, Khan K (eds). Clinical Sports Medicine. 3rd ed. Sydney: McGraw-Hill Professional, 2007: 900-911.
2. Harris MD, Terrio J, Miser WF, Yetter JF III. High-altitude medicine. Am Fam Physician 1998 Apr 15;57(8):1907-1914, 1924-1926.

200. A 20-year-old female collegiate hockey player comes into your office with symptoms of fever, sore throat, and "swollen glands" in her neck for the last several days. In addition to collecting a throat swab for strep, of the following tests, which is the next best test to order at this time?

   A. Epstein-Barr nuclear antigen
   B. EBV IgG
   C. EBV IgM
   D. Heterophile antibody
   E. Erythrocyte sedimentation rate (ESR)

Correct Answer: C

In a patient with symptoms of pharyngitis, it is important to rule out acute infectious mononucleosis (IM). The best test for ruling out acute IM is an EBV IgM titer, which will be elevated early in the disease process and clear within four to six weeks. EBV IgG will elevate early, but will persist for life and would be helpful in determining if the patient had IM previously. Heterophile antibody, also known as the monospot test, has a sensitivity and specificity of 87% and 91%, respectively, but has higher false negatives in the first week, can be elevated in other infectious disease states and in some people may never elevate. EBNA does not increase until two to four months after symptoms present. ESR may be elevated, but is nonspecific and does not assist with the diagnosis.

   1. Epstein-Barr virus infectious mononucleosis. Centers for Disease Control and Prevention. Accessed December 6, 2011 at www.cdc.gov/ncidod/diseases/ebv.htm.
   2. Ebell MH. Epstein-Barr virus infectious mononucleosis. Am Fam Physician 2004 Oct 1;70(7):1279-1287.

Appendix:
Sports Medicine Fellow In-Training Exam Score Distribution

Compare your number correct on each practice test with the class of primary care sports medicine fellows. The raw score is located on the x-axis, and the frequency of achieving that score is on the y-axis.

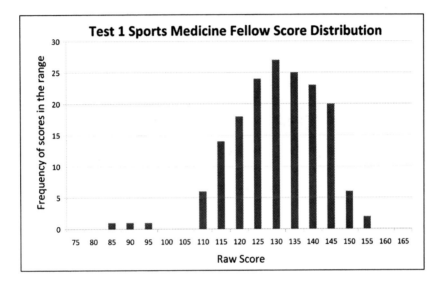

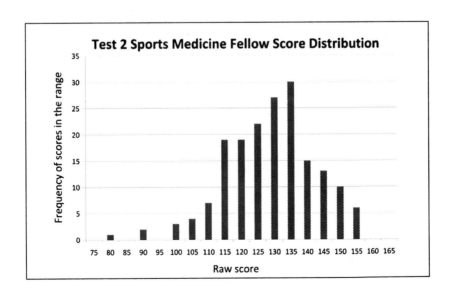

About the Editors

Stephen Paul, M.D., CAQSM, is an assistant professor at the University of Arizona. He is program director for the University of Arizona Sports Medicine Fellowship, coordinator for sports medicine at Campus Health Services, and assistant team physician for intercollegiate sports medicine at the University of Arizona. He graduated from the University of Texas Health Science Centers at Houston in 1987. He completed his fellowship in sports medicine at the Center for Sports Medicine and Orthopedics in Phoenix in 1996. He is board-certified in family medicine and holds a Certificate of Added Qualification in Sports Medicine. Paul has worked with professional, intercollegiate, club sports, and recreational athletes. He has published in *Athletic Training & Sports Health Care, Sports Health, The 5-Minute Sports Medicine Consult, Clinical Journal of Sport Medicine,* and *Saunder's Manual of Medical Practice.* He worked with the AMSSM to develop the first sports medicine In-Training Exam and is co-chair of the AMSSM In-Training Exam subcommittee. He lives in Tucson, Arizona, with his wife Janice and children Nika and Stryder.

Scott Rand, M.D., FAAFP, CAQSM, is an assistant clinical professor in family and community medicine with Weill Cornell Medical College and is the director of the Primary Care Sports Medicine Fellowship for the Methodist Hospital System in Houston, Texas. He graduated from the University of South Dakota Sanford School of Medicine in 1989 and completed his family medicine training with the U.S. Navy in Pensacola, Florida. He is board-certified in family medicine and completed his Certificate of Added Qualification in Sports Medicine in 1999. He has published articles in *American Family Physician, Journal of Family Practice, Family Practice Management,* and *Current Sports Medicine Reports.* He is currently a team physician for Rice University and USA Weightlifting along with multiple Texas high schools and Houston-area club sports. He is co-chair of the AMSSM In-Training Exam subcommittee and was instrumental in the development of the testing process for the test that is now used by virtually all primary care sports medicine fellowships in the country. He is an avid distance runner, loving husband, and father of two grown children.

Mark Stovak, M.D., FAAFP, FACSM, CAQSM, is the program director for both the Family Medicine Residency and the Sports Medicine Fellowship programs at the University of Kansas School of Medicine-Wichita (KUSM-W) and Via Christi Hospitals. He is also the medical director for sports medicine at Via Christi Hospitals and an associate professor in the Department of Family and Community Medicine at KUSM-W. He is on the AMSSM board of directors and is the chair of the AMSSM Fellowship Committee. He was a team physician for Team USA at the 2007 Pan-American Games in Rio de Janeiro, Brazil and for the 2008 USA Paralympic team at the Paralympics in Beijing, China. He is the head team physician at Wichita State University and the medical director for the Wichita State University Athletic Training Education Program.

Marc P. Hilgers, M.D., Ph.D., is an associate assistant professor at the University of South Florida. He is a clinical educator for the University of Tampa. He is the team physician for the University of Tampa and for local high schools. He served as team physician for Team Germany and for Team New Zealand at the 2009 World Championship of American Football. He graduated from the Heinrich Heine University in Duesseldorf, Germany in 1997 and completed a residency program consisting of a year each of anesthesiology, orthopaedic surgery, and internal medicine/endocrinology before coming to the United States. He completed a second residency program in family medicine at the Saint Joseph Regional Medical Center in South Bend, Indiana. He is board-certified and a diplomate for family medicine. He received his Certificate of Added Qualification after completing a Primary Care Sports Medicine Fellowship at the renowned Cleveland Clinic in Cleveland, Ohio. Hilgers has been working with athletes of all levels. He has been writing articles in peer-reviewed publications and has written chapters for sports medicine books. He is a requested lecturer throughout the state. He is also active as a physician for Divers Alert Network. He has been contributing to the sports medicine In-Training Exam since its beginning and is a member of the international, educational, and In-Training Exam subcommittees for the AMSSM. He lives in Tampa, Florida, where he works at the Florida Orthopaedic Institute.

About the Contributors

Robert J. Baker, M.D., Ph.D., FACSM, FAAFP
Program Director, Primary Care Sports Medicine Fellowship
MSU, Kalamazoo Center for Medical Studies
Professor, Clinical Medicine, Michigan State University
Team Physician, Western Michigan University

David T. Bernhardt, M.D.
Professor, Pediatrics and Orthopedics/Rehabilitation
Division of Sports Medicine
University of Wisconsin School of Medicine and Public Health

Kenneth Bielak, M.D., FACSM, CAQSM
Associate Professor, Program Director
Primary Care Sports Medicine
Department of Family Medicine
University of Tennessee

Blake Boggess, D.O., FAAFP
Assistant Professor
Team Physician, Duke Sports Medicine Center
Associate Director, Sports Medicine Fellowship
Department of Orthopedic Surgery, Duke University Medical Center

Anne S. Boyd, M.D., FAAFP, FACSM
LifeWellness Institute
San Diego, California

David Carfagno, D.O., CAQSM
Scottsdale Sports Medicine Institute

Terence M. Chang, M.D.
Clinical Assistant Professor
Memorial Family Medicine Residency Program, Houston/Sugar Land, Texas
Texas A&M Health Science Center, College of Medicine

Joseph Chorley, M.D.
Associate Professor of Pediatrics, Baylor College of Medicine
Fellowship Director, Baylor College of Medicine Primary Care Sports Medicine Fellowship
Team Physician, University of Houston and Texas Southern University

Rachel A. Coel, M.D., Ph.D., FAAP, CAQSM
Co-Medical Director, Sports Medicine for Young Athletes, Children's Hospital Colorado
Assistant Professor, University of Colorado

Nailah Coleman, M.D., FAAP
Assistant Professor of Pediatrics and Orthopaedics, The George Washington University
    Medical Center
Children's National Medical Center
Washington, DC

Kara D. Cox, M.D., FAAFP
Via Christi Medical Associates
Clinical Assistant Professor
Department of Family and Community Medicine
University of Kansas School of Medicine-Wichita

James M. Daniels II, M.D., MPH, FAAFP, FACOEM, FACPM
Program Director, Sports Medicine Fellowship
Professor of Family and Community Medicine
Adjunct Professor, Orthopedic Surgery
Southern Illinois University School of Medicine

Jim Dhanoa, M.D.
Fremont Orthopaedic and Rehabilitative Medicine
Fremont, California

Laura Dunne, M.D., FAAFP, CAQSM
OAA Orthopaedic Specialists

Nicholas M. Edwards, M.D., MPH
Assistant Professor of Pediatrics, Division of Sports Medicine
Cincinnati Children's Hospital Medical Center and University of Cincinnati
Cincinnati, Ohio

Mark I. Ellen M.D., FABPMR, CAQSM
Clinical Associate Professor
University of Alabama-Birmingham
Birmingham VAMC

Ted A. Farrar, M.D.
Associate Director, Primary Care Sports Medicine Fellowship
University of South Florida College of Medicine/Morton Plant Mease Healthcare

Jeffrey P. Feden, M.D.
Assistant Professor of Emergency Medicine
Alpert Medical School of Brown University
Providence, Rhode Island

Mark E. Halstead, M.D.
Assistant Professor, Departments of Pediatrics and Orthopedics
Washington University in St. Louis

J. Paul Hansen, M.D.
Utah Emergency Physicians

George D. Harris, M.D., M.S., FABFM, CAQSM
Professor, Assistant Dean, University of Missouri-Kansas City School of Medicine
Associate Director, Sports Medicine Fellowship

Benjamin A. Hasan, M.D.
Program Director, Primary Care Sports Medicine Fellowship
University of Chicago (North Shore)
Glenview, Illinois

Marc P. Hilgers, M.D., Ph.D.
Florida Orthopaedic Institute
Tampa, Florida

Crystal L. Hnatko, D.O.
Family and Sports Medicine
Kaiser Permanente
Vacaville, California

Garry Wai Keung Ho, M.D., CAQSM
Assistant Program Director, VCU/Fairfax Family Practice Sports Medicine Fellowship
    Program
Fairfax, Virginia
Assistant Professor, Department of Family Medicine, VCU School of Medicine
Richmond, Virginia

Gene Hong, M.D., CAQSM, FAAFP
Chief, Division of Sports Medicine
Department of Family, Community, and Preventive Medicine
Drexel University College of Medicine

Thomas M. Howard, M.D., FACSM
Program Director, Sports Medicine Fellowship
Fairfax Family Practice
Fairfax, Virginia

Jon Humphrey, M.D., CAQSM
Associate Director, Sports Medicine Fellowship
Assistant Professor, Southern Illinois University Family Medicine Residency
Carbondale, Illinois

Arthur Islas, M.D., MPH
Texas Tech Family Medicine

Robert L. Jones, M.D.
Team Physician, University of North Carolina at Charlotte
Director, Primary Care Sports Medicine Fellowship
Carolinas Medical Center
Charlotte, North Carolina

Sakina Kadakia, M.D.
Clinical Instructor, University of Michigan, Division of Pediatric Orthopedics

Barry E. Kenneally, M.D., CAQSM
Sports Medicine Specialist, Rothman Institute, Jefferson Medical College
Philadelphia, Pennsylvania

Morteza Khodaee, M.D., MPH
Assistant Professor, Department of Family Medicine
University of Colorado School of Medicine

K. Michele Kirk, M.D.
Assistant Director, JPS Sports Medicine Fellowship
Department of Family Medicine

Jennifer Scott Koontz, M.D., MPH, FAAFP
Pinnacle Sports Medicine and Orthopaedics
University of Kansas School of Medicine-Wichita

Charles A. Lascano, M.D., CAQSM
Staff Physician, OrthoNOW, Immediate Orthopedic Care
Clinical Assistant Professor, Florida International University, College of Medicine
Adjunct Faculty and Approved Clinical Instructor, Florida International University Athletic
    Training Education Program

Mark Lavallee, M.D.
Memorial Sports Medicine Institute
South Bend, Indiana

Lee A. Mancini, M.D., CSCS*D, CSN
Assistant Professor, University of Massachusetts-Amherst Medical School
Faculty, University of Massachusetts-Amherst Primary Care Sports Medicine Fellowship
Sports Medicine Physician, University of Massachusetts-Amherst

Damion A. Martins, M.D.
Director of Internal Medicine, New York Jets
Director of Sports Medicine and Orthopedics, Atlantic Health System
Program Director, Sports Medicine Fellowship, Atlantic Sports Health
Morristown, New Jersey

Jason Matuszak, M.D.
Excelsior Orthopedics
Amherst, New York

Christopher McGrew, M.D.
Department of Family and Community Medicine
Director, Primary Care Sports Medicine Fellowship
University of New Mexico Health Sciences Center
Albuquerque, New Mexico

Laura McIntosh, M.D.
Saint Vincent Sports Medicine
Erie, Pennsylvania

Michael D. Milligan, M.D., CAQSM
Head Team Physician/Medical Director, University of Nevada-Las Vegas Athletics
Program Director, University of Nevada School of Medicine, Sports Medicine Fellowship
Las Vegas, Nevada

David T. Millward, M.D., M.Sc.
Assistant Team Physician, University of Arizona
Tucson, Arizona

Jennifer J. Mitchell, M.D., FAAFP
Professor/Sports Medicine Fellowship Director, Texas Tech University Health Sciences
    Center
Lubbock, Texas

Ryan Modlinski, M.D.
Primary Care Sports Medicine
Texas Orthopedic Specialists
Dallas, Texas

Gaetano P. Monteleone, M.D.
Director, Primary Care Sports Medicine Fellowship
West Virginia University School of Medicine

Brian F. Morris, M.D., FAAFP
Sigma Sports Medicine
West Lafayette, Indiana

Grant Morrison, M.D.
Assistant Professor, Department of Family Medicine and Community Health
Division of Sports Medicine, University of Minnesota Medical School

John Munyak, M.D.
Program Director, NSUH Sports Medicine

Melissa Nayak, M.D.
Center for Athletic Medicine
Henry Ford Health System
Detroit, Michigan

Doug Okay, M.D.
Family and Sports Medicine, St. Francis
Midlothian, Virginia

Richard A. Okragly, M.D.
Program Director, TriHealth/Bethesda Primary Care Sports Medicine Fellowship
Cincinnati, Ohio

Ross Osborn, M.D.
Center for Health and Sports Medicine
Jacksonville, Florida

Luis E. Palacio, M.D.
Director, Sports Medicine
Northern Nevada Medical Group
Sparks, Nevada

Stacey Pappas, M.D.
Primary Care Sports Medicine Physician, Mologne Cadet Health Clinic at the United
  States Military Academy at West Point

Amit Parikh, D.O.
Houston Center for Family Practice and Sports Medicine
Cypress, Texas

Stephen Paul, M.D.
Director, University of Arizona Sports Medicine Fellowship
Coordinator, Sports Medicine Campus Health Service
Assistant Team Physician, University of Arizona
Tucson, Arizona

Randolph L. Pearson, M.D., FAAFP, FACSM
Professor, Department of Family Medicine
Sports Medicine Fellowship Director
Michigan State University

Matthew Pecci, M.D.
Boston University Family Medicine

David M. Peck, M.D., FACSM
Research/Education Director, Providence Athletic Medicine Fellowship Program

Bernadette Pendergraph, M.D.
Associate Professor, David Geffen School of Medicine
Department of Family Medicine

Mitchell Pratte, D.O.
Utah Valley Sports Medicine Fellowship
Head Team Physician, Brigham Young University
Intermountain Healthcare

Scott E. Rand, M.D., FAAFP, CAQSM
Director, Primary Care Sports Medicine Fellowship
Methodist Center for Orthopedic Surgery and Sports Medicine at Willowbrook
Houston, Texas

Tony S. Reed, M.D., MBA
Director, Sports Medicine Christiana Care Health System
Wilmington, Delaware
Assistant Professor of Family Medicine, Jefferson Medical College
Philadelphia, Pennsylvania

Alysia Robichau, M.D., CAQSM
Primary Care Sports Medicine
Memorial Hermann Medical Group
The Woodlands, Texas

Cherise Russo, D.O.
Primary Care Sports Medicine Physician, Northwestern Orthopaedic Institute
Clinical Instructor, Northwestern University, Feinberg School of Medicine

Todd S. Shatynski, M.D.
Capital Region Orthopaedics
Albany, New York

John Shelton, M.D.
Program Director, Sports Medicine Fellowship
Halifax FMRP
Daytona Beach, Florida

M. Kyle Smoot, M.D.
Program Director, Sports Medicine Fellowship
University of Iowa Hospitals and Clinics
Iowa City, Iowa

Mark Stovak, M.D., FACSM, FAAFP
Program Director, University of Kansas School of Medicine-Wichita Family Medicine
Residency and Sports Medicine Fellowship Programs, Via Christi Hospitals Wichita
Medical Director, Via Christi Sports Medicine
Associate Professor, Department of Family and Community Medicine, KUSM-W

W. Bradley Strauch, M.D.
Adena Bone and Joint Center
Chillicothe, Ohio

John K. Su, M.D., MPH, FAAFP
Associate Program Director, Kaiser Permanente
Los Angeles Sports Medicine Fellowship

Poonam P. Thaker, M.D., CAQSM
Director, Primary Care Sports Medicine Fellowship
Resurrection Medical Center
Chicago, Illinois

Thomas H. Trojian, M.D.
Director, UCHC Sports Medicine Fellowship
NEMSI Director of Injury Prevention and Sports Outreach

Priscilla Tu, D.O., CAQSM
Medical Instructor, Department of Community and Family Medicine, Duke University
    Medical Center
Team Physician, Duke Sports Medicine Center

Philipp Underwood, M.D., FAAEM, FACEP, FAAFP
Associate Program Director, Sports Medicine Fellowship
Department of Emergency Medicine, North Shore University Hospital
Manhasset, New York
Assistant Professor, Emergency Medicine
Hofstra North Shore-LIJ School of Medicine

Marissa Vasquez, M.D., CAQSM, FAAFP
Clinical Faculty, Family Medicine Residency Program and Division of Sports Medicine
Kaiser Permanente Los Angeles Medical Center
Clinical Instructor of Sports Medicine, Occidental College

Kevin D. Walter, M.D., FAAP
Assistant Professor, Departments of Orthopaedic Surgery and Pediatrics
Medical College of Wisconsin

Anna L. Waterbrook, M.D., CAQSM
Assistant Professor, University of Arizona
Associate Program Director, University of Arizona Sports Medicine Fellowship

David Westerdahl, M.D., FAAFP
Cleveland Clinic Florida, Department of Orthopaedics

Nancy White, M.D.
Henry Ford Health System, Departments of Orthopedics and Family Medicine

Russell D. White, M.D., FACSM, CAQSM, CAQAM
Professor of Medicine, Professor of Orthopedic Surgery
Director, Sports Medicine Fellowship Program
Medical Director, Sports Medicine Center
Head Team Physician, UMKC NCAA Division I Athletic Program
University of Missouri-Kansas City

Jason P. Womack, M.D.
Assistant Professor of Family Medicine
UMDNJ, Robert Wood Johnson

Craig Young, M.D.
Professor of Orthopaedic Surgery and Community and Family Medicine
Medical Director of Sports Medicine
Medical College of Wisconsin

Eliot Young, M.D.
Director, CHRISTUS Santa Rosa Primary Care Sports Medicine Fellowship
San Antonio, Texas

1. Ⓐ Ⓑ Ⓒ Ⓓ Ⓔ	35. Ⓐ Ⓑ Ⓒ Ⓓ Ⓔ	69. Ⓐ Ⓑ Ⓒ Ⓓ Ⓔ
2. Ⓐ Ⓑ Ⓒ Ⓓ Ⓔ	36. Ⓐ Ⓑ Ⓒ Ⓓ Ⓔ	70. Ⓐ Ⓑ Ⓒ Ⓓ Ⓔ
3. Ⓐ Ⓑ Ⓒ Ⓓ Ⓔ	37. Ⓐ Ⓑ Ⓒ Ⓓ Ⓔ	71. Ⓐ Ⓑ Ⓒ Ⓓ Ⓔ
4. Ⓐ Ⓑ Ⓒ Ⓓ Ⓔ	38. Ⓐ Ⓑ Ⓒ Ⓓ Ⓔ	72. Ⓐ Ⓑ Ⓒ Ⓓ Ⓔ
5. Ⓐ Ⓑ Ⓒ Ⓓ Ⓔ	39. Ⓐ Ⓑ Ⓒ Ⓓ Ⓔ	73. Ⓐ Ⓑ Ⓒ Ⓓ Ⓔ
6. Ⓐ Ⓑ Ⓒ Ⓓ Ⓔ	40. Ⓐ Ⓑ Ⓒ Ⓓ Ⓔ	74. Ⓐ Ⓑ Ⓒ Ⓓ Ⓔ
7. Ⓐ Ⓑ Ⓒ Ⓓ Ⓔ	41. Ⓐ Ⓑ Ⓒ Ⓓ Ⓔ	75. Ⓐ Ⓑ Ⓒ Ⓓ Ⓔ
8. Ⓐ Ⓑ Ⓒ Ⓓ Ⓔ	42. Ⓐ Ⓑ Ⓒ Ⓓ Ⓔ	76. Ⓐ Ⓑ Ⓒ Ⓓ Ⓔ
9. Ⓐ Ⓑ Ⓒ Ⓓ Ⓔ	43. Ⓐ Ⓑ Ⓒ Ⓓ Ⓔ	77. Ⓐ Ⓑ Ⓒ Ⓓ Ⓔ
10. Ⓐ Ⓑ Ⓒ Ⓓ Ⓔ	44. Ⓐ Ⓑ Ⓒ Ⓓ Ⓔ	78. Ⓐ Ⓑ Ⓒ Ⓓ Ⓔ
11. Ⓐ Ⓑ Ⓒ Ⓓ Ⓔ	45. Ⓐ Ⓑ Ⓒ Ⓓ Ⓔ	79. Ⓐ Ⓑ Ⓒ Ⓓ Ⓔ
12. Ⓐ Ⓑ Ⓒ Ⓓ Ⓔ	46. Ⓐ Ⓑ Ⓒ Ⓓ Ⓔ	80. Ⓐ Ⓑ Ⓒ Ⓓ Ⓔ
13. Ⓐ Ⓑ Ⓒ Ⓓ Ⓔ	47. Ⓐ Ⓑ Ⓒ Ⓓ Ⓔ	81. Ⓐ Ⓑ Ⓒ Ⓓ Ⓔ
14. Ⓐ Ⓑ Ⓒ Ⓓ Ⓔ	48. Ⓐ Ⓑ Ⓒ Ⓓ Ⓔ	82. Ⓐ Ⓑ Ⓒ Ⓓ Ⓔ
15. Ⓐ Ⓑ Ⓒ Ⓓ Ⓔ	49. Ⓐ Ⓑ Ⓒ Ⓓ Ⓔ	83. Ⓐ Ⓑ Ⓒ Ⓓ Ⓔ
16. Ⓐ Ⓑ Ⓒ Ⓓ Ⓔ	50. Ⓐ Ⓑ Ⓒ Ⓓ Ⓔ	84. Ⓐ Ⓑ Ⓒ Ⓓ Ⓔ
17. Ⓐ Ⓑ Ⓒ Ⓓ Ⓔ	51. Ⓐ Ⓑ Ⓒ Ⓓ Ⓔ	85. Ⓐ Ⓑ Ⓒ Ⓓ Ⓔ
18. Ⓐ Ⓑ Ⓒ Ⓓ Ⓔ	52. Ⓐ Ⓑ Ⓒ Ⓓ Ⓔ	86. Ⓐ Ⓑ Ⓒ Ⓓ Ⓔ
19. Ⓐ Ⓑ Ⓒ Ⓓ Ⓔ	53. Ⓐ Ⓑ Ⓒ Ⓓ Ⓔ	87. Ⓐ Ⓑ Ⓒ Ⓓ Ⓔ
20. Ⓐ Ⓑ Ⓒ Ⓓ Ⓔ	54. Ⓐ Ⓑ Ⓒ Ⓓ Ⓔ	88. Ⓐ Ⓑ Ⓒ Ⓓ Ⓔ
21. Ⓐ Ⓑ Ⓒ Ⓓ Ⓔ	55. Ⓐ Ⓑ Ⓒ Ⓓ Ⓔ	89. Ⓐ Ⓑ Ⓒ Ⓓ Ⓔ
22. Ⓐ Ⓑ Ⓒ Ⓓ Ⓔ	56. Ⓐ Ⓑ Ⓒ Ⓓ Ⓔ	90. Ⓐ Ⓑ Ⓒ Ⓓ Ⓔ
23. Ⓐ Ⓑ Ⓒ Ⓓ Ⓔ	57. Ⓐ Ⓑ Ⓒ Ⓓ Ⓔ	91. Ⓐ Ⓑ Ⓒ Ⓓ Ⓔ
24. Ⓐ Ⓑ Ⓒ Ⓓ Ⓔ	58. Ⓐ Ⓑ Ⓒ Ⓓ Ⓔ	92. Ⓐ Ⓑ Ⓒ Ⓓ Ⓔ
25. Ⓐ Ⓑ Ⓒ Ⓓ Ⓔ	59. Ⓐ Ⓑ Ⓒ Ⓓ Ⓔ	93. Ⓐ Ⓑ Ⓒ Ⓓ Ⓔ
26. Ⓐ Ⓑ Ⓒ Ⓓ Ⓔ	60. Ⓐ Ⓑ Ⓒ Ⓓ Ⓔ	94. Ⓐ Ⓑ Ⓒ Ⓓ Ⓔ
27. Ⓐ Ⓑ Ⓒ Ⓓ Ⓔ	61. Ⓐ Ⓑ Ⓒ Ⓓ Ⓔ	95. Ⓐ Ⓑ Ⓒ Ⓓ Ⓔ
28. Ⓐ Ⓑ Ⓒ Ⓓ Ⓔ	62. Ⓐ Ⓑ Ⓒ Ⓓ Ⓔ	96. Ⓐ Ⓑ Ⓒ Ⓓ Ⓔ
29. Ⓐ Ⓑ Ⓒ Ⓓ Ⓔ	63. Ⓐ Ⓑ Ⓒ Ⓓ Ⓔ	97. Ⓐ Ⓑ Ⓒ Ⓓ Ⓔ
30. Ⓐ Ⓑ Ⓒ Ⓓ Ⓔ	64. Ⓐ Ⓑ Ⓒ Ⓓ Ⓔ	98. Ⓐ Ⓑ Ⓒ Ⓓ Ⓔ
31. Ⓐ Ⓑ Ⓒ Ⓓ Ⓔ	65. Ⓐ Ⓑ Ⓒ Ⓓ Ⓔ	99. Ⓐ Ⓑ Ⓒ Ⓓ Ⓔ
32. Ⓐ Ⓑ Ⓒ Ⓓ Ⓔ	66. Ⓐ Ⓑ Ⓒ Ⓓ Ⓔ	100. Ⓐ Ⓑ Ⓒ Ⓓ Ⓔ
33. Ⓐ Ⓑ Ⓒ Ⓓ Ⓔ	67. Ⓐ Ⓑ Ⓒ Ⓓ Ⓔ	
34. Ⓐ Ⓑ Ⓒ Ⓓ Ⓔ	68. Ⓐ Ⓑ Ⓒ Ⓓ Ⓔ	

A copy of this answer sheet can be downloaded at http://www.amssmstore.com/download/AnswerSheet.pdf

101. Ⓐ Ⓑ Ⓒ Ⓓ Ⓔ	135. Ⓐ Ⓑ Ⓒ Ⓓ Ⓔ	169. Ⓐ Ⓑ Ⓒ Ⓓ Ⓔ
102. Ⓐ Ⓑ Ⓒ Ⓓ Ⓔ	136. Ⓐ Ⓑ Ⓒ Ⓓ Ⓔ	170. Ⓐ Ⓑ Ⓒ Ⓓ Ⓔ
103. Ⓐ Ⓑ Ⓒ Ⓓ Ⓔ	137. Ⓐ Ⓑ Ⓒ Ⓓ Ⓔ	171. Ⓐ Ⓑ Ⓒ Ⓓ Ⓔ
104. Ⓐ Ⓑ Ⓒ Ⓓ Ⓔ	138. Ⓐ Ⓑ Ⓒ Ⓓ Ⓔ	172. Ⓐ Ⓑ Ⓒ Ⓓ Ⓔ
105. Ⓐ Ⓑ Ⓒ Ⓓ Ⓔ	139. Ⓐ Ⓑ Ⓒ Ⓓ Ⓔ	173. Ⓐ Ⓑ Ⓒ Ⓓ Ⓔ
106. Ⓐ Ⓑ Ⓒ Ⓓ Ⓔ	140. Ⓐ Ⓑ Ⓒ Ⓓ Ⓔ	174. Ⓐ Ⓑ Ⓒ Ⓓ Ⓔ
107. Ⓐ Ⓑ Ⓒ Ⓓ Ⓔ	141. Ⓐ Ⓑ Ⓒ Ⓓ Ⓔ	175. Ⓐ Ⓑ Ⓒ Ⓓ Ⓔ
108. Ⓐ Ⓑ Ⓒ Ⓓ Ⓔ	142. Ⓐ Ⓑ Ⓒ Ⓓ Ⓔ	176. Ⓐ Ⓑ Ⓒ Ⓓ Ⓔ
109. Ⓐ Ⓑ Ⓒ Ⓓ Ⓔ	143. Ⓐ Ⓑ Ⓒ Ⓓ Ⓔ	177. Ⓐ Ⓑ Ⓒ Ⓓ Ⓔ
110. Ⓐ Ⓑ Ⓒ Ⓓ Ⓔ	144. Ⓐ Ⓑ Ⓒ Ⓓ Ⓔ	178. Ⓐ Ⓑ Ⓒ Ⓓ Ⓔ
111. Ⓐ Ⓑ Ⓒ Ⓓ Ⓔ	145. Ⓐ Ⓑ Ⓒ Ⓓ Ⓔ	179. Ⓐ Ⓑ Ⓒ Ⓓ Ⓔ
112. Ⓐ Ⓑ Ⓒ Ⓓ Ⓔ	146. Ⓐ Ⓑ Ⓒ Ⓓ Ⓔ	180. Ⓐ Ⓑ Ⓒ Ⓓ Ⓔ
113. Ⓐ Ⓑ Ⓒ Ⓓ Ⓔ	147. Ⓐ Ⓑ Ⓒ Ⓓ Ⓔ	181. Ⓐ Ⓑ Ⓒ Ⓓ Ⓔ
114. Ⓐ Ⓑ Ⓒ Ⓓ Ⓔ	148. Ⓐ Ⓑ Ⓒ Ⓓ Ⓔ	182. Ⓐ Ⓑ Ⓒ Ⓓ Ⓔ
115. Ⓐ Ⓑ Ⓒ Ⓓ Ⓔ	149. Ⓐ Ⓑ Ⓒ Ⓓ Ⓔ	183. Ⓐ Ⓑ Ⓒ Ⓓ Ⓔ
116. Ⓐ Ⓑ Ⓒ Ⓓ Ⓔ	150. Ⓐ Ⓑ Ⓒ Ⓓ Ⓔ	184. Ⓐ Ⓑ Ⓒ Ⓓ Ⓔ
117. Ⓐ Ⓑ Ⓒ Ⓓ Ⓔ	151. Ⓐ Ⓑ Ⓒ Ⓓ Ⓔ	185. Ⓐ Ⓑ Ⓒ Ⓓ Ⓔ
118. Ⓐ Ⓑ Ⓒ Ⓓ Ⓔ	152. Ⓐ Ⓑ Ⓒ Ⓓ Ⓔ	186. Ⓐ Ⓑ Ⓒ Ⓓ Ⓔ
119. Ⓐ Ⓑ Ⓒ Ⓓ Ⓔ	153. Ⓐ Ⓑ Ⓒ Ⓓ Ⓔ	187. Ⓐ Ⓑ Ⓒ Ⓓ Ⓔ
120. Ⓐ Ⓑ Ⓒ Ⓓ Ⓔ	154. Ⓐ Ⓑ Ⓒ Ⓓ Ⓔ	188. Ⓐ Ⓑ Ⓒ Ⓓ Ⓔ
121. Ⓐ Ⓑ Ⓒ Ⓓ Ⓔ	155. Ⓐ Ⓑ Ⓒ Ⓓ Ⓔ	189. Ⓐ Ⓑ Ⓒ Ⓓ Ⓔ
122. Ⓐ Ⓑ Ⓒ Ⓓ Ⓔ	156. Ⓐ Ⓑ Ⓒ Ⓓ Ⓔ	190. Ⓐ Ⓑ Ⓒ Ⓓ Ⓔ
123. Ⓐ Ⓑ Ⓒ Ⓓ Ⓔ	157. Ⓐ Ⓑ Ⓒ Ⓓ Ⓔ	191. Ⓐ Ⓑ Ⓒ Ⓓ Ⓔ
124. Ⓐ Ⓑ Ⓒ Ⓓ Ⓔ	158. Ⓐ Ⓑ Ⓒ Ⓓ Ⓔ	192. Ⓐ Ⓑ Ⓒ Ⓓ Ⓔ
125. Ⓐ Ⓑ Ⓒ Ⓓ Ⓔ	159. Ⓐ Ⓑ Ⓒ Ⓓ Ⓔ	193. Ⓐ Ⓑ Ⓒ Ⓓ Ⓔ
126. Ⓐ Ⓑ Ⓒ Ⓓ Ⓔ	160. Ⓐ Ⓑ Ⓒ Ⓓ Ⓔ	194. Ⓐ Ⓑ Ⓒ Ⓓ Ⓔ
127. Ⓐ Ⓑ Ⓒ Ⓓ Ⓔ	161. Ⓐ Ⓑ Ⓒ Ⓓ Ⓔ	195. Ⓐ Ⓑ Ⓒ Ⓓ Ⓔ
128. Ⓐ Ⓑ Ⓒ Ⓓ Ⓔ	162. Ⓐ Ⓑ Ⓒ Ⓓ Ⓔ	196. Ⓐ Ⓑ Ⓒ Ⓓ Ⓔ
129. Ⓐ Ⓑ Ⓒ Ⓓ Ⓔ	163. Ⓐ Ⓑ Ⓒ Ⓓ Ⓔ	197. Ⓐ Ⓑ Ⓒ Ⓓ Ⓔ
130. Ⓐ Ⓑ Ⓒ Ⓓ Ⓔ	164. Ⓐ Ⓑ Ⓒ Ⓓ Ⓔ	198. Ⓐ Ⓑ Ⓒ Ⓓ Ⓔ
131. Ⓐ Ⓑ Ⓒ Ⓓ Ⓔ	165. Ⓐ Ⓑ Ⓒ Ⓓ Ⓔ	199. Ⓐ Ⓑ Ⓒ Ⓓ Ⓔ
132. Ⓐ Ⓑ Ⓒ Ⓓ Ⓔ	166. Ⓐ Ⓑ Ⓒ Ⓓ Ⓔ	200. Ⓐ Ⓑ Ⓒ Ⓓ Ⓔ
133. Ⓐ Ⓑ Ⓒ Ⓓ Ⓔ	167. Ⓐ Ⓑ Ⓒ Ⓓ Ⓔ	
134. Ⓐ Ⓑ Ⓒ Ⓓ Ⓔ	168. Ⓐ Ⓑ Ⓒ Ⓓ Ⓔ	

A copy of this answer sheet can be downloaded at http://www.amssmstore.com/download/AnswerSheet.pdf

1. Ⓐ Ⓑ Ⓒ Ⓓ Ⓔ	35. Ⓐ Ⓑ Ⓒ Ⓓ Ⓔ	69. Ⓐ Ⓑ Ⓒ Ⓓ Ⓔ
2. Ⓐ Ⓑ Ⓒ Ⓓ Ⓔ	36. Ⓐ Ⓑ Ⓒ Ⓓ Ⓔ	70. Ⓐ Ⓑ Ⓒ Ⓓ Ⓔ
3. Ⓐ Ⓑ Ⓒ Ⓓ Ⓔ	37. Ⓐ Ⓑ Ⓒ Ⓓ Ⓔ	71. Ⓐ Ⓑ Ⓒ Ⓓ Ⓔ
4. Ⓐ Ⓑ Ⓒ Ⓓ Ⓔ	38. Ⓐ Ⓑ Ⓒ Ⓓ Ⓔ	72. Ⓐ Ⓑ Ⓒ Ⓓ Ⓔ
5. Ⓐ Ⓑ Ⓒ Ⓓ Ⓔ	39. Ⓐ Ⓑ Ⓒ Ⓓ Ⓔ	73. Ⓐ Ⓑ Ⓒ Ⓓ Ⓔ
6. Ⓐ Ⓑ Ⓒ Ⓓ Ⓔ	40. Ⓐ Ⓑ Ⓒ Ⓓ Ⓔ	74. Ⓐ Ⓑ Ⓒ Ⓓ Ⓔ
7. Ⓐ Ⓑ Ⓒ Ⓓ Ⓔ	41. Ⓐ Ⓑ Ⓒ Ⓓ Ⓔ	75. Ⓐ Ⓑ Ⓒ Ⓓ Ⓔ
8. Ⓐ Ⓑ Ⓒ Ⓓ Ⓔ	42. Ⓐ Ⓑ Ⓒ Ⓓ Ⓔ	76. Ⓐ Ⓑ Ⓒ Ⓓ Ⓔ
9. Ⓐ Ⓑ Ⓒ Ⓓ Ⓔ	43. Ⓐ Ⓑ Ⓒ Ⓓ Ⓔ	77. Ⓐ Ⓑ Ⓒ Ⓓ Ⓔ
10. Ⓐ Ⓑ Ⓒ Ⓓ Ⓔ	44. Ⓐ Ⓑ Ⓒ Ⓓ Ⓔ	78. Ⓐ Ⓑ Ⓒ Ⓓ Ⓔ
11. Ⓐ Ⓑ Ⓒ Ⓓ Ⓔ	45. Ⓐ Ⓑ Ⓒ Ⓓ Ⓔ	79. Ⓐ Ⓑ Ⓒ Ⓓ Ⓔ
12. Ⓐ Ⓑ Ⓒ Ⓓ Ⓔ	46. Ⓐ Ⓑ Ⓒ Ⓓ Ⓔ	80. Ⓐ Ⓑ Ⓒ Ⓓ Ⓔ
13. Ⓐ Ⓑ Ⓒ Ⓓ Ⓔ	47. Ⓐ Ⓑ Ⓒ Ⓓ Ⓔ	81. Ⓐ Ⓑ Ⓒ Ⓓ Ⓔ
14. Ⓐ Ⓑ Ⓒ Ⓓ Ⓔ	48. Ⓐ Ⓑ Ⓒ Ⓓ Ⓔ	82. Ⓐ Ⓑ Ⓒ Ⓓ Ⓔ
15. Ⓐ Ⓑ Ⓒ Ⓓ Ⓔ	49. Ⓐ Ⓑ Ⓒ Ⓓ Ⓔ	83. Ⓐ Ⓑ Ⓒ Ⓓ Ⓔ
16. Ⓐ Ⓑ Ⓒ Ⓓ Ⓔ	50. Ⓐ Ⓑ Ⓒ Ⓓ Ⓔ	84. Ⓐ Ⓑ Ⓒ Ⓓ Ⓔ
17. Ⓐ Ⓑ Ⓒ Ⓓ Ⓔ	51. Ⓐ Ⓑ Ⓒ Ⓓ Ⓔ	85. Ⓐ Ⓑ Ⓒ Ⓓ Ⓔ
18. Ⓐ Ⓑ Ⓒ Ⓓ Ⓔ	52. Ⓐ Ⓑ Ⓒ Ⓓ Ⓔ	86. Ⓐ Ⓑ Ⓒ Ⓓ Ⓔ
19. Ⓐ Ⓑ Ⓒ Ⓓ Ⓔ	53. Ⓐ Ⓑ Ⓒ Ⓓ Ⓔ	87. Ⓐ Ⓑ Ⓒ Ⓓ Ⓔ
20. Ⓐ Ⓑ Ⓒ Ⓓ Ⓔ	54. Ⓐ Ⓑ Ⓒ Ⓓ Ⓔ	88. Ⓐ Ⓑ Ⓒ Ⓓ Ⓔ
21. Ⓐ Ⓑ Ⓒ Ⓓ Ⓔ	55. Ⓐ Ⓑ Ⓒ Ⓓ Ⓔ	89. Ⓐ Ⓑ Ⓒ Ⓓ Ⓔ
22. Ⓐ Ⓑ Ⓒ Ⓓ Ⓔ	56. Ⓐ Ⓑ Ⓒ Ⓓ Ⓔ	90. Ⓐ Ⓑ Ⓒ Ⓓ Ⓔ
23. Ⓐ Ⓑ Ⓒ Ⓓ Ⓔ	57. Ⓐ Ⓑ Ⓒ Ⓓ Ⓔ	91. Ⓐ Ⓑ Ⓒ Ⓓ Ⓔ
24. Ⓐ Ⓑ Ⓒ Ⓓ Ⓔ	58. Ⓐ Ⓑ Ⓒ Ⓓ Ⓔ	92. Ⓐ Ⓑ Ⓒ Ⓓ Ⓔ
25. Ⓐ Ⓑ Ⓒ Ⓓ Ⓔ	59. Ⓐ Ⓑ Ⓒ Ⓓ Ⓔ	93. Ⓐ Ⓑ Ⓒ Ⓓ Ⓔ
26. Ⓐ Ⓑ Ⓒ Ⓓ Ⓔ	60. Ⓐ Ⓑ Ⓒ Ⓓ Ⓔ	94. Ⓐ Ⓑ Ⓒ Ⓓ Ⓔ
27. Ⓐ Ⓑ Ⓒ Ⓓ Ⓔ	61. Ⓐ Ⓑ Ⓒ Ⓓ Ⓔ	95. Ⓐ Ⓑ Ⓒ Ⓓ Ⓔ
28. Ⓐ Ⓑ Ⓒ Ⓓ Ⓔ	62. Ⓐ Ⓑ Ⓒ Ⓓ Ⓔ	96. Ⓐ Ⓑ Ⓒ Ⓓ Ⓔ
29. Ⓐ Ⓑ Ⓒ Ⓓ Ⓔ	63. Ⓐ Ⓑ Ⓒ Ⓓ Ⓔ	97. Ⓐ Ⓑ Ⓒ Ⓓ Ⓔ
30. Ⓐ Ⓑ Ⓒ Ⓓ Ⓔ	64. Ⓐ Ⓑ Ⓒ Ⓓ Ⓔ	98. Ⓐ Ⓑ Ⓒ Ⓓ Ⓔ
31. Ⓐ Ⓑ Ⓒ Ⓓ Ⓔ	65. Ⓐ Ⓑ Ⓒ Ⓓ Ⓔ	99. Ⓐ Ⓑ Ⓒ Ⓓ Ⓔ
32. Ⓐ Ⓑ Ⓒ Ⓓ Ⓔ	66. Ⓐ Ⓑ Ⓒ Ⓓ Ⓔ	100. Ⓐ Ⓑ Ⓒ Ⓓ Ⓔ
33. Ⓐ Ⓑ Ⓒ Ⓓ Ⓔ	67. Ⓐ Ⓑ Ⓒ Ⓓ Ⓔ	
34. Ⓐ Ⓑ Ⓒ Ⓓ Ⓔ	68. Ⓐ Ⓑ Ⓒ Ⓓ Ⓔ	

A copy of this answer sheet can be downloaded at http://www.amssmstore.com/download/AnswerSheet.pdf

101. Ⓐ Ⓑ Ⓒ Ⓓ Ⓔ	135. Ⓐ Ⓑ Ⓒ Ⓓ Ⓔ	169. Ⓐ Ⓑ Ⓒ Ⓓ Ⓔ
102. Ⓐ Ⓑ Ⓒ Ⓓ Ⓔ	136. Ⓐ Ⓑ Ⓒ Ⓓ Ⓔ	170. Ⓐ Ⓑ Ⓒ Ⓓ Ⓔ
103. Ⓐ Ⓑ Ⓒ Ⓓ Ⓔ	137. Ⓐ Ⓑ Ⓒ Ⓓ Ⓔ	171. Ⓐ Ⓑ Ⓒ Ⓓ Ⓔ
104. Ⓐ Ⓑ Ⓒ Ⓓ Ⓔ	138. Ⓐ Ⓑ Ⓒ Ⓓ Ⓔ	172. Ⓐ Ⓑ Ⓒ Ⓓ Ⓔ
105. Ⓐ Ⓑ Ⓒ Ⓓ Ⓔ	139. Ⓐ Ⓑ Ⓒ Ⓓ Ⓔ	173. Ⓐ Ⓑ Ⓒ Ⓓ Ⓔ
106. Ⓐ Ⓑ Ⓒ Ⓓ Ⓔ	140. Ⓐ Ⓑ Ⓒ Ⓓ Ⓔ	174. Ⓐ Ⓑ Ⓒ Ⓓ Ⓔ
107. Ⓐ Ⓑ Ⓒ Ⓓ Ⓔ	141. Ⓐ Ⓑ Ⓒ Ⓓ Ⓔ	175. Ⓐ Ⓑ Ⓒ Ⓓ Ⓔ
108. Ⓐ Ⓑ Ⓒ Ⓓ Ⓔ	142. Ⓐ Ⓑ Ⓒ Ⓓ Ⓔ	176. Ⓐ Ⓑ Ⓒ Ⓓ Ⓔ
109. Ⓐ Ⓑ Ⓒ Ⓓ Ⓔ	143. Ⓐ Ⓑ Ⓒ Ⓓ Ⓔ	177. Ⓐ Ⓑ Ⓒ Ⓓ Ⓔ
110. Ⓐ Ⓑ Ⓒ Ⓓ Ⓔ	144. Ⓐ Ⓑ Ⓒ Ⓓ Ⓔ	178. Ⓐ Ⓑ Ⓒ Ⓓ Ⓔ
111. Ⓐ Ⓑ Ⓒ Ⓓ Ⓔ	145. Ⓐ Ⓑ Ⓒ Ⓓ Ⓔ	179. Ⓐ Ⓑ Ⓒ Ⓓ Ⓔ
112. Ⓐ Ⓑ Ⓒ Ⓓ Ⓔ	146. Ⓐ Ⓑ Ⓒ Ⓓ Ⓔ	180. Ⓐ Ⓑ Ⓒ Ⓓ Ⓔ
113. Ⓐ Ⓑ Ⓒ Ⓓ Ⓔ	147. Ⓐ Ⓑ Ⓒ Ⓓ Ⓔ	181. Ⓐ Ⓑ Ⓒ Ⓓ Ⓔ
114. Ⓐ Ⓑ Ⓒ Ⓓ Ⓔ	148. Ⓐ Ⓑ Ⓒ Ⓓ Ⓔ	182. Ⓐ Ⓑ Ⓒ Ⓓ Ⓔ
115. Ⓐ Ⓑ Ⓒ Ⓓ Ⓔ	149. Ⓐ Ⓑ Ⓒ Ⓓ Ⓔ	183. Ⓐ Ⓑ Ⓒ Ⓓ Ⓔ
116. Ⓐ Ⓑ Ⓒ Ⓓ Ⓔ	150. Ⓐ Ⓑ Ⓒ Ⓓ Ⓔ	184. Ⓐ Ⓑ Ⓒ Ⓓ Ⓔ
117. Ⓐ Ⓑ Ⓒ Ⓓ Ⓔ	151. Ⓐ Ⓑ Ⓒ Ⓓ Ⓔ	185. Ⓐ Ⓑ Ⓒ Ⓓ Ⓔ
118. Ⓐ Ⓑ Ⓒ Ⓓ Ⓔ	152. Ⓐ Ⓑ Ⓒ Ⓓ Ⓔ	186. Ⓐ Ⓑ Ⓒ Ⓓ Ⓔ
119. Ⓐ Ⓑ Ⓒ Ⓓ Ⓔ	153. Ⓐ Ⓑ Ⓒ Ⓓ Ⓔ	187. Ⓐ Ⓑ Ⓒ Ⓓ Ⓔ
120. Ⓐ Ⓑ Ⓒ Ⓓ Ⓔ	154. Ⓐ Ⓑ Ⓒ Ⓓ Ⓔ	188. Ⓐ Ⓑ Ⓒ Ⓓ Ⓔ
121. Ⓐ Ⓑ Ⓒ Ⓓ Ⓔ	155. Ⓐ Ⓑ Ⓒ Ⓓ Ⓔ	189. Ⓐ Ⓑ Ⓒ Ⓓ Ⓔ
122. Ⓐ Ⓑ Ⓒ Ⓓ Ⓔ	156. Ⓐ Ⓑ Ⓒ Ⓓ Ⓔ	190. Ⓐ Ⓑ Ⓒ Ⓓ Ⓔ
123. Ⓐ Ⓑ Ⓒ Ⓓ Ⓔ	157. Ⓐ Ⓑ Ⓒ Ⓓ Ⓔ	191. Ⓐ Ⓑ Ⓒ Ⓓ Ⓔ
124. Ⓐ Ⓑ Ⓒ Ⓓ Ⓔ	158. Ⓐ Ⓑ Ⓒ Ⓓ Ⓔ	192. Ⓐ Ⓑ Ⓒ Ⓓ Ⓔ
125. Ⓐ Ⓑ Ⓒ Ⓓ Ⓔ	159. Ⓐ Ⓑ Ⓒ Ⓓ Ⓔ	193. Ⓐ Ⓑ Ⓒ Ⓓ Ⓔ
126. Ⓐ Ⓑ Ⓒ Ⓓ Ⓔ	160. Ⓐ Ⓑ Ⓒ Ⓓ Ⓔ	194. Ⓐ Ⓑ Ⓒ Ⓓ Ⓔ
127. Ⓐ Ⓑ Ⓒ Ⓓ Ⓔ	161. Ⓐ Ⓑ Ⓒ Ⓓ Ⓔ	195. Ⓐ Ⓑ Ⓒ Ⓓ Ⓔ
128. Ⓐ Ⓑ Ⓒ Ⓓ Ⓔ	162. Ⓐ Ⓑ Ⓒ Ⓓ Ⓔ	196. Ⓐ Ⓑ Ⓒ Ⓓ Ⓔ
129. Ⓐ Ⓑ Ⓒ Ⓓ Ⓔ	163. Ⓐ Ⓑ Ⓒ Ⓓ Ⓔ	197. Ⓐ Ⓑ Ⓒ Ⓓ Ⓔ
130. Ⓐ Ⓑ Ⓒ Ⓓ Ⓔ	164. Ⓐ Ⓑ Ⓒ Ⓓ Ⓔ	198. Ⓐ Ⓑ Ⓒ Ⓓ Ⓔ
131. Ⓐ Ⓑ Ⓒ Ⓓ Ⓔ	165. Ⓐ Ⓑ Ⓒ Ⓓ Ⓔ	199. Ⓐ Ⓑ Ⓒ Ⓓ Ⓔ
132. Ⓐ Ⓑ Ⓒ Ⓓ Ⓔ	166. Ⓐ Ⓑ Ⓒ Ⓓ Ⓔ	200. Ⓐ Ⓑ Ⓒ Ⓓ Ⓔ
133. Ⓐ Ⓑ Ⓒ Ⓓ Ⓔ	167. Ⓐ Ⓑ Ⓒ Ⓓ Ⓔ	
134. Ⓐ Ⓑ Ⓒ Ⓓ Ⓔ	168. Ⓐ Ⓑ Ⓒ Ⓓ Ⓔ	

A copy of this answer sheet can be downloaded at http://www.amssmstore.com/download/AnswerSheet.pdf